Coronary Artery Disease

Editor

ALBERTO POLIMENI

CARDIOLOGY CLINICS

www.cardiology.theclinics.com

November 2020 • Volume 38 • Number 4

ELSEVIER

1600 John F. Kennedy Boulevard • Suite 1800 • Philadelphia, Pennsylvania, 19103-2899

http://www.theclinics.com

CARDIOLOGY CLINICS Volume 38, Number 4
November 2020 ISSN 0733-8651, ISBN-13: 978-0-323-77709-4

Editor: Joanna Collett
Developmental Editor: Julia McKenzie

Cardiology Clinics (ISSN 0733-8651) is published quarterly by Elsevier Inc., 360 Park Avenue South, New York, NY 10010-1710. Months of issue are February, May, August, and November. Business and Editorial Offices: 1600 John F. Kennedy Blvd., Ste. 1800, Philadelphia, PA 19103-2899. Customer Service Office: 3251 Riverport Lane, Maryland Heights, MO 63043. Periodicals post-age paid at New York, NY and additional mailing offices. Subscription prices are $352.00 per year for US individuals, $706.00 per year for US institutions, $100.00 per year for US students and residents, $432.00 per year for Canadian individuals, $885.00 per year for Canadian institutions, $466.00 per year for international individuals, $885.00 per year for international institutions, $100.00 per year for Canadian students/residents and $220.00 per year for international students/residents. To receive student/resident rate, orders must be accompanied by name of affiliated institution, data of term, and the *signature* of program/residency coordinator on institution letterhead. Orders will be billed at individual rate until proof of status is received. Foreign air speed delivery is included in all *Clinics* subscription prices. All prices are subject to change without notice. **POSTMASTER:** Send address changes to *Cardiology Clinics*, Elsevier Health Sciences Division, Subscription Customer Service, 3251 Riverport Lane, Maryland Heights, MO 63043. **Customer Service: 1-800-654-2452 (U.S. and Canada); 314-447-8871 (outside U.S. and Canada). Fax: 314-447-8029. E-mail: journalscus-tomerservice-usa@elsevier.com (for print support); journalsonlinesupport-usa@elsevier.com (for online support).**

Reprints. For copies of 100 or more, of articles in this publication, please contact the Commercial Reprints Department, Elsevier Inc., 360 Park Avenue South, New York, NY 10010-1710. Tel.: 212-633-3874; Fax: 212-633-3820; E-mail: reprints@elsevier.com.

Cardiology Clinics is also published in Spanish by McGraw-Hill Interamericana Editores S. A., P.O. Box 5-237, 06500, Mexico D. F., Mexico; in Portuguese by Reichmann and Alfonso Editores Rio de Janeiro, Brazil; and in Greek by Dimitrios P. Lagos, 8 Pondon Street, GR115-28 Ilissia, Greece.

Cardiology Clinics is covered in *MEDLINE/PubMed (Index Medicus), Excerpta Medica, The Cumulative Index to Nursing and Allied Health Literature* (CINAHL).

Contributors

MICHAEL BEHNES, MD
First Department of Medicine, University Medical Centre Mannheim (UMM), Faculty of Medicine Mannheim, University of Heidelberg, European Center for AngioScience (ECAS), DZHK (German Center for Cardiovascular Research) Partner Site Heidelberg/Mannheim, Mannheim, Germany

GIOVANNI BENFARI, MD
Section of Cardiology, University of Verona, Verona, Italy

MARTIN BORGGREFE, MD
First Department of Medicine, University Medical Centre Mannheim (UMM), Faculty of Medicine Mannheim, University of Heidelberg, European Center for AngioScience (ECAS), DZHK (German Center for Cardiovascular Research) Partner Site Heidelberg/Mannheim, Mannheim, Germany

GIANLUCA CAIAZZO, MD, PhD
ICCU, San Giuseppe Moscati Hospital, ASL CE, Aversa, Italy

PAOLO CALABRÒ, MD, PhD
Division of Clinical Cardiology, A.O.R.N. "Sant'Anna e San Sebastiano," Caserta, Italy; Department of Translational Medical Sciences, University of Campania "Luigi Vanvitelli," Naples, Italy

ANTON CAMAJ, MD, MS
The Zena and Michael A. Wiener Cardiovascular Institute, The Icahn School of Medicine at Mount Sinai, New York, New York, USA

ARTURO CESARO, MD
Division of Clinical Cardiology, A.O.R.N. "Sant'Anna e San Sebastiano," Caserta, Italy; Department of Translational Medical Sciences, University of Campania "Luigi Vanvitelli," Naples, Italy

SILVIO COLETTA, MD
Division of Clinical Cardiology, A.O.R.N. "Sant'Anna e San Sebastiano," Caserta, Italy; Department of Translational Medical Sciences, University of Campania "Luigi Vanvitelli," Naples, Italy

MATTEO CONTE, MD
Division of Clinical Cardiology, A.O.R.N. "Sant'Anna e San Sebastiano," Caserta, Italy; Department of Translational Medical Sciences, University of Campania "Luigi Vanvitelli," Naples, Italy

FRANCESCO COSTA, MD, PhD
Department of Clinical and Experimental Medicine, Policlinico "G. Martino," University of Messina, Interventional Cardiology Unit, Policlinico G. Martino, Messina, Italy

GIUSEPPE DE LUCA, MD, PhD
Division of Cardiology, Azienda Ospedaliera-Universitaria "Maggiore della Carità," Università del Piemonte Orientale, Novara, Italy

SALVATORE DE ROSA, MD, PhD
Division of Cardiology, Department of Medical and Surgical Sciences, Research Center for Cardiovascular Diseases, "Magna Graecia" University, Catanzaro, Italy

PIERLUIGI DEMOLA, MD
Structural Interventional Cardiology, Department of Clinical and Experimental Medicine, Careggi University Hospital, Florence, Italy

DARIO DI MAIO, MD
Division of Clinical Cardiology, A.O.R.N. "Sant'Anna e San Sebastiano, Caserta, Italy; Department of Translational Medical Sciences, University of Campania "Luigi Vanvitelli," Naples, Italy

CARLO DI MARIO, MD, PhD, FRCP, FSCAI, FESC, FACC
Structural Interventional Cardiology, Department of Clinical and Experimental Medicine, Careggi University Hospital, Florence, Italy

VINCENZO DIANA, MD
Division of Clinical Cardiology, A.O.R.N. "Sant'Anna e San Sebastiano," Caserta, Italy; Department of Translational Medical Sciences, University of Campania "Luigi Vanvitelli," Naples, Italy

CEREN EYILETEN, MD, PhD
Department of Experimental and Clinical Pharmacology, Medical University of Warsaw,

Center for Preclinical Research and
Technology CEPT, Warsaw, Poland

DIEGO FANTI, MD
Section of Cardiology, University of Verona,
Verona, Italy

MARCO FERRONE, MD
Department of Advanced Biomedical
Sciences, Federico II University of Naples,
Naples, Italy; Division of Invasive Cardiology,
Clinica Montevergine, Mercogliano (Avellino),
Italy

KRZYSZTOF J. FILIPIAK, MD, PhD
First Chair, Department of Cardiology, Medical
University of Warsaw, Warszawa, Poland

FABIO FIMIANI, MD
Division of Clinical Cardiology, A.O.R.N.
"Sant'Anna e San Sebastiano," Caserta, Italy;
Department of Translational Medical Sciences,
University of Campania "Luigi Vanvitelli,"
Naples, Italy

LUIGI FIMIANI, MD
Department of Clinical and Experimental
Medicine, Policlinico "G. Martino," University
of Messina, Italy

ALEX FITAS, MD
Department of Experimental and Clinical
Pharmacology, Medical University of Warsaw,
Center for Preclinical Research and
Technology CEPT, Warsaw, Poland

LARA FREDIANI, MD
Department of Cardiology, Livorno Hospital,
Azienda Usl Toscana Nord-Ovest, Ospedali
Riuniti di Livorno, Livorno, Italy

VICTORIA GARCIA-RUIZ, MD
UGC del Corazón, Servicio de Cardiología,
Hospital Clínico Universitario Virgen de la
Victoria, Málaga, Spain

GIUSEPPE GARGIULO, MD, PhD
Department of Advanced Biomedical
Sciences, Federico II University of Naples,
Naples, Italy

MARTIN GEYER, MD
Department of Cardiology, Cardiology I,
University Medical Center of the Johannes
Gutenberg University Mainz, Mainz, Germany

ROCCO GIOSCIA, MD
Division of Cardiology, Azienda Ospedaliera-
Universitaria "Maggiore della Carità,"
Università del Piemonte Orientale, Novara, Italy

GENNARO GIUSTINO, MD
Cardiology Fellow, The Zena and Michael A.
Wiener Cardiovascular Institute, The Icahn
School of Medicine at Mount Sinai, New York,
New York, USA

TOMMASO GORI, MD, PhD
Department of Cardiology, Cardiology I,
German Center for Cardiovascular Research
(DZHK), Partner Site Rhine Main, University
Medical Center of the Johannes Gutenberg
University Mainz, Mainz, Germany

FELICE GRAGNANO, MD
Division of Clinical Cardiology, A.O.R.N.
"Sant'Anna e San Sebastiano," Caserta, Italy;
Department of Translational Medical Sciences,
University of Campania "Luigi Vanvitelli,"
Naples, Italy

JONATHAN L. HALPERIN, MD
The Zena and Michael A. Wiener
Cardiovascular Institute, The Icahn School of
Medicine at Mount Sinai, New York, New York,
USA

BRUNILDA HAMITI, CRN
Research Nurse, Structural Interventional
Cardiology, Department of Clinical and
Experimental Medicine, Careggi University
Hospital, Florence, Italy

FEDERICA ILARDI, MD
Department of Advanced Biomedical
Sciences, Federico II University of Naples,
Mediterranea Cardiocentro, Naples, Italy

CIRO INDOLFI, MD
Chief, Division of Cardiology, Department of
Medical and Surgical Sciences, Research
Center for Cardiovascular Diseases, "Magna
Graecia" University, Catanzaro, Italy;
Mediterranea Cardiocentro, Naples, Italy

EVA JUNGER, MD
Department of Experimental and Clinical
Pharmacology, Medical University of Warsaw,
Center for Preclinical Research and
Technology CEPT, Warsaw, Poland

SEUNG-HYUN KIM, MD
First Department of Medicine, University Medical Centre Mannheim (UMM), Faculty of Medicine Mannheim, University of Heidelberg, European Center for AngioScience (ECAS), DZHK (German Center for Cardiovascular Research) Partner Site Heidelberg/Mannheim, Mannheim, Germany

JACEK KUBICA, MD, PhD
Department of Cardiology, Collegium Medicum, Nicolaus Copernicus University, Bydgoszcz, SIRIO MEDICINE Network, Poland

ALFONSO IELASI, MD
Clinical and Interventional Cardiology Unit, Istituto Clinico S. Ambrogio, Milan, Italy

ROBERTO LICORDARI, MD
Department of Clinical and Experimental Medicine, Policlinico "G. Martino," University of Messina, Italy

THOMAS MÜNZEL, MD
Department of Cardiology, Cardiology I, German Center for Cardiovascular Research (DZHK), Partner Site Rhine Main, University Medical Center of the Johannes Gutenberg University Mainz, Mainz, Germany

JOANNA SAMANTA MAKOWSKA, MD, PhD
Department of Rheumatology, Medical University of Lodz, Lodz, Poland

MARCIN MAKOWSKI, MD, PhD
Department of Interventional Cardiology, Medical University of Lodz, Central Clinical Hospital, Lodz, Poland

ALESSANDRO MALAGOLI, MD
Division of Cardiology, Nephro-Cardiovascular Department, "S. Agostino-Estense" Public Hospital, University of Modena and Reggio Emilia, Modena, Italy

MARCO MARCOLONGO, MD
Cardiologia e Unità Coronarica, Ospedale degli Infermi, ASL Biella, Biella, Italy

CARLO DI MARIO, MD, PhD, FRCP, FSCAI, FESC, FACC
Structural Interventional Cardiology, Department of Clinical and Experimental Medicine, Careggi University Hospital, Florence, Italy

GIULIA MASIERO, MD
Department of Cardiac, Thoracic, Vascular Sciences and Public Health, University of Padua, Padua, Italy

JUJI MATSUDA, MD
Department of Cardiac, Thoracic, Vascular Sciences and Public Health, University of Padua, Padua, Italy; Department of Cardiovascular Medicine, Graduate School of Medical and Dental Science, Tokyo Medical and Dental University, Bunkyo-ku, Tokyo, Japan

ALESSIO MATTESINI, MD
Structural Interventional Cardiology, Department of Clinical and Experimental Medicine, Careggi University Hospital, Florence, Italy

FRANCESCO MEUCCI, MD
Structural Interventional Cardiology, Department of Clinical and Experimental Medicine, Careggi University Hospital, Florence, Italy

MICHAEL S. MILLER, MSc
The Zena and Michael A. Wiener Cardiovascular Institute, The Icahn School of Medicine at Mount Sinai, New York, New York, USA

ANNALISA MONGIARDO, MD
Division of Cardiology, Department of Medical and Surgical Sciences, "Magna Graecia" University, Catanzaro, Italy

ELISABETTA MOSCARELLA, MD
Division of Clinical Cardiology, A.O.R.N. "Sant'Anna e San Sebastiano," Caserta, Italy; Department of Translational Medical Sciences, University of Campania "Luigi Vanvitelli," Naples, Italy

RITA LEONARDA MUSCI, MD
Department of Cardiology, Azienda Ospedaliera Bonomo, Andria, Italy

ELIANO PIO NAVARESE, MD, PhD, FESC, FACC
Department of Cardiology, Collegium Medicum, Nicolaus Copernicus University, Bydgoszcz, SIRIO MEDICINE Network, Poland; Faculty of Medicine, University of Alberta, Edmonton, Alberta, Canada

ALBERTO POLIMENI, MD, PhD, FISC
Division of Cardiology and Research
Center for Cardiovascular Diseases,
Department of Medical and Surgical
Sciences, "Magna Graecia" University,
Catanzaro, Italy

MAREK POSTULA, MD, PhD
Department of Experimental and Clinical
Pharmacology, Medical University of Warsaw,
Center for Preclinical Research and
Technology CEPT, Longevity Center, Warsaw,
Poland

SUNIL V. RAO, MD
Division of Cardiology, Duke University
Medical Center, Duke Clinical Research
Institute, Durham, North Carolina, USA

FLAVIO L. RIBICHINI, MD, PhD
Section of Cardiology, University of Verona,
Verona, Italy

FRANCESCA RISTALLI, MD
Structural Interventional Cardiology,
Department of Clinical and Experimental
Medicine, Careggi University Hospital,
Florence, Italy

GIULIO RODINÒ, MD
Department of Cardiac, Thoracic, Vascular
Sciences and Public Health, University of
Padua, Padua, Italy

ANDREA ROSSI, MD
Section of Cardiology, University of Verona,
Verona, Italy

JOLANDA SABATINO, MD, PhD
Division of Cardiology, Department of Medical
and Surgical Sciences, Research Center for
Cardiovascular Diseases, "Magna Graecia"
University, Catanzaro, Italy

ALESSANDRA SCHIAVO, MD
Division of Clinical Cardiology, A.O.R.N.
"Sant'Anna e San Sebastiano," Caserta, Italy;
Department of Translational Medical Sciences,
University of Campania "Luigi Vanvitelli,"
Naples, Italy

GIUSEPPE SERVILLO, MD
Department of Neurosciences, Reproductive
and Odontostomatological Sciences,
University of Naples "Federico II," Naples, Italy

JOLANTA M. SILLER-MATULA, MD, PhD
Department of Experimental and Clinical
Pharmacology, Medical University of Warsaw,
Center for Preclinical Research and
Technology CEPT, Warsaw, Poland;
Department of Internal Medicine II, Division of
Cardiology, Medical University of Vienna,
Vienna, Austria

SABATO SORRENTINO, MD, PhD
Division of Cardiology, Department of Medical
and Surgical Sciences, Research Center for
Cardiovascular Diseases, "Magna Graecia"
University, Catanzaro, Italy

CARMEN SPACCAROTELLA, MD
Division of Cardiology, Department of Medical
and Surgical Sciences, Research Center for
Cardiovascular Diseases, "Magna Graecia"
University, Catanzaro, Italy

GIUSEPPE TARANTINI, MD, PhD
Department of Cardiac, Thoracic, Vascular
Sciences and Public Health, University of
Padua, Padua, Italy

JULIA UMIŃSKA, MD, PhD
Department of Cardiology, Collegium
Medicum, Nicolaus Copernicus University,
Bydgoszcz, SIRIO MEDICINE Network,
Bydgoszcz, Poland

MONICA VERDOIA, MD, PhD
Cardiologia e Unità Coronarica, Interventional
Cardiologists and Research Fellow, Ospedale
degli Infermi, ASL Biella, Biella, Italy; Division of
Cardiology, Azienda Ospedaliera-Universitaria
"Maggiore della Carità," Università del
Piemonte Orientale, Novara, Italy

WOJCIECH WANHA, MD, PhD
Division of Cardiology and Structural Heart
Diseases, Medical University of Silesia, Kato,
Katowice, Poland

ZACHARY K. WEGERMANN, MD
Division of Cardiology, Duke University
Medical Center, Duke Clinical Research
Institute, Durham, North Carolina, USA

PHILIP WENZEL, MD
Department of Cardiology, Cardiology I, Center
for Thrombosis and Hemostasis, German
Center for Cardiovascular Research (DZHK),
Partner Site Rhine Main, University Medical

Center of the Johannes Gutenberg University Mainz, Mainz, Germany

ZOFIA WICIK, MD
Department of Experimental and Clinical Pharmacology, Medical University of Warsaw, Center for Preclinical Research and Technology CEPT, Warsaw, Poland; Centro de Matemática, Computação e Cognição, Universidade Federal do ABC, Alameda da Universidade, São Paulo, Brazil

JOHANNES WILD, MD
Department of Cardiology, Cardiology I, Center for Thrombosis and Hemostasis, University Medical Center of the Johannes Gutenberg University Mainz, Mainz, Germany

MARTA WOLSKA, MD
Department of Experimental and Clinical Pharmacology, Medical University of Warsaw, Center for Preclinical Research and Technology CEPT, Warsaw, Poland

MARZENNA ZIELIŃSKA, MD, PhD
Department of Interventional Cardiology, Medical University of Lodz, Central Clinical Hospital, Lodz, Poland

LUKASZ ZAREBA, MD
Department of Experimental and Clinical Pharmacology, Medical University of Warsaw, Center for Preclinical Research and Technology CEPT, Warsaw, Poland

Contents

In cases of suspected acute coronary syndrome (ACS), rapid and accurate diagnosis is essential to establish effective evidence-based medical treatment. Patients' history, clinical examination, 12-lead electrocardiogram, and cardiac biomarkers are cornerstones in initial management. Since high-sensitivity cardiac troponins were established, they have markedly expedited and revolutionized rule-in and rule-out pathways of patients with ACS and changed our everyday clinical practice. Thus, they have become an indispensable tool in daily routine in emergency units. This review focuses on historical and contemporary standards in laboratory biomarkers of myocardial injury and discusses their implication in the context of the updated universal definition of myocardial infarction.

Out-of-hospital bleeding is a common complication after percutaneous coronary intervention (PCI) due to the concomitant need for dual antiplatelet therapy. A significant proportion of patients undergoing PCI carry specific clinical characteristics posing them at high bleeding risk (HBR), increasing the risk of hemorrhagic complications secondary to antithrombotic therapy. Identifying patients at HBR and adjust antithrombotic therapy accordingly to optimize treatment benefits and risk is a challenge of modern cardiology. Recently, multiple definitions and tools have been provided to help clinicians with prognostic stratification and treatment decision making in this subgroup.

In patients with multivessel disease, complete revascularization (CR) is the most biologically plausible approach irrespective of definition or type or clinical setting (acute or chronic coronary syndrome [ACS or CCS]). It aims at minimizing residual ischemia, relieving symptoms and reducing the risk of future cardiovascular events. Large evidence supports CR benefits in ACS, predominantly ST-segment elevation myocardial infarction, except cardiogenic shock, although optimal assessment and timing remain debated. In patients with CCS, when revascularization is indicated, a functional CR should be attempted. Therefore, heart-team is crucial in selecting the ideal strategy for each patient to optimize decision-making.

The evolution of percutaneous coronary intervention (PCI) enables a complete revascularization of complex coronary lesions. However, simultaneously, patients are presenting nowadays with higher rates of comorbidities, which may lead to a lower physiologic tolerance for complex PCI. To avoid hemodynamic instability during PCI and achieve safe complete revascularization, protected PCI using mechanical circulatory support devices has been developed. However, which patients would benefit from the protected PCI is still in debate. Hence, this review provides practical approaches for the selection of patients by outlining current clinical data assessing utility of protected PCI in high-risk patients.

For more than 30 years, echocardiography, through the measurement of ejection fraction and wall motion assessment, has played a crucial role in the diagnosis and management of patients with acute and chronic ischemic heart disease. The introduction of myocardial strain, measured by speckle tracking echocardiography, is shifting this paradigm. Strain imaging catches something pathophysiologically deeper into myocardial function, facing a wide range of clinical applications. This review summarizes the basic concepts of strain imaging and its applicability in clinical practice for the evaluation of the ventricular and the left atrial function in ischemic cardiomyopathy.

Cardiogenic shock (CS) is a complex condition with a high risk for morbidity and mortality. Mechanical circulatory support (MCS) devices were developed to support patients with CS in cases refractory to treatment with vasoactive medications. Current devices include intra-aortic balloon pumps, intravascular microaxial pumps, percutaneous LVAD, percutaneous RVAD, and VA ECMO. Data from limited observational studies and clinical trials show a clear difference in the level of hemodynamic support offered by each device. However, at this point, there are insufficient clinical trial data to guide MCS selection and, until ongoing clinical trials are completed, use of the right device for the right patient depends largely on clinical judgment.

The recent technological evolution of coronary computed tomography angiography (CTA) with improved sensitivity and high negative predictive value has extended its potential applications as a gatekeeper test before invasive coronary angiography. However, the definition of the most accurate diagnostic algorithms comprising CTA as a first-line strategy for ruling out coronary artery disease and the correct management of the patients according to the results of imaging tests still warrant better definition.

Patients with atrial fibrillation who undergo percutaneous coronary intervention with drug-eluting stent implantation often require oral anticoagulation (OAC) and antiplatelet therapies. Triple antithrombotic therapy (OAC, a $P2Y_{12}$-receptor inhibitor, and aspirin) has been the default antithrombotic strategy. Evidence from randomized trials indicates, however, that a dual antithrombotic therapy strategy (OAC plus a $P2Y_{12}$-receptor inhibitor) reduces bleeding risk without increasing the risk of ischemic events. This review provides an overview of advancements in this field as well as European and North American guidelines and consensus documents to inform clinical decision making around antithrombotic therapies for patients with atrial fibrillation who undergo percutaneous coronary intervention.

Primary percutaneous coronary intervention is the preferred reperfusion strategy for the management of acute ST-segment elevation myocardial infarction. No reflow is characterized by the inadequate myocardial perfusion of a given segment without angiographic evidence of persistent mechanical obstruction of epicardial vessels. Both pharmacologic and device-based strategies have been tested to resolve coronary no reflow. This article provides an updated overview of the no-reflow phenomenon, discussing clinical evidence and ongoing investigations of existing and novel therapeutic strategies to counteract it.

Functionally significant coronary lesions identification is necessary for appropriate revascularization. This review aims to provide an overview of the available options for coronary stenosis physiologic evaluation with a focus on the latest developments in the field.

To overcome the not negligible metallic drug-eluting stents adverse events rate, the polymeric or metallic bioresorbable scaffolds were designed to provide early drug delivery and mechanical support followed by complete resorption. However, the long-term evidence, focusing on the leading Absorb BVS technology, showed higher events compared with drug-eluting stents. This review discusses the lights and shadows of the current bioresorbable scaffolds according to their mechanical properties and biodegradation profile and suggests possible perspective on these technologies. Improved scaffold design and deployment techniques might mitigate early bioresorbable scaffolds risk enhancing the late benefit of complete resorption.

Noncoding RNAs (ncRNAs), including long noncoding RNAs and microRNAs, play an important role in coronary artery disease onset and progression. The ability of ncRNAs to simultaneously regulate many target genes allows them to modulate various key processes involved in atherosclerosis, including lipid metabolism, smooth muscle cell proliferation, autophagy, and foam cell formation. This review focuses on the therapeutic potential of the most important ncRNAs in coronary artery disease. Moreover, various other promising microRNAs and long noncoding RNAs that attract substantial scientific interest as potential therapeutic targets in coronary artery disease and merit further investigation are presented.

Coronary artery calcifications are always challenging scenarios for interventional cardiologists. Calcium content in coronary tree directly correlates with male sex, age, Caucasian ethnicity, diabetes, and chronic kidney disease. Intracoronary imaging is useful and necessary to understand calcific lesion features and plan the best percutaneous coronary intervention strategy. Thus, accurate evaluation of patient and lesion characteristics is crucial. For this reason, definition of calcific arc, length, and thickness can suggest the best procedure before stenting and final optimization. In our modern era, different devices are available and all are surprisingly promising.

The article discusses pharmacologic and interventional therapeutic options for patients with refractory angina. Refractory angina refers to long-lasting symptoms (≥ 3 months) due to established reversible ischemia in the presence of obstructive coronary artery disease, which cannot be controlled by escalating medical therapy with second-line and third-line pharmacologic agents, bypass grafting, or stenting. Due to an aging population, increased number of comorbidities, and advances in coronary artery disease treatment, incidence of refractory angina is growing. Although the number of therapeutic options is increasing, there is a lack of randomized clinical trials that could help create recommendations for this group of patients.

Since their introduction in clinical practice in 1986, different types of coronary stents have been developed and become available for the treatment of coronary artery disease. Stent thrombosis (ST) is an uncommon but harmful complication after percutaneous coronary implantation, with a high occurrence of acute myocardial infarction and risk of mortality. Among several procedural and clinical predictors, the type of coronary stent is a strong determinant of ST. This article reviews the available evidence on the most used coronary stent types in the modern era and the related risk of ST.

CARDIOLOGY CLINICS

SERIES OF RELATED INTEREST

Cardiac Electrophysiology Clinics
Heart Failure Clinics
Interventional Cardiology Clinics

THE CLINICS ARE AVAILABLE ONLINE!
Access your subscription at:
www.theclinics.com

Preface
Advances in the Diagnosis and Treatment of Coronary Artery Disease

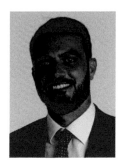

Alberto Polimeni, MD, PhD, FISC
Editor

Coronary artery disease (CAD) is a leading cause of death worldwide. Although the mortality from CAD has decreased in the last 4 decades in developed countries, it continues to cause approximately one-third of all deaths in people aged ≥35 years old.

Recently, several randomized clinical trials and new technologies have influenced international guidelines, changed the clinical practice, and improved the clinical care of patients with CAD.

The present issue of *Cardiology Clinics* aims to provide a modern and extensive review of all aspects of the management and treatment of patients with CAD. To achieve this, we have organized a team of highly talented physicians and research scientists. All authors have sought to provide evidence-based recommendations according to the latest clinical trials and discuss the innovations for the diagnosis and treatment of CAD.

The issue covers CAD from beginning to end, from noninvasive diagnostic tools (Echo strain imaging, CT angiography) to new transcatheter diagnostic techniques (fractional flow reserve, instantaneous wave-free ratio, and nonhyperemic physiologic indices). Articles focus on the management of pharmacologic therapies and new transcatheter technologies as well as future therapies (noncoding RNAs). Finally, the treatment and management of complex clinical scenarios were critically discussed and reviewed.

We hope you enjoy this issue of *Cardiology Clinics* and that the information provided enhances your medical knowledge and further improves the care of your patients with CAD.

Alberto Polimeni, MD, PhD, FISC
Division of Cardiology and Research
Center for Cardiovascular Diseases
Department of Medical and Surgical Sciences
"Magna Graecia" University
Viale Europa Snc, Catanzaro 88100, Italy

E-mail address:
polimeni@unicz.it

Cardiol Clin 38 (2020) xv
https://doi.org/10.1016/j.ccl.2020.08.001
0733-8651/20/© 2020 Published by Elsevier Inc.

State of the Art—High-Sensitivity Troponins in Acute Coronary Syndromes

Martin Geyer, MD[a],*, Johannes Wild, MD[a,b], Thomas Münzel, MD[a,c], Tommaso Gori, MD, PhD[a,c], Philip Wenzel, MD[a,b,c]

KEYWORDS

- High-sensitivity troponin • Acute coronary syndrome • Myocardial injury • Myocardial infarction
- Biomarker

KEY POINTS

- Because of limited sensitivity and accuracy of symptoms and electrocardiogram for the diagnosis of acute coronary syndrome, biomarkers have become an indispensable tool for diagnosis.
- Over the last years, high-sensitivity troponin (hsTN) assays have become ubiquitously available.
- The implementation of hsTN assays allows for the implementation of rapid rule-in and rule-out algorithms with a high negative predictive value.
- Because of their high sensitivity, a relevant number of positive troponin tests outside the setting of myocardial infarction is a frequent challenge to the clinician.
- The use of high-sensitivity troponins led to the redefinition of the term "myocardial injury," with clinical and prognostic implication for patient care.

INTRODUCTION

History: Biomarkers for the Diagnosis of Acute Myocardial Infarction—from Liver Enzymes to High-Sensitivity Troponin

Biomarkers indicating acute myocardial damage have become an indispensable cornerstone in diagnosis and risk stratification in emergency medicine in patients with suspected acute coronary syndrome (ACS), particularly for cases in which the accuracy of clinical parameters and electrocardiogram (ECG) changes is thought to be limited.[1,2] Only 60 years ago, biomarkers were established as a tool for the diagnosis of acute myocardial infarction (MI) for the first time in 1956[3] (**Fig. 1**). At that time, measurement of serum levels of aspartate transaminase was widely used, and the proof of elevated levels entered the first World Health Organization (WHO) definition of MI.[4] In the 1970s, lactate dehydrogenase (LDH), creatine kinase (CK), and myoglobin were introduced and further enhanced the available spectrum of blood markers in the context of the early differential diagnosis of MI.[5] Yet, a relevant lack of specificity of these markers limited their use. Later advances in electrophoresis allowed detection of cardiac-specific isoenzymes of CK and LDH (ie, CK-MB and LDH-1 and -2), which led to a modification of WHO criteria to rule out acute MI in 1979.[6] Although the high rate of false-positive results due to equally high positivity in

Funding: This work was supported by the German Federal Ministry of Education and Research (Bonn, Germany; grant number BMBF 01EO1503).

[a] Department of Cardiology, Cardiology I, University Medical Center of the Johannes Gutenberg University Mainz, Langenbeckstr. 1, 55131 Mainz, Germany; [b] Center for Thrombosis and Hemostasis, University Medical Center of the Johannes Gutenberg University Mainz, Langenbeckstr. 1, 55131 Mainz, Germany; [c] German Center for Cardiovascular Research (DZHK), Partner Site Rhine Main, University Medical Center of the Johannes Gutenberg University Mainz, Langenbeckstr. 1, 55131 Mainz, Germany

* Corresponding author. Universitätsmedizin Mainz, Zentrum für Kardiologie, Kardiologie 1, Langenbeckstr. 1, 55131 Mainz, Germany.

E-mail address: martin.geyer@unimedizin-mainz.de

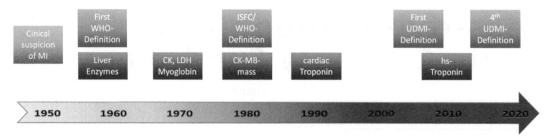

Fig. 1. Timeline of clinical definitions of myocardial infarction and development of cardiac biomarkers. For details, see text. CK, creatine kinase; hs, high-sensitivity; ISFC, International Society and Federation of Cardiology; LDH, lactate dehydrogenase; MI, myocardial infarction; UDMI, universal definition of myocardial infarction; WHO, World Health Organization. (*Data from* Garg P, Morris P, Fazlanie AL, et al. Cardiac biomarkers of acute coronary syndrome: from history to high-sensitivity cardiac troponin. Intern Emerg Med 2017;12:147-155. And Thygesen K, Alpert JS, Jaffe AS, et al. Fourth universal definition of myocardial infarction. Eur Heart J 2018;40:237-269.)

the setting of skeletal muscular injury relevantly impaired their diagnostic accuracy, CK and LDH played a crucial role in the diagnosis of MI up to the 1990s. Troponin—a protein component of myofibrils—had already been discovered in 1965.[7] In 1989, a reliable immunoassay to detect serum levels of cardiac troponin (cTN) levels as cardiospecific protein was developed.[8] In contrast to the contemporary approach, cTN measurements were initially only used in cases of ST-segment elevation MI (STEMI) to monitor infarct size.[9] In the context of acute MI, elevated cTN levels can be detected after 4 to 10 hours after onset of symptoms with a peak at 12 up to 48 hours and return to normal concentrations after 4 to 10 days. Test sensitivity of cTN measurements for MI was found to be as high as nearly 100% after 6 to 12 hours after symptom onset with these early assays.[10,11] Thus, guidelines of the early 2000s established a rule-out strategy for patients with ACS presenting without ST-segment elevation (NSTE-ACS) based on the sequential measurements of cTN levels, repeated after 6 to 12 hours (eg,[12]).

The Protein Troponin as Component of the Cardiomyocyte

The contractile apparatus of skeletal and cardiac myocytes is constructed as a sliding filament mechanism centered on the interaction between actin and myosin filaments. Their calcium-dependent activation is regulated by the troponin complex. The cardiac troponin complex is formed by 3 subunits: troponin C, T, and I. While troponin C harbors the calcium-binding site, troponin T attaches to the actin filament and troponin I works as inhibitor of interaction with myosin heads in the absence of calcium. Of these 3 subunits, cTNI and cTNT isoforms are specific to cardiac

myocytes, and thus, their level in serum can be used as surrogate for myocardial damage.[5,13]

Evolution of High-Sensitivity Cardiac Troponin Assays

High-sensitivity (hs) TN assays are capable to detect cTNI or cTNT concentrations 10- to 100-fold lower than conventional tests. Their superior sensitivity entails exact quantification of cTN levels in up to 95% of the healthy individuals.[14] With this development, an even more rapid rule-out strategy for patients with acute chest pain became generally available. Two ground-breaking trials were published in 2009 demonstrating an excellent diagnostic performance of hsTN assays to improve early diagnosis and risk stratification of patients with ACS.[15,16] In 2011, European Society of Cardiology (ESC) guidelines—in contrast to US guidelines—endorsed a 3-hour instead of 6-hour algorithm of repeated cTN measurements, if a hs-assay is available.[17,18]

DEFINITIONS

Over the last years, hsTN-essays have become ubiquitously available and found their way into everyday clinical practice. From a theoretic point of view, they might not only be capable to increase patients' safety by an expedited clinical diagnosis or rule-out of acute MI, but they are also fulfilling caregivers' demands of an economic management of stationary wards, allowing shorter delays to establish or exclude a diagnosis. Nevertheless, the wide-spread use of even more sensitive troponin testing over the last years also poses a challenge to the clinician—whether cardiologist or not—as in more and more cases questions arise about potential consequences and clinical implications of positive cTN tests, especially those derived outside the setting of suspected MI.

Accounting for this clinical dilemma, the ESC and the American College of Cardiology (ACC) updated their consensus statement on the "Fourth Universal Definition on Myocardial Infarction" in August 2018.[19] This position paper aims to solve the question how to discriminate between different entities, which were formerly all submersed under the prevailing definition of "myocardial infarction" based on elevated biomarkers in a setting of now commonly available hsTN tests. Although a classification into 5 different types of "MI" introduced before was adopted, a term of "myocardial injury" was newly redefined. It accounts for the circumstance that elevated levels of cardiac biomarkers—in particular hsTN—are highly sensitive to detect damage of cardiomyocytes but are not specific for the detection of a "classical" ischemic MI. Per definition, all conditions characterized by an elevation of serum troponin levels—that is, defined by exceeding the 99th percentile upper reference level (URL) of serum levels of the healthy population—are now summarized as "myocardial injury," independent of their underlying pathology. Although different biomarkers indicating myocardial damage have been frequently used in the past, the position paper restricts the diagnosis of "myocardial injury" solely to abnormal serum cTN values because of their superior specificity for myocardial tissue.

A chronic form of myocardial injury is to be discriminated from its acute variant based on repetitive serum cTN tests, as stated by the position paper's authors. A myocardial injury is considered as "acute" if cTN levels show a relevant kinetic in serial blood tests—regardless of increase or decrease—with at least one value higher than the 99th percentile URL (Fig. 2). Stable cTN values indicate for a chronic myocardial injury. Thresholds for determining a significant difference between two serial cTN values are assay dependent. Elevated cTN levels cannot identify their cause—including ischemic as well as nonischemic conditions. Thus, the diagnosis of acute or chronic myocardial injury per se does not primarily justify a specific treatment, for example, direct referral to heart catheterization, but should lead to a further thorough clinical investigation.

Acute Myocardial Injury, Myocardial Ischemia, and Acute Myocardial Infarction

Various causes can induce a liberation of intracellular proteins (cTN and other markers) from the cardiomyocytes by pathophysiological mechanisms including preload-induced mechanical stretch and physiologic stress even in healthy hearts. On a histologic base, this release might be mediated by increased cellular turnover as well as apoptosis, liberation of cTN-degradation products, increased cellular wall permeability, release of membranous blebs, and myocyte necrosis.[20] Because of its broad and heterogenous cause, myocardial injury has a relatively high clinical incidence, which poses a challenge to the clinician and—per se—has negative influence on patients' prognosis independent of its pathophysiology.[21,22] Clinicians will have to rule out between a variety of nonischemic causes of myocardial injury, including primary cardiac diseases, for example, myocarditis, or noncardiac pathologies, for example, renal failure, and ischemic forms in kind of 1 of the 5 subtypes of MI (for an overview, see **Fig. 2**, **Table 1**). A proof of myocardial ischemia in combination with elevated hsTN levels justifies the clinical diagnosis of an MI (see **Fig. 2**). Typical clinical presentation, electrocardiographic signs, as well as characteristic findings in cardiac imaging—for example, echocardiography or cardiac magnetic resonance tomography—are accepted clinical surrogates for myocardial ischemia qualifying for the diagnosis of MI (eg, type 1 or type 2). Notably, this definition does not distinguish among the different mechanisms of MI, which may be based on a primary coronary problem as plaque rupture, coronary spasm, embolism, or dissection, but may also follow systemic processes resulting in decreased coronary perfusion of the cardiomyocytes, for example, due to hemodynamic deterioration by relevant bradycardia, hypotension, or any form of shock, as well as also compromised systemic oxygenation by acute diseases of the respiratory system or anemia. Furthermore, any cause of increased aerobic metabolism, for example, tachycardia or hypertension, might result in myocardial ischemia.

Clinical Concept of Acute Coronary Syndrome as Working Diagnosis and Different Types of Acute Myocardial Infarction

The concept of ACS as working diagnosis in emergency medicine comprises a clinical pathway for optimal risk stratification in patients presenting with acute chest discomfort or other ischemic symptoms. To optimize the timing of treatment strategies such as reperfusion therapy, patients must receive a 12-lead electrocardiography performed within 10 minutes after first medical contact, which will allow allocation into a category with a working diagnosis of STEMI, based on typical electrocardiographic findings in kind of ischemic repolarization patterns demanding for

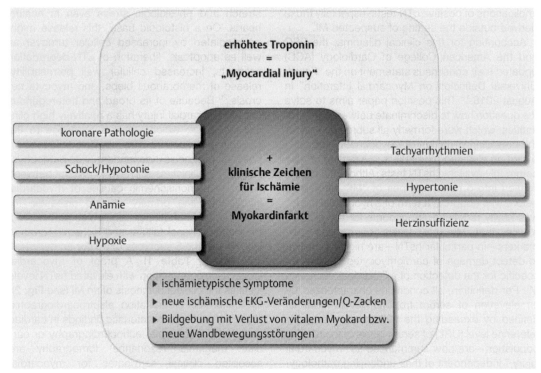

Fig. 2. Discrimination between the entities of myocardial injury and myocardial infarction. For details, see text. (*From* Wild J, Wenzel P: Myocardial Injury and myocardial infarction – consequences for clinical care in the light of current guidelines. Aktuel Kardiol 2019;8:193-198.)

urgent referral to heart catheterization or the group of patients without those typical ischemic ECG changes (working diagnosis of NSTE-ACS). For these, sequential cTN testing is essential for rule-in (or rule-out) of acute MI. In this context, it must be emphasized that a small subgroup of patients with NSTE-ACS also qualifies for an immediate invasive management in case of high-risk criteria as hemodynamic instability or refractory angina pectoris. Clinical pathways and timing of further diagnostic strategies in patients presenting with STEMI or NSTE-ACS are described in the specific guidelines.[17,18]

According to the "Universal Definition of MI" position paper, all of these clinical settings defining acute MI may be classified into 5 types, based on pathologic, clinical, and prognostic differences. This allocation to different types of MI grounded on their distinct pathophysiology might also justify different and individual treatment strategies.[1] MI type 1 is defined as the presence of atherothrombotic coronary artery disease resulting in an acute occlusion or relevant stenosis of a coronary vessel precipitated by atherosclerotic plaque disruption (rupture or erosion). Confirmation of the diagnosis is based on identification of a coronary thrombus

by angiography including intracoronary imaging or post mortem by autopsy.

Type 2 MI is also defined by the confirmation of acute myocardial ischemia, which—in contrast to type 1 MI—is not caused by an acute coronary plaque disruption but rather by an imbalance of myocardial oxygen supply and demand. Patients with type 2 MI might also suffer from known or presumed coronary artery disease and might thus be prone to ischemia in cases of additional acute stress such as hemorrhagic conditions with a relevant drop of hemoglobin or sustained heart rhythm disorders. Although coronary atherosclerosis is a common finding in type 2 MI, it has to be emphasized that the presence of coronary artery disease is not a mandatory precondition for every type 2 MI. Other potential causes comprise various pathologies including severe hypoxemia, shock, coronary artery dissection, or spasm and microvascular dysfunction, for instance. Interestingly, type 2 MI has worse short- and long-term outcomes as compared with type 1 MI. A large meta-analysis found a significantly higher intrahospital (15% vs 4.7%), 30 days (17.6% vs 5.3%) and 1-year mortality (27% vs 13%) and a higher rate of major adverse cardiovascular events

Table 1
Overview of variable causes resulting in elevations of cardiac troponins/myocardial injury

Cardiac Pathology	Noncardiac Pathology
Myocardial infarction/ischemia	SIRS or sepsis, infectious diseases
Heart failure	Renal failure or chronic kidney disease
(Peri-) myocarditis	Stroke or cerebral hemorrhage
Cardiomyopathies (of any type)	Pulmonary embolism, pulmonary hypertension
Valvular heart disease	Amyloidosis, sarcoidosis
Takotsubo syndrome	Cardiotoxicity, for example, chemotherapy
Cardiac procedures of any kind (PCI, intervention for structural or valvular heart disease, heart surgery, catheter ablation)	Shock, critically ill patients
	Extensive exercise training
Cardioversion/defibrillator shocks	
Cardiac contusion	

Abbreviations: PCI, percutaneous coronary intervention; SIRS, systemic inflammatory response syndrome.
  Data from Wild J, Wenzel P: Myocardial Injury and myocardial infarction – consequences for clinical care in the light of current guidelines. Aktuel Kardiol 2019;8:193-198. And Thygesen K, Alpert JS, Jaffe AS, et al. Fourth universal definition of myocardial infarction. Eur Heart J 2018;40:237-269.

(MACE; 20% vs 9%) in patients with type 2 versus type 1 MI. Moreover, a higher incidence of relevant cardiac and noncardiac comorbidities (diabetes mellitus, hypertension, renal failure, preexisting heart failure, chronic obstructive pulmonary disease) and a higher mean age of these patients seem to account for these findings, at least partially. As to be expected, only a minority of patients with type 2 MI (13.7%) who underwent invasive diagnostics were treated by percutaneous coronary intervention (PCI). Noncardiac surgery (20%), sepsis (19%), cardiac rhythm disturbances (19%), heart failure (15%), and anemia (12%) were identified as most probable causes for concomitant myocardial damage.[23] For definitions of MI types 3, 4a-c, and 5, see **Fig. 3**.

DISCUSSION
Type 2 Myocardial Infarction, Myocardial Injury, and Implications for Prognosis

Type 2 MI shares many of the prerequisites and diagnostic features of the rather broad definition of acute myocardial injury, and thus a clear-cut distinction between type 1 and type 2 MIs according to the contemporary definition will not always be possible. As outlined earlier, the diagnosis of type 2 MI based on the current classification additionally requires the clinical proof of myocardial ischemia—for example, by symptoms, dynamic changes in ECG, or cardiac imaging modalities besides elevated cTN levels. Thus, it might not be surprising that—with regard to prognosis—diagnoses of acute myocardial injury and type 2 MI are both correlated to a higher rate of adverse outcome in comparison to patients with type 1 MI: After a 1-year follow-up, mortality rates of 31% in type 2 MI

and 37% in myocardial injury were reported, compared with 16% in type 1 MI.[24,25] A Scottish monocentric registry including more than 2000 patients analogously reported on a doubled mortality in long-term follow-up of patients with noncardiac or multifactorial cause of myocardial injury and a similar rate of MACE compared with patients with type 1 MI.[26] A Danish cohort study with analogous design (approximately 1000 patients included) concluded that acute myocardial injury relevantly impaired prognosis when the cause was not primarily associated to cardiac diseases such as, for example, valvular heart disease or other causes of heart failure.[22] Based on these studies, the relatively high mortality after type 2 MI and myocardial injury might be mainly influenced by noncardiac comorbidities.[22,26,27]

Definition of a Proper Threshold for "Normal" cTN Values in the Context of High-Sensitivity Assays

As in all cases of all tests allowing hs-diagnostics, a proper interpretation of elevated serum hsTN indicating for AMI becomes more and more challenging—especially in cases with mild aberrance from normal values. As shown earlier, elevated cTN levels can be found in patients with a variety of cardiac coronary and noncoronary, as well as noncardiac disorders. Although the cut-off value (99th percentile URL) has been adopted by the guidelines as soon as 2007,[12] the definition of this threshold for determination in "normal" and "pathologic" findings is still under debate. The high negative predictive value of hsTN assays allows for a safe and time-efficient rule-out of most of the patients presenting with chest discomfort.

Clinical Classification of Myocardial Infarction

Type 1:   Myocardial infarction due to coronary plaque rupture/erosion (with occlusive or non-occlusive thrombus)

Type 2:   Myocardial infarction due to imbalance in oxygen supply/demand without evidence of coronary plaque disrupture

Type 3:   cardiac death with symptoms suggestive of myocardial ischemia (death before biomarkers could be obtained), or myocardial ischemia detected by auptosy examination

Type 4:   Myocardial infarction related to previous coronary intervention
4a: after PCI   4b: due to Stent/scaffold thrombosis
4c: due to restenosis

Type 5:   Myocardial infarction associated to coronary artery bypass grafting

Fig. 3. Clinical classification of different subtypes of acute myocardial infarction. PCI, percutaneous coronary intervention. For details, see text. (*Data from* Thygesen K, Alpert JS, Jaffe AS, et al. Fourth universal definition of myocardial infarction. Eur Heart J 2018;40:237-269.)

On the other hand, more patients will be found at putatively pathologic cTN levels using hsTN over conventional assays. A study on 3327 consecutive patients admitted to the Chest Pain Unit of the University of Heidelberg reported that in up to 69% of the patients the finding of an elevated hsTNT level could finally not be correlated to an ACS.[28] Recently, a large Scottish multicenter trial on more than 48,000 patients found that implementation of an hsTN assay in patients presenting as ACS in emergency departments led to a reclassification in kind of an additional increase of patients meeting criteria of myocardial injury or acute MI by 17% in comparison to conventional cTN testing; yet, the incidence of MI or cardiovascular death after 1 year could not be reduced by using hsTN over the conventional assay.[29] The controversy about a proper cut-off level for normal findings of hsTN has been heated up further by the fact that physiologic cTN levels are influenced by a variety of causes, for example, renal failure, gender, stroke, obesity, age,[30] and even circadian rhythm.[31] Up to now, the implementation of adapted thresholds, for example, sex-specific or dependent on renal function,[32] are not recommended by current guidelines. Nevertheless, as discussed earlier, there is solid evidence that any clinical situation with a documented increase of cTN levels higher than the defined threshold levels conveys important prognostic implications for the patients, regardless of the cause of this finding—MI or any other clinical setting of myocardial injury—and demands further evaluation [for example, [28,33]].

Future Developments in Clinical Risk Stratification Based on Cardiac Biomarkers

The implementation of hs-assays has expedited clinical algorithm for the management of ACS. More sensitive troponin tests allow for the detection of smaller myocardial injury and thus, swifter and safer diagnostics in confirmation or rule-out of acute MI. In the future, further progress and evidence in biomarker testing might unleash further potential for acceleration without a loss of diagnostic accuracy. At the moment, European Guidelines endorse a fast 0/3 hours strategy as standard algorithm if hsTN testing is available or an even swifter 0/1 hours rule-out strategy if validated hsTN assays are used. Contemporarily this is applicable to the kits of many vendors; nevertheless, even lower hsTN thresholds (in comparison to the "regular" cut-off level of 99th percentile URL) have to be applied for this expedited diagnostic workup. Even more, a "direct" rule-out pathway has been introduced, allowing for a negative predictive value of more than 99% if initial hsTN levels are less than the limit of detection at admission.[17] It is important to emphasize that these rapid rule-out strategies are not recommended in "very early presenters" (onset of symptoms < 3 hours) due to a potential time-shift in cTN release. A "dual marker strategy," including the measurement of Copeptin (a fragment of vasopressin) might enable an even higher diagnostic accuracy in rapid algorithms. Furthermore, the implementation of clinical scores (eg, GRACE-Score) is strongly recommended before discharge.[34] Future developments might lead to superior biomarker tests, facilitating ambulatory "point of care" diagnostics at highest safety. This might be a further aid to the clinician in the emergency department having to distinguish between the high-risk patient requiring for urgent treatment and low-risk patients, of which some will have to be discharged rapidly. In this context, dedicated emergency units specialized for the evaluation of patients presenting with chest pain, so called chest pain units (CPU), have been established in many countries. There is evidence that a concept of CPUs undergoing standardized certification process entail a better adherence to guidelines[35] and might influence survival positively.[36] In this regard, the Acute Cardiovascular Care Association of the ESC has published a position paper endorsing standardized implementations of CPUs in emergency departments.[37]

SUMMARY

Because of a rather limited specificity and predictive value of symptoms and other clinical findings including ECG in the context of MI, biomarkers have become an indispensable tool for daily diagnostic and risk stratification. Among a variety of blood tests available, cTN levels may serve as best surrogates for myocardial damage up to now. The implementation of hsTN assays in clinical practice has expedited rule-out pathways for MI due to a higher negative predictive value in comparison to conventional cTN tests. Yet, higher sensitivity of markers for myocardial damage may result in a higher number of patients "ruled-in." In 2018, the updated "Fourth Universal Definition on Myocardial Infarction" was published as ESC/ACC consensus statement, defining the term of "myocardial injury" comprising all nonischemic and ischemic causes of myocardial damage, including MI. Whereas the diagnosis of myocardial injury is based on cTN testing, the confirmation of MI requires the clinical proof of cardiac ischemia. Myocardial injury is a heterogenous entity that can be caused by a large variety of cardiac as well as extracardiac disorders; furthermore, it exceeds "classical" type 1 MI in mortality. As a matter of fact, abnormal biomarker values are always to be interpreted within their clinical context; serial samplings can be helpful in ruling-in and -out

strategies. Of many biomarkers used, hsTN assays are one of those that have truly proved the potential diagnostic power of blood tests in emergency medicine. They have not only changed our diagnostic strategy in ACS but also allow superior risk stratification in the context of noncardiac disorders. In the future, potentially superior and tailored biomarkers might allow quickest optimal diagnostic and therapeutic guidance to identify patients at risk for future cardiovascular events.

CLINICS CARE POINTS

- Clinical symptoms as typical angina pectoris and ECG compatible with cardiac ischemia are a frequent cause for admission to emergency units, but only have limited predictive value for the prevalence of significant coronary stenoses
- Biomarkers for myocardial damage have become an indispensable tool for diagnostics in settings of acute coronary syndromes
- Over the last years, hs-cardiac troponin (hsTN) assays have become ubiquitously available
- Because of high sensitivity, hsTN testing has expedited rule-in and -out algorithms
- In 2018, the fourth universal definition on MI was published, which redefined the condition of myocardial injury
- Myocardial injury is diagnosed by elevated troponin serum levels even in the absence of myocardial ischemia and is characterized by impaired prognosis that may even exceed that of type 1 MI
- Clinical implications based on elevations of serum troponin must always be validated in their clinical context
- The diagnosis of MI requires clinical proof of myocardial ischemia in the addition of elevated cardiac troponin levels
- hsTN assays allow safe and economic therapeutic guidance for the clinician in the emergency unit

DISCLOSURE

The authors have nothing to disclose.

REFERENCES

1. Faranoff AC, Rymer JA, Goldstein SA, et al. Does this patient with chest pain have acute coronary syndrome? JAMA 2015;314:1955–65.
2. Carton EW, Than M, Cullen L, et al. Chest pain typicality in suspected acute coronary syndromes and the impact of clinical experience. Am J Med 2015; 128:1109–16.

3. LaDue JS, Wroblewski F, Karmen A. Serum glutamic oxaloacetic transaminase activity in human acute transmural myocardial infarction. Science 1954; 120:497–9.

4. HYPERTENSION and coronary heart disease: classification and criteria for epidemiological studies. World Health Organ Tech Rep Ser 1959;58(168): 1–28.

5. Garg P, Morris P, Fazlanie AL, et al. Cardiac biomarkers of acute coronary syndrome: from history to high-sensitivity cardiac troponin. Intern Emerg Med 2017;12:147–55.

6. World Health Organization. Report of the Joint International Society and Federation of Cardiology/World Health Organization Task Force on Standardization of clinical nomenclature. Nomenclature and criteria for diagnosis of ischemic heart disease. Circulation 1979;59:607–9.

7. Ebashi S, Kodama A. A new protein factor promoting aggregation of tropomyosin. J Biochem 1965; 58:107–8.

8. Katus HA, Remppis A, Looser S, et al. Enzyme linked immuno assay of cardiac troponin T for the detection of acute myocardial infarction in patients. J Mol Cell Cardiol 1989;21:1349–53.

9. Katus HA, Giannitsis E. Biomarkers in cardiology. Clin Res Cardiol 2018;107:S10–5.

10. Jaffe AS, Landt Y, Parvin CA, et al. Comparative sensi- tivity of cardiac troponin I and lactate dehydrogenase isoenzymes for diagnosing acute myocardial infarction. Clin Chem 1996;42:1770–6.

11. Balk EM, Ioannidis JP, Salem D, et al. Accuracy of biomarkers to diagnose acute cardiac ischemia in the emergency department: a meta-analysis. Ann Emerg Med 2001;37:478–94.

12. Bassand JP, Hamm CW, Ardissino D, et al. Guidelines for the diagnosis and treatment of non-ST-segment elevation acute coronary syndromes. Eur Heart J 2007;28:1598–660.

13. Ooi DS, Isotalo PA, Veinot JP. Correlation of antemortem serum creatinine kinase, creatinine kinase-MB, troponin I, and troponin T with cardiac pathology. Clin Chem 2000;46:338–44.

14. Apple FS, Ler R, Murakami MM. Determination of 19 cardiac troponin I and T assay 99th percentile values from a common presumably healthy population. Clin Chem 2012;58:1574–81.

15. Reichlin T, Hochholzer W, Bassetti S, et al. Early Diagnosis of Myocardial Infarction with sensitive cardiac troponin assays. N Engl J Med 2009;361:858–67.

16. Keller T, Zeller T, Peetz D, et al. Sensitive troponin I assay in early diagnosis of acute myocardial infarction. N Engl J Med 2009;361:868–77.

17. Roffi M, Patrono C, Collet JP, et al. 2015 ESC Guidelines for the management of acute coronary syndromes in patients presenting without persistent ST-segment elevation. Eur Heart J 2015;37:267–315.

18. Amsterdam EA, Wenger NK, Brindis RG, et al. 2014 AHA/ACC Guideline for the management of patients with non-ST-elevation acute coronary syndromes. J Am Coll Cardiol 2014;64:2645–87.

19. Thygesen K, Alpert JS, Jaffe AS, et al. Fourth universal definition of myocardial infarction. Eur Heart J 2018;40:237–69.

20. White HD. Pathobiology of troponin elevations: do elevations occur with myocardial ischemia as well as necrosis? J Am Coll Cardiol 2011;57:2406–8.

21. Sarkisian L, Saaby L, Poulsen TS, et al. Clinical characteristics and outcomes of patients with myocardial infarction, myocardial injury, and nonelevated troponins. Am J Med 2016;129:446.e5-e21.

22. Sarkisian L, Saaby L, Poulsen TS, et al. Prognostic impact of myocardial injury related to various cardiac and noncardiac conditions. Am J Med 2016; 129:506–14.

23. Gupta S, Vaidya SR, Arora S, et al. Type 2 versus type 1 myocardial infarction: a comparison of clinical characteristics and outcomes with a meta-analysis of observational studies. Cardiovasc Diagn Ther 2017;7:348–58.

24. Chapman AR, Adamson PD, Mills NL. Assessment and classification of patients with myocardial injury and infarction in clinical practice. Heart 2017;103:10–8.

25. Javed U, Aftab W, Ambrose JA, et al. Frequency of elevated troponin I and diagnosis of acute myocardial infarction. Am J Cardiol 2009;104:9–13.

26. Chapman AR, Shah AS, Lee KK, et al. Long-term outcomes in patients with type 2 myocardial infarction and myocardial injury. Circulation 2018;137: 1236–45.

27. Lambrecht S, Sarkisian L, Saaby L, et al. Different causes of death in patients with myocardial infarction type 1, type 2, and myocardial injury. Am J Med 2018;131:548–54.

28. Mueller M, Varaie M, Biener M, et al. Cardiac Troponin T – from diagnosis of myocardial infarction to cardiovascular risk prediction. Circ J 2013;77:1654–61.

29. Shah AS, Anand A, Strachan FE, et al. High-sensitivity troponin in the evaluation of patients with suspected acute coronary syndrome: a stepped-wedge, cluster-randomised controlled trial. Lancet 2018;392:919–28.

30. Nishimura M, Brann A, Chang KW, et al. The confounding effects of non-cardiac pathologies on the interpretation of cardiac biomarkers. Curr Heart Fail Rep 2018;15:239–49.

31. Fournier S, Iten L, Marques-Vidal P, et al. Circadian rhythm of blood cardiac troponin T concentration. Clin Res Cardiol 2017;106:1026–32.

32. Twerenbold R, Wildi K, Jaeger C, et al. Optimal cutoff levels of more sensitive cardiac troponin assays for the ealy diagnosis of myocardial infarction in patients with renal dysfunction. Circulation 2015;131: 2041–50.

33. Celik S, Giannitsis E, Wollert KC, et al. Cardiac troponin t concentrations above the 99th percentile value as measured by a new high-sensitivity assay predict long-term prognosis in patients with acute coronary syndromes undergoing routine early invasive strategy. Clin Res Cardiol 2011;100:1077–85.

34. Mockel M, Searle J, Hamm C, et al. Early discharge using single cardiac troponin and co-peptin testing in patients with suspected acute coronary syndrome (ACS): a randomized, controlled clinical process study. Eur Heart J 2015;36:369–76.

35. Ross MA, Amsterdam E, Peacock WF, et al. Chest pain center accreditation is associated with better perfomance of centers for medicare and medicaid services core measures for acute myocardial infarction. Am J Cardiol 2008;102:120–4.

36. Keller T, Post F, Tzikas S, et al. Improved outcome in acute coronary syndrome by establishing a chest pain unit. Clin Res Cardiol 2010; 99:149–55.

37. Claeys MJ, Ahrens I, Sinnaeve P, et al. The organization of chest pain units: position statement of the Acute Cardiovascular Care Association. Eur Heart J Acute Cardiovasc Care 2017;6:203–11.

The High Bleeding Risk Patient with Coronary Artery Disease

Francesco Costa, MD, PhD[a,b,*], Victoria Garcia-Ruiz, MD[c], Roberto Licordari, MD[a], Luigi Fimiani, MD[a]

KEYWORDS

- PCI • Coronary • Stent • DAPT • PRECISE-DAPT • Bleeding • Risk • Score

KEY POINTS

- Reducing bleeding complications has become a priority in modern cardiology.
- Bleeding carries a significant prognostic impact that could equate or surpass ischemic events.
- Specific tools and definitions to identify and treat high bleeding risk patients are now available and could support decisions for antiplatelet therapy duration selection.

INTRODUCTION

The role of antithrombotic therapy in the treatment of acute ischemic heart disease has been established for more than 40 years.[1] Discoveries linking myocardial infarction (MI) to coronary thrombosis have prompted research in the field of thrombocardiology, pushing boundaries for more effective and prolonged treatments to reduce recurrences of vascular thrombosis.[2] Dual antiplatelet therapy (DAPT), consisting of a combination of aspirin and a P2Y12 platelet receptor inhibitor, is mandatory after percutaneous coronary intervention (PCI) to reduce the risk of stent-related and non–stent-related coronary ischemic events.[3] Yet, the introduction of more potent or prolonged courses of treatment has invariably increased the rate of bleeding events.[4–6] Similar to coronary ischemic events, bleeding events could have a negative impact on prognosis, especially among individuals at high bleeding risk (HBR).[7] For this reason, identifying HBR patients is key to optimizing outcomes. Prognostic tools and standardized definitions recently have been proposed with this scope and have been endorsed by specialty guidelines.[8,9] This report provides a summary of the current available evidence regarding HBR-PCI and a description of the current tools to identify and individualize treatment in this subgroup.

PROGNOSTIC IMPACT OF BLEEDING EVENTS AFTER PERCUTANEOUS CORONARY INTERVENTION OR ACUTE CORONARY SYNDROME

In the past 2 decades, ischemic events after PCI halved, reduced from 18.4% to 9.1%, and out-of-hospital bleeding doubled, increasing from 2.5% in the period 1995 to 2000 to approximately 5% in the period 2013 to 2016.[10] Bleeding prevention has become a priority in modern cardiology.[11] Hemorrhagic events during antithrombotic treatment could occur at multiple organs (**Fig. 1**). In the ADAPT-DES study, 61.7% of out-of-hospital bleeding occurred in the gastrointestinal tract, 12.2% were peripheral, 8.6% were genitourinary, 7.4% were in the central nervous system, 7.0% were from the vascular access site, and 3.2%

Funding: No external funding was used for this article.
[a] Department of Clinical and Experimental Medicine, Policlinico "G. Martino", University of Messina, Via C Valeria 1, Messina 98100, Italy; [b] Interventional Cardiology Unit, Policlinico G. Martino, Via C Valeria 1, Messina 98100, Italy; [c] UGC del Corazón, Servicio de Cardiología, Hospital Clínico Universitario Virgen de la Victoria, Málaga 29010, Spain
* Corresponding author.
E-mail address: dottfrancescocosta@gmail.com

cardiology.theclinics.com

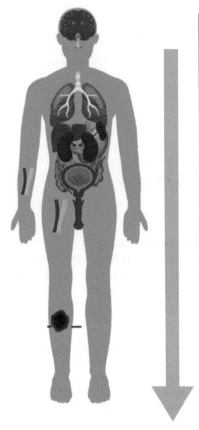

Site of bleeding	Incidence	Suggestion to prevent or to treat
Gastrointestinal	61,7%	- Use of proton-pump inhibitors - Avoid NSAIDs - Before elective PCI consider gastroscopy or colonoscopy if active bleeding is suspected
Peripheral	12,2%	- Local haemostatic measures - Cold water rinse - Tranexamic acid if mucosal bleed
Genitourinary	8,6%	- Urine cytology, imaging for diagnosis and treatment - Consider hormonal or local therapy for menometrorrhagia
Central Nervous System	7,4%	- Consider short DAPT in patients at risk of intracranial bleeding - Blood pressure management
Access site	7.0%	- Prefer radial access - Echo-guided puncture if femoral artery is needed
Retroperitoneal	3.2%	- Look for signs and symptoms - Make early diagnosis

When severe or life threatening bleeding consider:
- Surgical or endoscopic treatment of bleeding source if possible
- Fluid replacement
- Red blood cells transfusion
- Platelet transfusion

Fig. 1. Bleeding risk after PCI and bleeding avoidance strategies.

were retroperitoneal.[12] Depending on their location and severity, the prognostic impact of major bleeding could be similar or even worse compared with recurrent MI.[7] Even when not associated directly with worse outcomes, bleeding episodes are linked to poor drug adherence and deterioration in quality of life.[13–15]

HIGH BLEEDING RISK DEFINITION AND RISK STRATIFICATION

Proper identification of HBR patients is key to recognizing and then individualizing treatment.

In a survey published in 2015, advanced age, chronic renal failure, anemia, and a positive history of past bleeding events were considered the most important markers of HBR after PCI.[16]

Risk stratification tools previously have been proposed to improve in-hospital outcomes and quality metrics,[17] although most bleeding events related to DAPT after coronary stenting occur in the out-of-hospital setting. Only recently, multiple risk stratification tools have been proposed to measure this risk.

The PARIS score is a set of 2 prediction tools focused on ischemic and bleeding risk prediction after discharge.[18] These tools have been developed from a real-world cohort of 4190 patients undergoing drug-eluting stent (DES) implantation. The integer risk score developed for major bleeding at 2 years included 6 clinical features: age, body mass index, current smoking, anemia, renal impairment (ie, with a creatinine clearance <60 mL/min), and triple antithrombotic therapy at discharge.[18] The predicted risk of Bleeding Academic Research Consortium (BARC) type 3 or 5 bleeding at 2 years was 1.80% among patients at low bleeding risk, 3.90% in the intermediate risk, and 10.0% in the HBR patients.[18]

The PRECISE-DAPT is a risk score focused on out-of-hospital bleeding events among patients treated with PCI and assigned to DAPT.[19] It has been developed from a collaborative data set of 8 randomized clinical trials, including 14,963 patients. The risk score developed for major bleeding at 1 year included 5 clinical and laboratory variables: age, a history of prior bleeding, hemoglobin, white blood cell count, and creatinine clearance. An alternative score excluding white blood cell count also was developed and validated.[19,20] A history of prior bleeding was the most important contributor to the model. The score has been validated in 2 different external cohorts from a large randomized controlled trial and from a large real-world registry.[4,21] High-risk patients carried a predicted risk of thrombosis in MI (TIMI) major or minor bleeding at 1 year greater than 1.85%.[19]

Score discrimination was decent in both the derivation cohort (C statistic = 0.73) and in the validation cohort from the PLATO trial (C statistic = 0.70); it was modest in the validation cohort from the Bern PCI registry (C statistic = 0.66).

Recently the HBR Academic Research Consortium (HBR-ARC) provided a consensus-based definition of HBR after PCI. HBR patients were defined as those with an estimated risk of major bleeding (ie, according to the standardized definition of the BARC 3 and 5) of at least 4% per year or a risk of intracranial bleeding of at least 1% year.[22] This threshold has been selected by consensus based on data from HBR-PCI trial literature, selecting a meaningful and clinical sound limit of events. The task force also listed a series of 20 clinical or laboratory criteria that could be used for identifying patients at HBR. These are divided in major or minor criteria of HBR, qualifying as HBR if at least 1 major criterion or 2 minor criteria are present in the single patient (**Fig. 2**). This definition has been independently validated in CREDO-Kyoto register.[23] In this population, HBR patients were associated with a significant increase of GUSTO moderate or severe bleeding at 1-year (10.4% vs 3.4%, respectively) and at 5-year follow-up (18.9% vs 6.6%, respectively; P <.0001). The presence of multiple risk criteria was associated with a linear increase in bleeding risk (no criteria: 6.6%; ≥2 minor criteria: 14.7%; 1 major criterion: 18.5%; 2 major criteria: 30.6%; and ≥3 major criteria: 49.9%, P<.0001).[23]

Another external validation of this definition recently has been provided from the Bern PCI registry.[24] In this population of all-comer patients treated with PCI in a single, large-volume tertiary center in Switzerland, a total of 39.4% of patients were deemed at HBR. As expected, HBR patients were associated to a significantly higher risk of BARC type 3 or 5 bleeding (6.4% vs 1.9%, respectively; P<.001). An increasing number of bleeding criteria was associated to a proportional higher risk of bleeding, which was greater than 10% at 12 months if greater than or equal to 3 major criteria were present.[24]

The criteria proposed by the HBR-ARC initiative have a robust literature confirming their link to a higher risk of bleeding. Oral anticoagulant (OAC) treatment is considered a major criterion in the HBR-ARC definition. The combination of OAC and antiplatelet therapy after PCI is associated with a 3-fold to 5-fold increase of bleeding risk.[25,26] Use of OAC is mandatory to reduce stroke and systemic thromboembolism in a series of conditions, including high-risk atrial fibrillation (AF). In PCI patients with need for long-term OAC for AF, implementation of direct OACs (DOACs), instead of vitamin K antagonists, and implementation of dual antithrombotic therapy, instead of triple antithrombotic therapy (ie, by excluding aspirin from the antithrombotic strategy), early after stenting is associated with a reduction of bleeding events[26]; yet, the rates of bleeding also with DOACs and single antiplatelet therapy with a P2Y12 inhibitor remain high, requiring a closer follow-up in this group of patients.[27]

Malignancy, defined as a diagnosis of active cancer in the previous 12 months before PCI or an ongoing illness on actual treatment, is considered a major criterion of HBR. Cancer poses patients at both higher risk of bleeding and thrombosis. It generally is associated with a hypercoagulable state with increased platelet activation and aggregation, despite a high prevalence of thrombocytopenia.[28,29] Hence, malignancy could be associated with major bleeding due to both blood dyscrasia or direct bleeding from the malignant tissue. In a prior report from the Bern PCI registry, a history of malignancy was a strong predictor of novel gastrointestinal bleeding, with a more than 2-fold higher risk.[21]

Moderate or severe thrombocytopenia (<100,000 elements per mm^3) is considered a major HBR-ARC criterion. Patients with chronic thrombocytopenia undergoing PCI have a more than doubled risk of postprocedural bleeding and greater postprocedural complications, with the risk of bleeding proportional to the degree of thrombocytopenia.[30,31] This also is associated with higher intrahospital mortality.[32] The association between thrombocytopenia and bleeding

MAJOR
Anticipated use of long-term oral anticoagulation
Severe or end-stage CKD (eGFR <30 mL/min)
Hemoglobin < 11 g / dL
Spontaneous bleeding requiring hospidalization or trasfusion in the past 6 mo or any time, if recurrent
Moderate or severe baseline thrombocytopenia (platelet < 100 x 10⁹/L)
Chronic bleeding diathesis
Liver cirrhosis with portal hypertension
Active malignancy
Previous spontaneous ICH, previous traumatic ICH within the past 12 mo, Presence of bAVM, Moderate or severe ischemic stroke (National Institutes of Health Stroke Scale score ≥ 5) within the past 6 mo
Nondeferrable major surgery on DAPT
Recent major surgery or major trauma within 30 day before PCI

MINOR
Age ≥ 75 y
Moderate CKD (eGFR 30-59 mL/min)
Hemoglobin 11-12,9 g/dL for men, 11-11,9 g/dL for women
Spontaneous bleeding requiring hospidalization or trasfusion in the past 12 mo not meeting the major criterion
Long term use of oral NSAIDs or steroids
Any ischemic stroke at any time not meeting the major criterion

Fig. 2. Major and minor criteria for HBR after PCI according to HBR-ARC. Hb, hemoglobin; ICH, intracranial hemorrhage; PLT, platelet.

may be direct, owing to the limited platelet number or secondary to other comorbidities.

A history of spontaneous bleeding or blood transfusion is an important predictor of future bleeding events and is considered a major criterion, if occurring in the 6 months prior to PCI, or minor, if occurring 6 months to 12 months earlier. In addition, a prior history of recurrent bleeding any time before PCI, which have not been resolved, accounts as a major criterion of bleeding risk. Prior bleeding was the single variable associated most strongly with an increased risk of bleeding in several clinical studies.[19,33]

Brain arteriovenous malformations (bAVMs), a history of previous intracranial hemorrhage, and ischemic stroke in the 6 months prior to PCI (with National Institutes of Health Stroke Scale ≥5 scale at the clinical presentation) represent major HBR criterion. There is a paucity of evidence informing the best antithrombotic strategy in patients with bAVMs; hence, in the absence of robust evidence, a conservative treatment seems the most reasonable option in this group of patients.

Anemia is another pivotal marker of higher bleeding risk. Anemia is considered a major criterion, if the baseline hemoglobin value is less than 11 g/dL, or a minor criterion, if it is between 11 g/dL and 12.9 g/dL in men and 11 g/dL and 11.9 g/dL in women. Anemia frequently is found among patients with cardiovascular diseases and significantly affects the prognosis in patients with either heart failure or coronary artery disease undergoing PCI.[34] Anemia may represent a sign of a silent, nonclinically overt bleeding or more generally represent a marker of comorbidity and frailty, which indirectly influence the bleeding risk.

Renal function also is a major determinant of bleeding risk after PCI.[35,36] The HBR-ARC proposed severe or end-stage chronic kidney disease (CKD) (estimated glomerular filtration rate [eGFR] <30 mL/min) as a major criterion and moderate CKD (eGFR 30–59 mL/min) as a minor criterion. Multiple reasons place CKD patients at higher risk of bleeding, including the unpredictable pharmacokinetics of antithrombotic agents with the risk of accumulation and overdose.

Long-term treatment with nonsteroidal anti-inflammatory drugs (NSAIDs) and corticosteroids (≥4 d/wk) is considered a minor HBR criterion. The use of these drugs is associated with a dose-dependent increase in gastrointestinal bleeding risk.

Finally, advanced age is one of the most recognized factors of HBR after PCI.[37] Advanced age has been the most common inclusion criteria among HBR-PCI stent trials.[38,39] It is, however, controversial whether advanced age qualifies per se as a marker of major bleeding risk, because many elderly patients without significant comorbidities do not necessarily qualify in this category.[24] Yet, on absolute terms, elderly patients are more likely to have comorbidities, which pose increased bleeding risk for them, reducing the benefit of prolonged or more potent antithrombotic treatments. In the TRITON trial, patients older than 75 years did not benefit from prasugrel, 10 mg, and showed a significant increase in bleeding events.[5] Similarly, in the PRODIGY study, elderly patients treated with DAPT for 24 months were associated with an excess of BARC 2, 3, and 5 bleeding events, compared with those undergoing DAPT for 6 months, with a higher absolute bleeding risk increase compared with younger patients.[40]

DUAL ANTIPLATELET THERAPY DURATION INDIVIDUALIZATION AMONG PATIENTS AT HIGH BLEEDING RISK

DAPT duration selection lies on the equilibrium between the risk of ischemia and bleeding and could be informed by various clinical and procedural elements (**Fig. 3**).[41–43] Prolonged DAPT has been shown to reduce the risk of stent thrombosis and coronary ischemic events after PCI, but it is associated with a higher risk of bleeding,[44–46] whereas a shorter-term DAPT is associated with a reduction in bleeding events.[47] The overall neutral impact on death makes the optimal risk/benefit balance unclear.[47,48]

Importantly, the risk/benefit balance can be very different in HBR patients, in which the higher baseline risk of bleeding and the higher severity of these events may outweigh the benefit of prolonged antithrombotic treatments.

Using algorithms to identify HBR patients and inform DAPT duration decision making recently has been proposed. The advantage of these tools lies in the objective estimate of the clinical risks.[49,50] A subjective evaluation tends to overestimate the ischemic and bleeding risk in low-risk patients and to underestimate it in high-risk patients.[51]

The first attempt to provide an objective stratification of the bleeding risk to guide DAPT decisions was proposed in a retrospective analysis of the PRODIGY trial, which randomized all-comer patients after PCI to 6 months versus 24 months of DAPT.[52] In this study, the population was stratified according to the CRUSADE score, which accounts for 8 clinical variables: female gender, signs of heart failure, diabetes and peripheral artery disease, hematocrit, creatinine clearance, heart rate, systolic pressure.[17] HBR patients (ie, with a CRUSADE score >40), which represented the 15.7% of the overall PRODIGY population, were associated with a more than 3-fold increased risk of BARC type 3 or 5 bleeding when treated with 24 months compared with 6 months' DAPT (9.7% vs 3.7%, respectively; $P = .04$). In contrast, patients at low bleeding risk (ie, with a CRUSADE ≤40) were not exposed to a significant increase of bleeding complications after a longer DAPT.[52] The risk of ischemic events, a composite of death, MI, or cerebrovascular accident, was similar for a 24-month compared with 6-month DAPT, irrespective of the baseline bleeding risk. Hence, patients at HBR were not deemed suitable for a longer treatment with DAPT given the exaggerated risk of bleeding. Yet, the CRUSADE score was developed to predict in-hospital bleeding, and for this reason its ability to be applied to long-term treatment decisions was suboptimal.

The DAPT score[53] was the first dedicated tool to inform decision making for DAPT duration after PCI. This algorithm developed within the DAPT study could be calculated after 12 months of uneventful DAPT to identify candidates who could benefit from prolonged treatment with DAPT beyond 12 months. The score includes age, smoking, diabetes mellitus, MI at presentation, previous MI or PCI, paclitaxel-eluting stent implantation, stent diameter less than 3 mm, heart failure or ejection fraction less than 30%, and stenting of a venous graft. The DAPT score was designed to evaluate the net benefit between ischemic and hemorrhagic endpoints for patients treated with a prolonged DAPT: those with a score less than 2 points are considered at higher bleeding than ischemic risk, whereas those with a score of 2

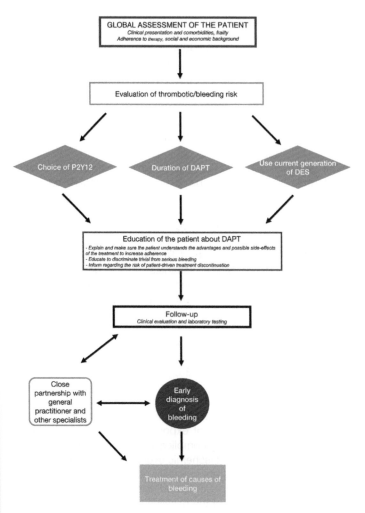

Fig. 3. Management of HBR patient after PCI. Patient-centered approach.

points are considered at higher ischemic than bleeding risk. Patients with scores less than 2 had a greater than 2-fold increase in bleeding events, with a prolonged DAPT beyond 12 months. Therefore, prolonged DAPT is not advantageous in this subset of patients. On the contrary, patients with a score of 2 points or more were associated with a reduction of ischemic events, without a significant increase in bleeding complications after prolonged DAPT.

At difference with the DAPT score, the PRECISE-DAPT score[19] provides a tool for decision making at the time of PCI. After PCI, patients were assigned to DAPT with aspirin and a P2Y12 inhibitor, whereas patients with OAC were excluded. In the subgroup of 10,081 patients assigned to a randomized duration of the DAPT (12–24 months' long or 3–6 months' short), the impact of the duration of DAPT was assessed within the risk categories defined by the score.

Patients in the higher-risk quartile (PRECISE-DAPT ≥25 points) were considered HBR, whereas those with very low risk, low risk, or moderate risk were considered non-HBR. In this analysis, patients defined as HBR were associated with a significant increase in TIMI major or minor bleeding when assigned to a prolonged DAPT (absolute risk increase 2.59% [95% CI, +0.82 to +4.34]) whereas low-risk patients were not associated with a significant increase in bleeding events when treated with prolonged DAPT. Similarly, only not-HBR patients gained benefit in the composite endpoint of ischemia (MI, stent thrombosis, stroke, and target vessel revascularization) from prolonged DAPT (absolute risk reduction 1.53% [95% CI, −2.64 to −0.41]), but not those at HBR at baseline.

The early selection of a treatment duration of 3 months or 6 months in HBR patients (PRECISE-DAPT score ≥25) could avoid exposing patients to a risk of excessive bleeding, whereas in non-HBR patients (PRECISE-DAPT score <25), standard (12-month) or prolonged (>12-month) treatment, if tolerated, could guarantee a further reduction of ischemic events without an excessive risk of bleeding complications. This algorithm has been further validated within the subgroup of HBR patients undergoing complex angioplasty,[54] which are associated with a high ischemic risk.[55,56]

Hence, international guidelines endorse the use of validated risk scores for DAPT decision making.[8,57,58] The PRECISE-DAPT score can be evaluated at the time of PCI, with clinical and laboratory values calculated in close proximity to the PCI. Instead, the DAPT score should be calculated among patients who already have been treated with DAPT without ischemic and bleeding events during the first 12 months to decide whether extend treatment up to 30 months or stop treatment.

The type of stent used (ie, DES vs bare-metal stent [BMS]) during the coronary interventional procedure traditionally has been linked to decisions regarding DAPT duration, but in modern practice should no more be a driver of treatment decisions.[59] BMSs, once considered safer than first-generation DESs during short DAPT strategy,[60–62] have been progressively limited in their use with the implementation of second-generation and third-generation DESs that proved safer and more biocompatible, even when a short DAPT strategy was necessary.[59] The first study assessing the impact of second-generation DES versus BMS in suboptimal candidates for DES was the ZEUS trial.[63] In the ZEUS, 1606 patients were randomized to DES with zotarolimus-eluting stent (Endeavor) or BMS. The primary outcome, including cardiovascular adverse events at 12 months (death from all causes, MI, or target vessel revascularization), was reduced in the DES group (17.5%) compared with the BMS group (22.1%); the bleeding risk in 2 arms was similar (TIMI major/minor bleeding: 1.7% vs 2.1%, respectively; $P = .72$). A large proportion of the patients included in the study were assigned to a very short DAPT (30 days) due to their HBR. In this subset of patients, the use of DES was associated with a reduction in the rate of major cardiovascular events of 25%, largely due to a significant reduction in MI and the need for revascularization of the treated vessel.[61]

These results were confirmed later in other 2 randomized trials in which BMSs were compared with bioresorbable polymer[38] or polymer-free[60] stents. More recent trials also have confirmed the role of novel-generation DES with a permanent polymer in patients managed with a short DAPT strategy.[39]

BMS is associated with an increased rate of restenosis and revascularization independently of the diameter of the treated vessel.[44] Therefore, multiple revascularizations in patients assigned to BMS potentially can lead to a paradoxically higher total exposure to DAPT than DES. For this reason, the use of BMSs in HBR patients no longer should be considered the gold standard for safety,[64] and the routine use of DES, regardless of DAPT duration and bleeding risk, is recommended.[9] In addition, the use of drug-eluting balloon is developing as a promising alternative to stent in patients with HBR[65] or with small diameter vessels.[66]

In conclusion, the identification of HBR patients should prompt the selection of treatment strategies aiming at reducing the bleeding risk and optimizing the secondary prevention of ischemic events with lipid-lowering drugs.[67] The most common bleeding events after PCI occur in the gastrointestinal tract,[12] and the use of drugs, such as proton pump inhibitors, that can reduce these complications should be liberal.[68,69]

SUMMARY

Patients at HBR represent a large proportion of the current population treated with PCI and undergoing DAPT. The clinical consequences and the prognostic impact of bleeding events is relevant. Focusing on HBR patients with correct risk stratification and individualized treatment is key to improving outcomes in modern practice.

REFERENCES

1. Willard JE, Lange RA, Hillis LD. The use of aspirin in ischemic heart disease. N Engl J Med 1992;327(3): 175–81.
2. Braunwald E. An important step for thrombocardiology. N Engl J Med 2017;377(14):1387–8.
3. Valgimigli M, Bueno H, Byrne RA, et al. 2017 ESC focused update on dual antiplatelet therapy in coronary artery disease developed in collaboration with EACTS: the Task Force for dual antiplatelet therapy in coronary artery disease of the European Society of Cardiology (ESC) and of the European Association for Cardio-Thoracic Surgery (EACTS). Eur Heart J 2018;39(3):213–60.
4. Wallentin L, Becker RC, Budaj A, et al. Ticagrelor versus clopidogrel in patients with acute coronary syndromes. N Engl J Med 2009;361(11): 1045–57.
5. Wiviott SD, Braunwald E, McCabe CH, et al. Prasugrel versus clopidogrel in patients with acute

coronary syndromes. N Engl J Med 2007;357(20): 2001–15.

6. Eikelboom JW, Connolly SJ, Bosch J, et al. Rivaroxaban with or without aspirin in stable cardiovascular disease. N Engl J Med 2017;377(14):1319–30.

7. Valgimigli M, Costa F, Lokhnygina Y, et al. Trade-off of myocardial infarction vs. bleeding types on mortality after acute coronary syndrome: lessons from the Thrombin Receptor Antagonist for Clinical Event Reduction in Acute Coronary Syndrome (TRACER) randomized trial. Eur Heart J 2017;38(11):804–10.

8. Marquis-Gravel G, Metha S, Valgimigli M, et al. A critical comparison of Canadian and international guidelines recommendations for antiplatelet therapy in coronary artery disease. Can J Cardiol 2020. S0828-282X(19)31526-0.

9. Collet JP, Roffi M, Byrne RA, et al. Case-based implementation of the 2017 ESC focused update on dual antiplatelet therapy in coronary artery disease. Eur Heart J 2018;39(3):e1–33.

10. Simonsson M, Wallentin L, Alfredsson J, et al. Temporal trends in bleeding events in acute myocardial infarction: insights from the SWEDEHEART registry. Eur Heart J 2020;41(7):833–43.

11. Valgimigli M, Ariotti S, Costa F. Duration of dual antiplatelet therapy after drug-eluting stent implantation: will we ever reach a consensus? Eur Heart J 2015; 36(20):1219–22.

12. Genereux P, Giustino G, Witzenbichler B, et al. Incidence, predictors, and impact of post-discharge bleeding after percutaneous coronary intervention. J Am Coll Cardiol 2015;66(9):1036–45.

13. Mehran R, Baber U, Steg PG, et al. Cessation of dual antiplatelet treatment and cardiac events after percutaneous coronary intervention (PARIS): 2 year results from a prospective observational study. Lancet 2013;382(9906):1714–22.

14. Amin AP, Bachuwar A, Reid KJ, et al. Nuisance bleeding with prolonged dual antiplatelet therapy after acute myocardial infarction and its impact on health status. J Am Coll Cardiol 2013;61(21):2130–8.

15. Valgimigli M, Garcia-Garcia HM, Vrijens B, et al. Standardized classification and framework for reporting, interpreting, and analysing medication non-adherence in cardiovascular clinical trials: a consensus report from the Non-adherence Academic Research Consortium (NARC). Eur Heart J 2019;40(25):2070–85.

16. Valgimigli M, Costa F, Byrne R, et al. Dual antiplatelet therapy duration after coronary stenting in clinical practice: results of an EAPCI survey. Eurointervention 2015;11(1):68–74.

17. Subherwal S, Bach RG, Chen AY, et al. Baseline risk of major bleeding in non-ST-segment-elevation myocardial infarction: the CRUSADE (Can Rapid risk stratification of Unstable angina patients Suppress ADverse outcomes with Early implementation of the ACC/AHA Guidelines) Bleeding Score. Circulation 2009;119(14):1873–82.

18. Baber U, Mehran R, Giustino G, et al. Coronary thrombosis and major bleeding after PCI with drug-eluting stents: risk scores from PARIS. J Am Coll Cardiol 2016;67(19):2224–34.

19. Costa F, van Klaveren D, James S, et al. Derivation and validation of the predicting bleeding complications in patients undergoing stent implantation and subsequent dual antiplatelet therapy (PRECISE-DAPT) score: a pooled analysis of individual-patient datasets from clinical trials. Lancet 2017; 389(10073):1025–34.

20. Costa F, van Klaveren D, Colombo A, et al. A 4-item PRECISE-DAPT score for dual antiplatelet therapy duration decision-making. Am Heart J 2020;223: 44–7.

21. Koskinas KC, Raber L, Zanchin T, et al. Clinical impact of gastrointestinal bleeding in patients undergoing percutaneous coronary interventions. Circ Cardiovasc Interv 2015;8(5):e002053.

22. Urban P, Mehran R, Colleran R, et al. Defining high bleeding risk in patients undergoing percutaneous coronary intervention. Circulation 2019;140(3): 240–61.

23. Natsuaki M, Morimoto T, Shiomi H, et al. Application of the academic research Consortium high bleeding risk criteria in an all-comers registry of percutaneous coronary intervention. Circ Cardiovasc Interv 2019; 12(11):e008307.

24. Ueki Y, Bar S, Losdat S, et al. Validation of bleeding risk criteria (ARC-HBR) in patients undergoing percutaneous coronary intervention and comparison with contemporary bleeding risk scores. Eurointervention 2020. EIJ-D-20-00052.

25. Lamberts M, Gislason GH, Lip GY, et al. Antiplatelet therapy for stable coronary artery disease in atrial fibrillation patients taking an oral anticoagulant: a nationwide cohort study. Circulation 2014;129(15): 1577–85.

26. Ando G, Costa F. Double or triple antithrombotic therapy after coronary stenting and atrial fibrillation: a systematic review and meta-analysis of randomized clinical trials. Int J Cardiol 2020;302: 95–102.

27. van Rein N, Heide-Jorgensen U, Lijfering WM, et al. Major bleeding rates in atrial fibrillation patients on single, dual, or triple antithrombotic therapy. Circulation 2019;139(6):775–86.

28. Blann AD, Dunmore S. Arterial and venous thrombosis in cancer patients. Cardiol Res Pract 2011; 2011:394740.

29. Costa F, Valgimigli M. Long-term use of ticagrelor in patients with prior myocardial infarction. N Engl J Med 2015;373(13):1271–2.

30. Valgimigli M, Costa F. Chronic thrombocytopenia and percutaneous coronary intervention: the virtue

of prudence. JACC Cardiovasc Interv 2018;11(18): 1869–71.

31. Adamo M, Ariotti S, Costa F, et al. Phosphate- or citrate-buffered tirofiban versus unfractionated heparin and its impact on thrombocytopenia and clinical outcomes in patients with acute coronary syndrome: a post hoc analysis from the PRISM trial. JACC Cardiovasc Interv 2016;9(16):1667–76.

32. Ayoub K, Marji M, Ogunbayo G, et al. Impact of chronic thrombocytopenia on in-hospital outcomes after percutaneous coronary intervention. JACC Cardiovasc Interv 2018;11(18):1862–8.

33. Raposeiras-Roubin S, Faxen J, Iniguez-Romo A, et al. Development and external validation of a post-discharge bleeding risk score in patients with acute coronary syndrome: the BleeMACS score. Int J Cardiol 2018;254:10–5.

34. Reinecke H, Trey T, Wellmann J, et al. Haemoglobin-related mortality in patients undergoing percutaneous coronary interventions. Eur Heart J 2003; 24(23):2142–50.

35. Guedeney P, Sorrentino S, Vogel B, et al. Assessing and minimizing the risk of percutaneous coronary intervention in patients with chronic kidney disease. Expert Rev Cardiovasc Ther 2018; 16(11):825–35.

36. Crimi G, Leonardi S, Costa F, et al. Incidence, prognostic impact, and optimal definition of contrast-induced acute kidney injury in consecutive patients with stable or unstable coronary artery disease undergoing percutaneous coronary intervention. insights from the all-comer PRODIGY trial. Catheterization Cardiovasc interventions 2015; 86(1):E19–27.

37. Costa F, Windecker S, Valgimigli M. Dual antiplatelet therapy duration: reconciling the inconsistencies. Drugs 2017;77(16):1733–54.

38. Varenne O, Cook S, Sideris G, et al. Drug-eluting stents in elderly patients with coronary artery disease (SENIOR): a randomised single-blind trial. Lancet 2018;391(10115):41–50.

39. Windecker S, Latib A, Kedhi E, et al. Polymer-based or polymer-free stents in patients at high bleeding risk. N Engl J Med 2020;382(13):1208–18.

40. Piccolo R, Magnani G, Ariotti S, et al. Ischaemic and bleeding outcomes in elderly patients undergoing a prolonged versus shortened duration of dual antiplatelet therapy after percutaneous coronary intervention: insights from the PRODIGY randomised trial. Eurointervention 2017;13(1):78–86.

41. Costa F, Brugaletta S. Antithrombotic therapy in acute coronary syndrome: striking a happy medium. Rev Esp Cardiol (Engl Ed) 2018;71(10):782–6.

42. Costa F, Vranckx P, Leonardi S, et al. Impact of clinical presentation on ischaemic and bleeding outcomes in patients receiving 6- or 24-month duration of dual-antiplatelet therapy after stent implantation: a pre-specified analysis from the PRODIGY (Prolonging Dual-Antiplatelet Treatment after Grading Stent-Induced Intimal Hyperplasia) trial. Eur Heart J 2015;36(20):1242–51.

43. Costa F, Adamo M, Ariotti S, et al. Left main or proximal left anterior descending coronary artery disease location identifies high-risk patients deriving potentially greater benefit from prolonged dual antiplatelet therapy duration. Eurointervention 2016; 11(11):e1222–30.

44. Caracciolo A, Mazzone P, Laterra G, et al. Antithrombotic therapy for percutaneous cardiovascular interventions: from coronary artery disease to structural heart interventions. J Clin Med 2019;8(11):2016.

45. Costa F, Valgimigli M. The optimal duration of dual antiplatelet therapy after coronary stent implantation: to go too far is as bad as to fall short. Cardiovasc Diagn Ther 2018;8(5):630–46.

46. Udell JA, Bonaca MP, Collet JP, et al. Long-term dual antiplatelet therapy for secondary prevention of cardiovascular events in the subgroup of patients with previous myocardial infarction: a collaborative meta-analysis of randomized trials. Eur Heart J 2016;37(4):390–9.

47. Navarese EP, Andreotti F, Schulze V, et al. Optimal duration of dual antiplatelet therapy after percutaneous coronary intervention with drug eluting stents: meta-analysis of randomised controlled trials. BMJ 2015;350:h1618.

48. Costa F, Adamo M, Ariotti S, et al. Impact of greater than 12-month dual antiplatelet therapy duration on mortality: drug-specific or a class-effect? A meta-analysis. Int J Cardiol 2015;201:179–81.

49. Ferlini M, Rossini R, Musumeci G, et al. Perceived or calculated bleeding risk and their relation with dual antiplatelet therapy duration in patients undergoing percutaneous coronary intervention. Circ Cardiovasc Interv 2019;12(6):e007949.

50. Ando G, Costa F. Bleeding risk stratification in acute coronary syndromes. Is it still valid in the era of the radial approach? Postepy Kardiol Interwencyjnej 2015;11(3):170–3.

51. Chew DP, Junbo G, Parsonage W, et al. Perceived risk of ischemic and bleeding events in acute coronary syndromes. Circ Cardiovasc Qual Outcomes 2013;6(3):299–308.

52. Costa F, Tijssen JG, Ariotti S, et al. Incremental value of the CRUSADE, ACUITY, and HAS-BLED risk scores for the prediction of hemorrhagic events after coronary stent implantation in patients undergoing long or short duration of dual antiplatelet therapy. J Am Heart Assoc 2015;4(12):e002524.

53. Yeh RW, Secemsky EA, Kereiakes DJ, et al. Development and validation of a prediction rule for benefit and harm of dual antiplatelet therapy beyond 1 Year after percutaneous coronary intervention. Jama 2016;315(16):1735–49.

54. Costa F, Van Klaveren D, Feres F, et al. Dual anti-platelet therapy duration based on ischemic and bleeding risks after coronary stenting. J Am Coll Cardiol 2019;73(7):741–54.

55. Giustino G, Costa F. Characterization of the individual patient risk after percutaneous coronary intervention: at the crossroads of bleeding and thrombosis. JACC Cardiovasc Interv 2019;12(9):831–4.

56. Giustino G, Chieffo A, Palmerini T, et al. Efficacy and safety of dual antiplatelet therapy after complex PCI. J Am Coll Cardiol 2016;68(17):1851–64.

57. Valgimigli M, Bueno H, Byrne RA, et al. 2017 ESC focused update on dual antiplatelet therapy in coronary artery disease developed in collaboration with EACTS. Kardiol Pol 2017;75(12):1217–99.

58. Levine GN, Bates ER, Bittl JA, et al. 2016 ACC/AHA guideline focused update on duration of dual antiplatelet therapy in patients with coronary artery disease: a report of the American College of Cardiology/American Heart Association task force on clinical practice guidelines. J Am Coll Cardiol 2016;68(10):1082–115.

59. Ariotti S, Costa F, Valgimigli M. Coronary stent selection and optimal course of dual antiplatelet therapy in patients at high bleeding or thrombotic risk: navigating between limited evidence and clinical concerns. Curr Opin Cardiol 2015;30(4):325–32.

60. Urban P, Meredith IT, Abizaid A, et al. Polymer-free drug-coated coronary stents in patients at high bleeding risk. N Engl J Med 2015;373(21):2038–47.

61. Ariotti S, Adamo M, Costa F, et al. Is bare-metal stent implantation still justifiable in high bleeding risk patients undergoing percutaneous coronary intervention?: a pre-specified analysis from the ZEUS trial. JACC Cardiovasc Interv 2016;9(5):426–36.

62. Crimi G, Leonardi S, Costa F, et al. Role of stent type and of duration of dual antiplatelet therapy in patients with chronic kidney disease undergoing percutaneous coronary interventions. Is bare metal stent implantation still a justifiable choice? A post-hoc analysis of the all comer PRODIGY trial. Int J Cardiol 2016;212:110–7.

63. Valgimigli M, Patialiakas A, Thury A, et al. Zotarolimus-eluting versus bare-metal stents in uncertain drug-eluting stent candidates. J Am Coll Cardiol 2015;65(8):805–15.

64. Piccolo R, Bonaa KH, Efthimiou O, et al. Drug-eluting or bare-metal stents for percutaneous coronary intervention: a systematic review and individual patient data meta-analysis of randomised clinical trials. Lancet 2019;393(10190):2503–10.

65. Rissanen TT, Uskela S, Eranen J, et al. Drug-coated balloon for treatment of de-novo coronary artery lesions in patients with high bleeding risk (DEBUT): a single-blind, randomised, non-inferiority trial. Lancet 2019;394(10194):230–9.

66. Jeger RV, Farah A, Ohlow MA, et al. Drug-coated balloons for small coronary artery disease (BASKET-SMALL 2): an open-label randomised non-inferiority trial. Lancet 2018;392(10150):849–56.

67. Sabouret P, Angoulvant D, Pathak A, et al. A look beyond statins and ezetimibe: a review of other lipid-lowering treatments for cardiovascular disease prevention in high-risk patients. Int J Cardiol 2020.

68. Gargiulo G, Costa F, Ariotti S, et al. Impact of proton pump inhibitors on clinical outcomes in patients treated with a 6- or 24-month dual-antiplatelet therapy duration: insights from the PROlonging Dual-antiplatelet treatment after Grading stent-induced Intimal hyperplasia studY trial. Am Heart J 2016;174:95–102.

69. Bhatt DL, Cryer BL, Contant CF, et al. Clopidogrel with or without omeprazole in coronary artery disease. N Engl J Med 2010;363(20):1909–17.

Complete Revascularization in Acute and Chronic Coronary Syndrome

Federica Ilardi, MD[a,b], Marco Ferrone, MD[a,c], Marisa Avvedimento, MD[a], Giuseppe Servillo, MD[d], Giuseppe Gargiulo, MD, PhD[a,*]

KEYWORDS

- Multivessel coronary artery disease (MVD) • Complete revascularization (CR)
- Incomplete revascularization (IR) • Culprit-only revascularization
- Percutaneous coronary intervention (PCI) • Coronary artery bypass graft (CABG)
- Acute coronary syndrome (ACS) • Chronic coronary syndrome (CCS)

KEY POINTS

- Multivessel coronary artery disease (MVD) is a common finding both in acute (ACS) and chronic coronary syndrome (CCS) and poses challenges to revascularization strategy.
- Complete revascularization (CR) has been based on anatomic or functional definitions, both in ACS and CCS.
- In ACS, mainly ST-segment elevation myocardial infarction, CR improves prognosis, but how define significant nonculprit lesions and when treating them still remain highly debated.
- In CCS, when myocardial revascularization (percutaneous coronary intervention or coronary artery bypass graft) is deemed beneficial, a functionally guided CR should be encouraged.
- Heart-team is essential to personalize strategies and reach balanced and optimized decision-making.

INTRODUCTION

Multivessel coronary artery disease (MVD) is a common finding both in acute (ACS) and chronic coronary syndrome (CCS) and poses challenges to revascularization strategy.

Despite the question of whether patients with MVD should undergo complete (CR) versus incomplete revascularization (IR) has been investigated in several studies, this issue still remains debated. This is attributable to conflicting results in clinical studies as well as to an evolved definition of coronary artery disease (CAD) over time, with a shift toward pursuing functional CR. Indeed, various definitions of CR exist and, to date, there is no consensus.[1,2] Although the anatomic-based definition has been the most widely used classification, in contemporary practice, a functional/physiological approach is encouraged.[3–5] Moreover, in the acute setting, the identification of nonculprit lesions (NCLs) poses relevant questions on their management. Finally, the optimal timing for

---

Federica Ilardi and Marco Ferrone equally contributed to this article.

[a] Department of Advanced Biomedical Sciences, Federico II University of Naples, Via S. Pansini 5, Naples 80131, Italy; [b] Mediterranea Cardiocentro, Via Orazio 2, Naples 80122, Italy; [c] Division of Invasive Cardiology, Clinica Montevergine, Via Mario Malzoni, 5, Mercogliano (Avellino) 83013, Italy; [d] Department of Neurosciences, Reproductive and Odontostomatological Sciences, Federico II University of Naples, Via S. Pansini 5, Naples 80131, Italy

* Corresponding author.

E-mail addresses: peppegar83@libero.it; giuseppe.gargiulo1@unina.it

reaching CR, in particular in acute presentations, and type of revascularization strategy also remain critical issues to be fully clarified. In this review, we provide an overview of recent evidence and current indication to perform a CR in patients with ACS or CCS and MVD.

COMPLETE REVASCULARIZATION IN ACUTE CORONARY SYNDROME

The identification of NCL is frequent in both ST-segment elevation myocardial infarction (STEMI) and non-ST-segment elevation ACS (NSTE-ACS). Although in the latter setting there are no dedicated prospective studies on the revascularization strategy with MVD, there are relevant randomized trials for STEMI. In patients with STEMI, primary percutaneous coronary intervention (PCI) to treat the infarct related artery (IRA) or culprit lesion is essential to reduce myocardial damage and prevent reperfusion injury.[6] However, up to half of patients with STEMI show additional significant stenosis.[7,8] In this setting, the optimal management of NCL and whether to perform a CR has been a matter of discussion for years. Indeed, if on one hand most NCLs are asymptomatic or induce limited myocardial ischemia, conversely, it has been demonstrated that MVD following primary PCI associates with worse outcome than single-vessel disease.[7,8] This worse prognosis could be attributable to an increased disease burden, or a pan-coronary process of vulnerable plaque development, responsible for multiple plaque rupture even distant from the culprit lesion throughout the coronary tree.[9] One option could be a culprit-only revascularization with initial medical therapy followed by eventual further revascularization guided by recurrent symptoms. Alternatively, NCL revascularization (anatomically or functionally guided) may be performed immediately during the index procedure or as staged procedure, and the latter, in turn, could be performed during the index hospitalization or on a subsequent readmission. Thus, main open issues are as follows: (1) Is CR really beneficial? (2) If yes, how to optimally define NCLs needing revascularization? (3) Which is the optimal timing for NCL revascularization?

Clinical Evidence

Some randomized trials investigated the preferred strategy for patients with STEMI with MVD (CR vs IRA-only PCI), and also the optimal timing for CR (during index procedure or staged) (**Table 1**). In a small single-center trial, IRA-only PCI was associated with the highest risk of repeat unplanned revascularization, rehospitalization, and in-

hospital death at 2.5-years compared with CR (at index PCI or staged).[10] The Preventive Angioplasty in Acute Myocardial Infarction (PRAMI) trial randomized 465 patients with STEMI with MVD to treatment of IRA lesion alone (n = 231) or revascularization of all obstructive (>50% angiographic stenosis) non-IRA lesions during the index procedure (n = 234).[11] Recruitment was stopped prematurely due to highly significant benefit of preventive PCI that at a mean of 23 months significantly reduced the composite of cardiac death or nonfatal myocardial infarction (MI) or refractory angina, as well as cardiac death and nonfatal MI, whereas cardiac death alone did not differ significantly. Interestingly, the benefit was evident within 6 months and maintained thereafter. Similarly, the Complete versus Lesion-only Primary PCI trial (CvLPRIT) (n = 269) showed that CR (>70% angiographic stenosis or 50% in 2 orthogonal views) during index hospitalization significantly reduced death, reinfarction, heart failure, or ischemia-driven revascularization, compared with IRA-only PCI.[12,13] There was a 40% reduction of primary endpoint after 5.6-year median follow-up, with most of the benefit occurring early. The composite of all-cause mortality and MI was also significantly lower in CR, whereas no significant difference was observed in individual components, although all were numerically lower in the CR group. Both the PRAMI and the CvLPRIT trial used the anatomic definition of significant stenosis to guide the CR, and did not evaluate the role of Fractional Flow Reserve (FFR) for MVD. Conversely, 2 randomized trials have proposed FFR to guide NCL revascularization.[14,15] The Third Danish Study of Optimal Acute Treatment of Patients with STEMI: Primary PCI in Multivessel Disease (DANAMI-3 PRIMULTI) trial (n = 627) showed a reduction in composite endpoint (all-cause mortality, reinfarction and ischemia-driven revascularization) with FFR-guided CR versus IRA-PCI only after a mean follow-up of 27 months, although this benefit was mainly driven by reduction of reintervention.[14] Notably, a recent cardiac magnetic resonance substudy on 280 patients showed that CR had no impact on left ventricle function and remodeling, nor on final infarct size, whereas a large but not significant increase of new nonculprit MI, related to periprocedural MI occurring during nonculprit intervention, was observed.[16] The Comparison Between FFR Guided Revascularization versus Conventional Strategy in Acute STEMI Patients with MVD (COMPARE-ACUTE) enrolled 885 patients who were assigned (2:1) to receive IRA-only PCI or FFR-guided CR.[15] Again, FFR-guided CR significantly reduced the composite of all-cause death, nonfatal MI, revascularization, or

Table 1
Overview of randomized clinical trials in patients with acute STEMI with MVD comparing complete revascularization with culprit-only PCI

Characteristics	Politi et al.	PRAMI	DANAMI-3-PRIMULTI	CvLPRIT	Compare-Acute	COMPLETE
Inclusion period	2003–2007	2008–2013	2011–2014	2011–2013	2011–2015	2013–2017
Trial registration	None	ISRCTN73028481	NCT01960933	ISRCTN70913605	NCT01399736	NCT01740479
Multicenter	No	Yes	Yes	Yes	Yes	Yes
Population	214	465	627	296	885	4041
Mean age	65	62	63	65	61	62
Lesion criteria	>70% stenosis	≥50% stenosis	>50%	≥70% or >50% in 2 orthogonal views	≥50% + FFR ≤0.80	≥70% or FFR ≤0.80
FFR measurement of NCL	No	No	Yes	No	Yes	Yes
Timing complete revascularization	2 CR groups randomized to index procedure vs staged revascularization	Index procedure	Index hospitalization	Index procedure or index hospitalization	Index procedure	Index hospitalization or after hospital discharge (no later than 45 d)
Median time from randomization to 2nd procedure (d)	0 (index procedure, n = 65) or 56.8 (staged, n = 65)	0 (index procedure)	2	<2	0 (index procedure)	1 (during admission, n = 1285) or 23 (after discharge, n = 596)
Primary endpoint	CV or all-death, in-hospital death, MI, rehospitalization for ACS, RR	CV death, MI, refractory angina	All-death, MI, RR or non-IRA	Death, reinfarction, HF, any RR	Death from any cause, MI, revascularization, cerebrovascular events	1) CV death or new MI; 2) CV death, new non-fatal MI or ischemia-driven revascularization
Blinded adjudication of clinical events	No	Yes	Yes	Yes	Yes	Yes
FUP, mo	30	23	27	12 (primary) and 66	12	36

(continued on next page)

Table 1
(continued)

Characteristics	Politi et al.	PRAMI	DANAMI-3-PRIMULTI	CvLPRIT	Compare-Acute	COMPLETE
Main results	20% in CR staged, 23.1% in CR index vs 50% in IR (staged HR: 0.37; 95% CI: 0.19–0.69; P = .002; index HR: 0.41; 95% CI: 0.22–0.74; P = .003)	9% in CR vs 23% in IR (HR: 0.35; 95% CI: 0.21–0.58; P<.001)	13% in CR vs 22% in IR (HR: 0.56, 95% CI: 0.38–0.83; P = .004)	At 1y: 10% in CR vs 21.2% in IR (HR: 0.45; 95% CI: 0.24–0.84; P = .009); At 5.6 y: 24% in CR vs 37.7% in IR (HR: 0.57; 95% CI: 0.37–0.87; P = .008)	7.8% in CR vs 20.5% in IR (HR: 0.35; 95% CI: 0.22–0.55; P<.001)	7.8% in CR vs 10.5% in IR (HR: 0.74; 95% CI: 0.60–0.91; P = .004)

Abbreviations: ACS, acute coronary syndrome; CI, confidence interval; CR, complete revascularization; CV, cardiovascular; FFR, fractional flow reserve; FUP, follow-up; HF, heart failure; HR, hazard ratio; IR, incomplete revascularization; IRA, infarct-related artery; MACE, major adverse cardiac event; MI, myocardial infarction; MVD, multivessel coronary artery disease; NCL, nonculprit lesion; PCI, percutaneous coronary intervention; RR, repeat revascularization; STEMI, ST-segment elevation myocardial infarction.

cerebrovascular events at 12 months, mainly driven by lower reinterventions. Importantly, FFR-guided revascularizations were performed in 83.6% of cases during the index procedure and elective revascularizations of non-IRA performed within 45 days after primary PCI for clinical evaluations were not counted, as events in the group receiving IRA-only PCI (occurred in 10% of this group).

The most recent Complete versus Culprit-Only Revascularization to Treat Multivessel Disease After Primary PCI for STEMI (COMPLETE) trial was the first powered for hard outcomes (composite of death or MI and the composite of cardiovascular death, MI, or revascularization).[17] A total of 4041 patients who had NCL with at least 70% stenosis or FFR ≤0.80 were randomly assigned (1:1) to CR or IRA-only PCI. At a median of 3 years, cardiovascular death or new MI was lower in CR, mainly driven by lower MI. The decision to perform preventive revascularization during the index hospitalization or after discharge (within 45 days after randomization) was specified by investigator before randomization. Interestingly, the benefit of CR was independent of timing of NCL-PCI (Pinteraction = 0.62) and a landmark analysis demonstrated that CR benefit of cardiovascular death or new MI emerged mostly over the long-term,

with continued divergence of Kaplan–Meier curves for several years.[18] In an optical coherence tomography substudy, NCLs were in large proportion characterized by thin-cap fibroatheroma, thus, contributing to explain the benefit associated with multivessel revascularization.

Therefore, COMPLETE, the largest trial on the topic, confirmed that CR in patients with STEMI is associated with a significant reduction of the need for repeated revascularization and recurrence of MI. It remained, however, unclear if the lack of benefit in terms of cardiovascular and all-cause mortality was related to unpowered sample size, or to patient characteristics. Indeed, patients were relatively young and with a low mean SYNTAX (Synergy between PCI with Taxus and Cardiac Surgery) score, that could not reflect the clinical setting, often characterized by sicker patients with more diffuse and complex CAD.

All individual trials were underpowered for cardiovascular mortality. A recent meta-analysis included all of them with 6528 patients with STEMI with MVD (3139 CR vs 3389 culprit-only) demonstrating that CR significantly reduced cardiovascular mortality, as well as recurrent MI and repeated revascularization (**Fig. 1**).[19] Notably, CR was not associated with a significant increase of acute kidney injury (AKI), suggesting no

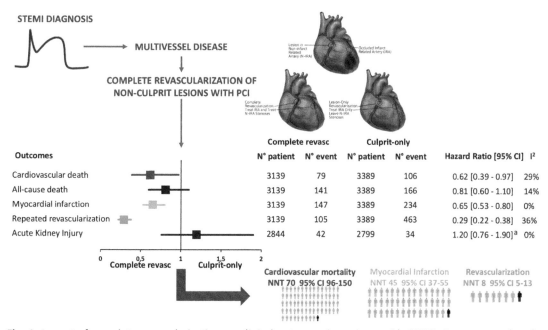

Fig. 1. Impact of complete revascularization on clinical outcomes in patients with STEMI. Summary results of a meta-analysis of 6 trials comparing CR versus culprit-only. CI, confidence interval; NNT, number needed to treat. [a] Risk ratio [95% CI]. (*Data from* Pavasini R, Biscaglia S, Barbato E et al. Complete revascularization reduces cardiovascular death in patients with ST-segment elevation myocardial infarction and multivessel disease: systematic review and meta-analysis of randomized clinical trials. Eur Heart J 2019.)

complications for this strategy; however, this outcome should be interpreted with caution considering that it was available in a limited number of patients and affected by heterogeneous definitions used. There was no benefit on all-cause mortality, likely related to low-risk population, or to length of follow-up. Conversely, a significant reduction in both all-cause mortality and MI was demonstrated in a previous meta-analysis in which the greater benefit was observed in CR performed during index PCI, suggesting that also timing of NCL treatment could affect prognosis.[20]

Data on patients with NSTE-ACS with MVD derive mainly form retrospective studies. In contrast with STEMI, in this setting to identify the culprit lesion is often difficult. Despite limited, some data indicate that CR might improve prognosis even in NSTE-ACS,[21–23] and a randomized trial showed that CR performed in a single procedure seems better than multistage PCI.[24] However, the long-term benefit of CR has to be balanced with the periprocedural risk of pursuing CR, mainly in those patients with complex coronary anatomy or chronic total occlusion (CTO).[25]

Practical Considerations and Future Perspectives

According to European Society of Cardiology (ESC) guidelines for STEMI, revascularization of NCL should be completed before hospital discharge (class IIa, level A).[6] Latest evidence will be incorporated in future recommendations and could change clinical practice. However, the decision whether to perform CR or not, and when/how, should take into account several factors, and data supporting benefits of CR should be interpreted with caution and in light of relevant considerations:

- COMPLETE showed small benefit in terms of cardiovascular mortality that instead was greater in older and smaller trials.
- There was huge variation in trial design, mainly on NCL evaluation (angio vs functional) and when CR was achieved (index vs staged PCI during same or subsequent hospitalization). In COMPLETE, treatment of NCL was mainly based on visual estimation, but nearly 60% of lesions had at least 80% stenosis, thus not requiring FFR. Therefore, beyond those lesions angiographically significant, FFR or instantaneous wave-free ratio (iwFR) may still be important in diagnosing intermediate lesions (50%–69%), and whether CR of such intermediate lesions further reduces the hard endpoints of death or MI at long-term remains unclear. Contrarily, some concerns on

the value of functional assessment in the early phase of STEMI are related to concomitant microvascular dysfunction.[26]

- Different antiplatelet regimens may have influenced the findings described among studies conducted in different time periods. In a recent subanalysis of the TRITON-TIMI38 trial a more potent therapy with prasugrel reduced nonculprit MI compared with clopidogrel.[27] This supports that CR in patients with ACS should be attempted to prevent future events, but it could also be speculated that CR might influence the decision-making on the intensity of the antiplatelet therapy (ie, a more potent P2Y12 inhibitor should be always prioritized in patients with ACS, and deescalation to clopidogrel should not be considered in patients not receiving CR).
- Risks related to CR (including AKI and periprocedural MI) may have been underestimated and should never be forgotten because they can negatively impact on prognosis. Some concerns are related to perform CR during the index PCI; indeed, not rarely, an initial thrombotic burden, a nonoptimal IRA reperfusion result, or a significant coronary spasm that would cause inaccurate stent size, can occur and represent potential challenges to CR. Also the potential risk of AKI that may occur in some patients during primary PCI should be taken into account and could induce to decide for a staged approach. On the other hand, an advantage of CR during the index hospitalization is to avoid that patients after discharge do not return to complete procedure.
- Clinical factors always should be considered (patient's age and comorbidities, like chronic kidney disease), to avoid futile complex procedures in frail and old patients. Overall, patients participating in trials are generally less sick than those in the real world, and extending the results to patients with a greater risk of complications may not be safe. Yet, trials had specific exclusions criteria and were not designed to address the specific setting of cardiogenic shock in which MVD is frequent and associated with higher mortality. Guidelines recommended CR of all angiographic significant lesions during the index procedure (class IIa, level C),[6] but the recent CULPRIT shock trial, the largest randomized controlled trial in cardiogenic shock complicating MI (62% STEMI), showed that IRA-only PCI significantly reduced death or renal-replacement therapy at 30 days, and the difference was mainly driven by significantly

lower all-cause mortality. At 1-year, however, mortality did not differ significantly, suggesting that the benefit of culprit-only PCI was confined to the early period during which death in patients with cardiogenic shock mainly occurs.[28] Therefore, a subsequent document stated that in patients with cardiogenic shock complicating MI, primary PCI should be restricted to the IRA, whereas multivessel PCI should be limited to cases in which IRA is difficult to identify or incorrectly defined initially or when multiple culprit lesions are identified.[29]

In patients with NSTE-ACS, given the paucity of data, guidelines suggest to tailor CR to age, general patient condition and comorbidities, and to select a CR during a single procedure or with staged procedures based on clinical presentation, comorbidities, complexity of coronary anatomy, ventricular function, and revascularization modality.[30,31]

Available evidence supports NCL revascularization in patients with STEMI; however, the optimal tool(s) to guide NCL revascularization (which NCL to revascularize?) and the optimal timing for this (NCL assessment and revascularization) remain unsolved. Ongoing randomized trials will provide important insights in the future and are summarized in **Table 2**.

COMPLETE REVASCULARIZATION IN CHRONIC CORONARY SYNDROME

CAD is a chronic and frequently progressive disease that can present long, stable periods but can also become unstable at any time. Because of its dynamic nature, CAD can have different clinical presentations, including ACS or CCS. The latter group includes several clinical scenarios sharing the risk, although variable, of future cardiovascular events (mortality or MI).[32] Together with appropriate lifestyle modifications and optimal medical therapy (OMT), successful myocardial revascularization is crucial to reduce such risk.[30,32] OMT is essential to reduce symptoms, limit atherosclerosis progression, and prevent atherothrombotic events in patients with CCS, but on top of it (without supplanting it), myocardial revascularization (PCI or CABG) is fundamental for 2 main reasons: symptom relief and/or prognosis improvement. Huge evidence has shown that when compared with OMT alone, revascularization is effective in relieving angina, reducing the need for antianginal drugs, and improving exercise capacity and quality of life, as well as reducing the risk of major acute cardiovascular events, including MI and cardiovascular death.[30,32] A practical approach to the indication to revascularization in patients with CCS according to ESC guidelines is summarized in **Fig. 2**.

Selecting PCI or CABG remains a matter of ongoing discussion, but this is beyond our scope and is detailed elsewhere.[30,32–36] However, CR is key for both strategies; indeed, the benefit of CABG versus PCI has been attributed, in part, to greater degree of CR, and relevant evidence has demonstrated worse prognosis with IR compared with CR, either with PCI or CABG.[37–41]

Clinical Evidence

Most data evaluating the impact of CR is based on anatomic definition derived from studies comparing long-term outcomes of PCI versus CABG in MVD patients. In 2 pivotal trials, CR was more frequently reached with CABG, and the benefit of CR over IR was significant in patients with PCI but not in those with CABG.[42–44] Notably, they included PCI using bare-metal stents (BMS) or first-generation drug-eluting stents (DES, paclitaxel-eluting stent). More contemporary data on PCI with new-generation DES, specifically everolimus-eluting stents, showed that among 15,046 patients with MVD, CR was obtained in 30% and significantly reduced cardiovascular events including death compared with IR, and most relevant predictors of IR were the number of vessels diseased and the presence of a CTO.[39] Yet, data from 6539 patients demonstrated that surgical IR had negative impact on long-term survival, and this was strongly associated with age (higher mortality in <60 years but not in older patients).[45] A large meta-analysis on 89,883 patients comparing CR versus IR in MVD confirmed that CR was more often achieved with CABG than PCI and was associated with significantly better long-term mortality, MI, and repeat revascularization.[37] Remarkably, CR benefit was present in both PCI and CABG, and was independent of study design and definition. Similarly, in a pooled analysis of 3 trials including 3212 patients, CR rate was 61.7% (57.2% with PCI and 66.8% with CABG) and CR-PCI was associated with similar survival to CR-CABG at a median of 4.9 years.[46] Moreover, PCI resulting in IR had a higher risk of all-cause death and the composite of death/MI/ stroke than CR-CABG. Importantly, these findings were consistent in subgroup analysis of MVD, high SYNTAX score (>32), and diabetes.

Overall, much evidence supports that CR improves outcomes, irrespective of whether achieved through PCI or CABG.

Table 2
Overview of ongoing randomized clinical trials on NCL management in STEMI and/or ACS as reported on clinicaltrials.gov

	FULL REVASC	iMODERN	FLOWER-MI	Safe STEMI for Seniors	FRAME-AMI	MULTISTARS AMI	BIOVASC	FIRE
Trial registration	NCT02862119	NCT03298659	NCT02943954	NCT02933976	NCT02715518	NCT03135275	NCT03621501	NCT03772743
Official title	Ffr-gUidance for compLete Non-cuLprit REVASCularizAtion - a Registry-based Randomized Clinical Trial	Instantaneous Wave-free Ratio Guided Multi-vessel revascularizatiOn During Percutaneous Coronary intervEntion for Acute myocaRdial iNfarction	FLOW Evaluation to Guide Revascularization in Multi-vessel ST-elevation Myocardial Infarction	Study of Access Site for Enhancing PCI in STEMI for Seniors	Comparison of Clinical Outcomes Between FFR-guided Strategy and Angiography-guided Strategy in Treatment of Non-Infarction Related Artery Stenosis in Patients With Acute MI	MULTivessel Immediate vs STAged RevaScularization in Acute MI	Percutaneous Complete Revascularization Strategies Using Sirolimus Eluting Biodegradable Polymer Coated Stents in Patients Presenting With ACS and MVD	Functional vs Culprit-only Revascularization in Elderly Patients With MI and MVD
Estimated N	4052	1146	1170	875	1292	700	1525	1385
Type of patients	STEMI	STEMI	STEMI	STEMI	STEMI	STEMI	STEMI and NSTE-ACS	Elderly (>74y) STEMI and NSTEMI
Study start date	Aug 2016	Dec 2017	Dec 2016	Aug 2017	Aug 2016	Jan 2017	Jun 2018	Jul 2019
Estimated primary completion date	Jun 2021	Jan 2021	Dec 2019	Oct 2022	June 2020	Jun 2020	Dec 2020	Dec 2021

	FFR-guided PCI of NCL(s) during index hospital admission	iFR-guided revascularization of NCL with >50% diameter stenosis and iFR ≤0.89 during index procedure or index hospitalization	Angiography-guided PCI of NCL	iFR-guided revascularization of NCL	Angiography-guided PCI of NCL during index procedure or index hospitalization	Staged CR PCI (new hospitalization after 19–45 d, to complete the coronary revascularization)	Staged CR PCI (within 6 wk after index procedure)	Functionally-guided CR PCI
Intervention	FFR-guided PCI of NCL(s) during index hospital admission	iFR-guided revascularization of NCL with >50% diameter stenosis and iFR ≤0.89 during index procedure or index hospitalization	Angiography-guided PCI of NCL	iFR-guided revascularization of NCL	Angiography-guided PCI of NCL during index procedure or index hospitalization	Staged CR PCI (new hospitalization after 19–45 d, to complete the coronary revascularization)	Staged CR PCI (within 6 wk after index procedure)	Functionally-guided CR PCI
Alternative intervention	Initial conservative management of NCL	Adenosine stress perfusion CMR scan within 6 wk after STEMI, with revascularization of NCL associated with perfusion defects	FFR-guided PCI of NCL	Initial conservative management of NCL	FFR-guided PCI of NCL during index procedure or index hospitalization	Immediate CR PCI	Immediate CR PCI	Initial conservative management of NCL
Primary endpoint	all-cause mortality and MI during follow-up of minimum 1y	All-cause death, recurrent MI and hospitalization for heart failure at 1y	death, MI and unplanned hospitalization leading to urgent revascularization at 1y	cardiac death, infarct artery target-vessel MI, or ischemia-driven index IRA revascularization at 1y	Any death and any MI at 2 y	all-cause death, non-fatal MI, unplanned ischemia-driven revascularization, hospitalization for heart failure, and stroke at 1y	all-cause mortality, nonfatal type 1 MI, any unplanned revascularization, and cerebrovascular events at 1y	all-cause death, any MI, any stroke, any coronary revascularization at 1y

Abbreviations: ACS, acute coronary syndrome; CMR, cardiac magnetic resonance; CR, complete revascularization; FFR, fractional flow reserve; FUP, follow-up; HF, heart failure; iFR, instantaneous-wave free ratio; IRA, infarct-related artery; MI, myocardial infarction; NCL, nonculprit lesion; NSTE-ACS, non–ST-segment elevation ACS; NSTEMI, non–ST-segment elevation MI; PCI, percutaneous coronary intervention; STEMI, ST-segment elevation MI.

Data from NIH. National Library of Medicine. Clinicaltrials.gov.

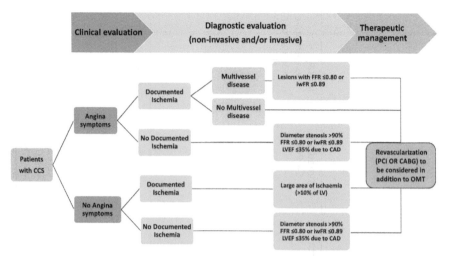

Fig. 2. Algorithm for patients undergoing invasive coronary angiography. CAD, coronary artery disease; FFR, fractional flow reserve; iwFR, instantaneous wave-free ratio; LV, left ventricle; LVEF, left ventricular ejection fraction; OMT, optimal medical therapy. (*Data from* Knuuti J, Wijns W, Saraste A et al. 2019 ESC Guidelines for the diagnosis and management of chronic coronary syndromes. Eur Heart J 2020;41:407-477.)

Since IR has been considered a surrogate marker of greater burden on anatomic coronary complexity and associated with worse outcome,[21] the residual SYNTAX score after PCI has been proposed as an objective measure of residual stenosis and indicator of clinical outcome.[47] In the PCI group of SYNTAX, a residual SYNTAX score greater than 8 was associated with increased long-term mortality and death/MI/stroke, whereas a residual SYNTAX ≤8 was associated with long-term mortality comparable with CR-PCI. This finding introduced the concept of "reasonable IR," which implies that an acceptable burden of obstructive CAD postrevascularization is associated with similar outcomes than CR.

Although the anatomy-based definition of CR has been the most widely used in previous studies and practice, optimized decision-making on myocardial revascularization should also account for vessel size, angiographic and functional/physiologic severity of lesions, and myocardial viability. In the past decade, functional-based definition of CR has reached great clinical relevance and attention. Functional CR is accomplished when all lesions causing resting or stress-induced ischemia are treated by either PCI or CABG.

A pivotal trial investigating the impact of functionally guided decision in CCS was the Clinical Outcomes Utilizing Revascularization and AGgressive drug Evaluation (COURAGE) study in which PCI (with BMS) plus OMT had apparently similar all-cause death and MI than OMT alone in 2287 patients with significant coronary lesions and evidence of myocardial ischemia, after a

median of 4.6 years. This inevitably led to the conclusion that OMT is as effective as PCI in CCS.[48] However, a nuclear imaging substudy, despite underpowered for prognosis, provided insights into the importance of functional evaluation, indeed, reduction of ≥5% of myocardial ischemia was associated with significantly lower rates of death and MI, and this level of ischemia reduction was achieved more frequently with PCI, suggesting that CR might have developed a larger proportion of patients reaching a significant reduction of residual ischemia.[49] As an alternative to noninvasive stress-imaging, FFR provides a validated and recommended method for ischemia detection. In the Fractional Flow Reserve versus Angiography for Multivessel Evaluation (FAME) study, FFR-guided PCI in patients with MVD (cutoff FFR 0.80) was associated with a significant reduction of death, nonfatal MI, or repeat revascularization at 1 year,[50] and mortality plus MI at 2 years.[51] Furthermore, it was cost-saving and cost-effective, being associated with lower use of stents and contrast medium, compared with angiographically guided PCI.[52] In FAME-2, FFR-guided PCI of functional relevant lesions was superior to OMT in preventing urgent revascularization.[5] These results were confirmed at 3 and 5 years with a significant reduction of major adverse cardiac events (MACE), including death, MI, and urgent revascularization.[53,54] These important findings led to propose an FFR-guided SYNTAX score (so-called, "functional SYNTAX score") in patients with PCI with MVD. It showed a better predictive accuracy for MACE than classic

SYNTAX score and also led to decrease by 32% the number of higher-risk patients.[55] Further evidence supporting the functional CR concept rather than angiographic CR alone derived by FAME analysis showed that residual angiographic lesions not functionally significant did not predict poorer outcomes.[56]

A special setting of patients with CCS with MVD is characterized by those with CTO. CTO influences CR and can have an impact on the decision between PCI or CABG. Despite limited evidence from large trials, data from registries and small trials show encouraging results in favor of CTO revascularization (probably due to optimal CR), that improves angina symptoms, quality of life, exercise capacity, and left ventricular function; reduces the risk of ventricular arrhythmias; and improves clinical outcomes.[57]

Recent studies have questioned revascularization value in CCS and generated huge debate. The Objective Randomized Blinded Investigation with optimal medical Therapy of Angioplasty in stable angina (ORBITA) was the first trial to investigate the influence of PCI in a sham-controlled fashion on angina symptoms and exercise time.[58] Despite all included patients had anatomically and/or functionally significant stenosis, PCI failed to improve exercise times or chest pain frequency. However, this was a small study (n = 200) with relevant limitations that should be interpreted with caution when considering daily practice.[59] The recent International Study of Comparative Health Effectiveness With Medical and Invasive Approaches (ISCHEMIA) trial represents an important additional piece of evidence (**Fig. 3**, **Box 1**). ISCHEMIA questioned whether in stable patients with at least moderate ischemia on a stress test, there is a benefit to adding cardiac catheterization and, if feasible, revascularization to OMT.[60] The primary endpoint did not differ at 4 years between conservative and invasive strategy.

Practical Considerations and Future Perspectives

Large evidence and practice guidelines support the role of the heart team to consider myocardial revascularization, whether with PCI or CABG, in patients with CCS with symptoms and/or documented ischemia and MVD, based on a functional/physiologic approach (see **Fig. 2**). Therefore, reflecting contemporary practice of ischemia-based revascularization, a physiologic/ functional approach (FFR or iwFR) is considered

ISCHEMIA Trial Design and Results

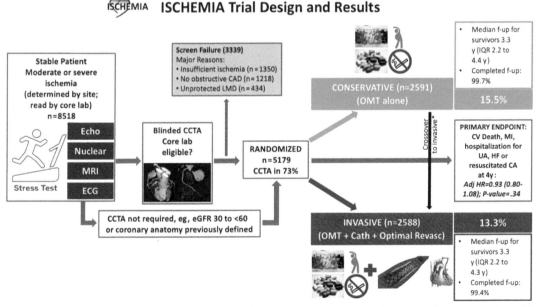

Fig. 3. Design and main results of the ISCHEMIA trial. CCTA, coronary computed tomography angiography; ECG, electrocardiogram; eGFR, estimated glomerular filtration rate; f-up, follow-up; HF, heart failure; HR, hazard ratio; IQR, interquartile range. *At 4 years, indications for cath in CON: 25.8% cumulative incidence 28%): suspected/ confirmed event 13.8%; OMT failure 3.9%; nonadherence 8.1%, and revascularization in CON: 16% (cumulative incidence 23%). CA, cardiac arrest; CAD, coronary artery disease; Cath, cathererization; CV, cardiovascular; LMD, left main disease; MI, myocardial infarction; MRI, magnetic resonance imaging; OMT, optimal medical therapy; UA, unstable angina.

Box 1
Eligibility criteria of the ISCHEMIA (International Study of Comparative Health Effectiveness With Medical and Invasive Approaches) trial

Clinical and Stress Test Eligibility Criteria

Inclusion criteria

Age $\geq$21 years

Moderate or severe ischemia[a]:

- Nuclear $\geq$10% left ventricular ischemia (summed difference score $\geq$7)
- Echo $\geq$3 segments stress-induced moderate or severe hypokinesis, or akinesis
- Cardiac Magnetic Resonance:
  - Perfusion: $\geq$12% myocardium ischemic, and/or
  - Wall motion: $\geq$3/16 segments with stress-induced severe hypokinesis or akinesis

Exercise Tolerance Testing (ETT) >1.5 mm ST depression in greater than 2 leads or >2 mm ST depression in single lead at less than 7 METS, with angina

Major exclusion criteria

New York Heart Association Class III-IV heart failure

Unacceptable angina despite medical therapy

Left ventricular ejection fraction <35%

Acute coronary syndrome within 2 months

Percutaneous coronary intervention or coronary artery bypass grafting within 1 year

Estimated glomerular filtration rate less than 30 mL/min or on dialysis (ISCHEMIA chronic kidney disease study)

Coronary Computed Tomography Angiography Eligibility Criteria

Inclusion criteria

$\geq$50% stenosis in a major epicardial vessel (stress imaging participants)

$\geq$70% stenosis in a proximal or mid vessel (ETT participants)

Major exclusion criteria

$\geq$50% stenosis in unprotected left main

[a] Ischemia eligibility determined by sites. All stress tests interpreted at core laboratories.

---

more reasonable and should be encouraged for appropriate CR.

In past years the so-called "hybrid" revascularization approach in patients with MVD has emerged as alternative to PCI or CABG alone with the aim to achieve CR by reducing the risks of a conventional CABG. Hybrid CR is characterized by the graft of internal mammary artery to the left anterior descending coronary artery through a small thoracotomy and then PCI with DES to other diseased vessels. Promising data support this approach, although potential limitations are also present (technically demanding, bleeding risks related to dual antiplatelet therapy in the immediate postoperative setting). Current ESC guidelines state that hybrid procedures may be considered in specific patient subsets at experienced centers (class IIb, level B).[30] Future studies will offer new insights (NCT03089398).

Despite small and inconclusive, ORBITA highlights that patients with CCS should be carefully evaluated before PCI. Yet, ISCHEMIA results overcome the previous COURAGE limitations (eg, PCI with new-generation DES, revascularization including both PCI and CABG) and reinforce the concept that probably not all patients with CCS with demonstrated ischemia/lesions should undergo revascularization. While waiting for its results be digested by the scientific community and incorporated into guidelines, some considerations can be made:

- Coronary computed tomography angiography reinforced its role in screening patients with suspected CAD, confirming the extent of disease and excluding left main disease.
- OMT and lifestyle changes are essential to all patients.
- Results cannot be extended to all patients with CCS (main exclusion criteria were ACS within 2 months, highly symptomatic patients, left main stenosis, and heart failure or left ventricular ejection fraction <35%).
- In people with chest pain symptoms, revascularization improved symptoms better than conservative strategy and the more symptomatic the patient was, the more symptoms improved after revascularization.
- Procedural MI was increased with an invasive strategy, but spontaneous MI was reduced.
- There were very low rates of procedure-related stroke and death, and all-cause death was low in both groups.
- During follow-up, a not negligible proportion of conservative patients required invasive management.
- Data on CR are not yet available.

SUMMARY

In patients with MVD, CR is the most biologically plausible approach irrespective of definition (anatomic or functional) or type (PCI or CABG) or clinical setting (ACS or CCS). It aims at minimizing residual ischemia, relieving symptoms and reducing the risk of future cardiovascular events. Large evidence supports CR benefits in ACS, predominantly STEMI, except cardiogenic shock, although the optimal tool to evaluate NCL and timing for achieving it remain to be clarified. In CCS, when revascularization is deemed appropriate, a functional CR should be attempted. Therefore, the heart-team plays a crucial role in the individualization of therapies aimed at selecting the ideal strategy for each patient to optimize decision-making. Ongoing studies will further inform our current knowledge.

DISCLOSURE

The authors have nothing to disclose.

REFERENCES

1. Sandoval Y, Brilakis ES, Canoniero M, et al. Complete versus incomplete coronary revascularization of patients with multivessel coronary artery disease. Curr Treat Options Cardiovasc Med 2015;17:366.
2. Ong AT, Serruys PW. Complete revascularization: coronary artery bypass graft surgery versus percutaneous coronary intervention. Circulation 2006; 114:249–55.
3. Tonino PA, Fearon WF, De Bruyne B, et al. Angiographic versus functional severity of coronary artery stenoses in the FAME study fractional flow reserve versus angiography in multivessel evaluation. J Am Coll Cardiol 2010;55:2816–21.
4. Pijls NH, van Schaardenburgh P, Manoharan G, et al. Percutaneous coronary intervention of functionally nonsignificant stenosis: 5-year follow-up of the DEFER Study. J Am Coll Cardiol 2007;49: 2105–11.
5. De Bruyne B, Pijls NH, Kalesan B, et al. Fractional flow reserve-guided PCI versus medical therapy in stable coronary disease. N Engl J Med 2012;367: 991–1001.
6. Ibanez B, James S, Agewall S, et al. 2017 ESC Guidelines for the management of acute myocardial infarction in patients presenting with ST-segment elevation: the Task Force for the management of acute myocardial infarction in patients presenting with ST-segment elevation of the European Society of Cardiology (ESC). Eur Heart J 2018;39:119–77.
7. Sorajja P, Gersh BJ, Cox DA, et al. Impact of multivessel disease on reperfusion success and clinical outcomes in patients undergoing primary percutaneous coronary intervention for acute myocardial infarction. Eur Heart J 2007;28:1709–16.
8. Park DW, Clare RM, Schulte PJ, et al. Extent, location, and clinical significance of non-infarct-related coronary artery disease among patients with ST-elevation myocardial infarction. JAMA 2014;312: 2019–27.
9. Asakura M, Ueda Y, Yamaguchi O, et al. Extensive development of vulnerable plaques as a pan-coronary process in patients with myocardial infarction: an angioscopic study. J Am Coll Cardiol 2001; 37:1284–8.
10. Politi L, Sgura F, Rossi R, et al. A randomised trial of target-vessel versus multi-vessel revascularisation in ST-elevation myocardial infarction: major adverse cardiac events during long-term follow-up. Heart 2010;96:662–7.
11. Wald DS, Morris JK, Wald NJ, et al. Randomized trial of preventive angioplasty in myocardial infarction. N Engl J Med 2013;369:1115–23.
12. Gershlick AH, Khan JN, Kelly DJ, et al. Randomized trial of complete versus lesion-only revascularization in patients undergoing primary percutaneous coronary intervention for STEMI and multivessel disease: the CvLPRIT trial. J Am Coll Cardiol 2015;65:963–72.
13. Gershlick AH, Banning AS, Parker E, et al. Long-term follow-up of complete versus lesion-only revascularization in STEMI and multivessel disease: the CvLPRIT trial. J Am Coll Cardiol 2019;74:3083–94.
14. Engstrom T, Kelbaek H, Helqvist S, et al. Complete revascularisation versus treatment of the culprit lesion only in patients with ST-segment elevation myocardial infarction and multivessel disease (DANAMI-3-PRIMULTI): an open-label, randomised controlled trial. Lancet 2015;386:665–71.
15. Smits PC, Abdel-Wahab M, Neumann FJ, et al. Fractional flow reserve-guided multivessel angioplasty in myocardial infarction. N Engl J Med 2017;376: 1234–44.
16. Kyhl K, Ahtarovski KA, Nepper-Christensen L, et al. Complete revascularization versus culprit lesion only in patients with ST-segment elevation myocardial infarction and multivessel disease: a DANAMI-3-PRIMULTI Cardiac Magnetic Resonance Substudy. JACC Cardiovasc Interv 2019;12:721–30.
17. Mehta SR, Wood DA, Storey RF, et al. Complete revascularization with multivessel PCI for myocardial infarction. N Engl J Med 2019;381:1411–21.
18. Wood DA, Cairns JA, Wang J, et al. Timing of staged nonculprit artery revascularization in patients with ST-segment elevation myocardial infarction: COMPLETE trial. J Am Coll Cardiol 2019;74: 2713–23.
19. Pavasini R, Biscaglia S, Barbato E, et al. Complete revascularization reduces cardiovascular death in patients with ST-segment elevation myocardial infarction and multivessel disease: systematic

review and meta-analysis of randomized clinical trials. Eur Heart J 2019. https://doi.org/10.1093/eurheartj/ehz896.

20. Pasceri V, Patti G, Pelliccia F, et al. Complete revascularization during primary percutaneous coronary intervention reduces death and myocardial infarction in patients with multivessel disease: meta-analysis and meta-regression of randomized trials. JACC Cardiovasc Interv 2018;11:833–43.

21. Farooq V, Serruys PW, Garcia-Garcia HM, et al. The negative impact of incomplete angiographic revascularization on clinical outcomes and its association with total occlusions: the SYNTAX (Synergy between Percutaneous Coronary Intervention with Taxus and Cardiac Surgery) trial. J Am Coll Cardiol 2013;61:282–94.

22. Shishehbor MH, Lauer MS, Singh IM, et al. In unstable angina or non-ST-segment acute coronary syndrome, should patients with multivessel coronary artery disease undergo multivessel or culprit-only stenting? J Am Coll Cardiol 2007;49:849–54.

23. Rathod KS, Koganti S, Jain AK, et al. Complete versus culprit-only lesion intervention in patients with acute coronary syndromes. J Am Coll Cardiol 2018;72:1989–99.

24. Sardella G, Lucisano L, Garbo R, et al. Single-staged compared with multi-staged PCI in multivessel NSTEMI patients: the SMILE trial. J Am Coll Cardiol 2016;67:264–72.

25. Fox KA, Clayton TC, Damman P, et al. Long-term outcome of a routine versus selective invasive strategy in patients with non-ST-segment elevation acute coronary syndrome a meta-analysis of individual patient data. J Am Coll Cardiol 2010;55:2435–45.

26. van der Hoeven NW, Janssens GN, de Waard GA, et al. Temporal changes in coronary hyperemic and resting hemodynamic indices in nonculprit vessels of patients with ST-segment elevation myocardial infarction. JAMA Cardiol 2019;4(8):736–44.

27. Scirica BM, Bergmark BA, Morrow DA, et al. Nonculprit lesion myocardial infarction following percutaneous coronary intervention in patients with acute coronary syndrome. J Am Coll Cardiol 2020;75:1095–106.

28. Thiele H, Akin I, Sandri M, et al. One-year outcomes after PCI strategies in cardiogenic shock. N Engl J Med 2018;379:1699–710.

29. Ibanez B, Halvorsen S, Roffi M, et al. Integrating the results of the CULPRIT-SHOCK trial in the 2017 ESC ST-elevation myocardial infarction guidelines: viewpoint of the task force. Eur Heart J 2018;39:4239–42.

30. Neumann FJ, Sousa-Uva M, Ahlsson A, et al. 2018 ESC/EACTS guidelines on myocardial revascularization. Eur Heart J 2019;40:87–165.

31. Roffi M, Patrono C, Collet JP, et al. 2015 ESC guidelines for the management of acute coronary syndromes in patients presenting without persistent ST-segment elevation: task force for the management of acute coronary syndromes in patients presenting without persistent ST-segment elevation of the European Society of Cardiology (ESC). Eur Heart J 2016;37:267–315.

32. Knuuti J, Wijns W, Saraste A, et al. 2019 ESC guidelines for the diagnosis and management of chronic coronary syndromes. Eur Heart J 2020;41:407–77.

33. Capodanno D, Gargiulo G, Buccheri S, et al. Computing methods for composite clinical endpoints in unprotected left main coronary artery revascularization: a post hoc analysis of the DELTA Registry. JACC Cardiovasc Interv 2016;9:2280–8.

34. Gargiulo G, Tamburino C, Capodanno D. Five-year outcomes of percutaneous coronary intervention versus coronary artery bypass graft surgery in patients with left main coronary artery disease: an updated meta-analysis of randomized trials and adjusted observational studies. Int J Cardiol 2015;195:79–81.

35. Giacoppo D, Colleran R, Cassese S, et al. Percutaneous coronary intervention vs coronary artery bypass grafting in patients with left main coronary artery stenosis: a systematic review and meta-analysis. JAMA Cardiol 2017;2:1079–88.

36. Head SJ, Milojevic M, Daemen J, et al. Mortality after coronary artery bypass grafting versus percutaneous coronary intervention with stenting for coronary artery disease: a pooled analysis of individual patient data. Lancet 2018;391:939–48.

37. Garcia S, Sandoval Y, Roukoz H, et al. Outcomes after complete versus incomplete revascularization of patients with multivessel coronary artery disease: a meta-analysis of 89,883 patients enrolled in randomized clinical trials and observational studies. J Am Coll Cardiol 2013;62:1421–31.

38. Hannan EL, Racz M, Holmes DR, et al. Impact of completeness of percutaneous coronary intervention revascularization on long-term outcomes in the stent era. Circulation 2006;113:2406–12.

39. Bangalore S, Guo Y, Samadashvili Z, et al. Outcomes with complete versus incomplete revascularization in patients with multivessel coronary disease undergoing percutaneous coronary intervention with everolimus eluting stents. Am J Cardiol 2020;125:362–9.

40. Synnergren MJ, Ekroth R, Oden A, et al. Incomplete revascularization reduces survival benefit of coronary artery bypass grafting: role of off-pump surgery. J Thorac Cardiovasc Surg 2008;136:29–36.

41. Takagi H, Watanabe T, Mizuno Y, et al. A meta-analysis of adjusted risk estimates for survival from observational studies of complete versus incomplete revascularization in patients with multivessel disease undergoing coronary artery bypass

grafting. Interact Cardiovasc Thorac Surg 2014;18: 679–82.

42. van den Brand MJ, Rensing BJ, Morel MA, et al. The effect of completeness of revascularization on event-free survival at one year in the ARTS trial. J Am Coll Cardiol 2002;39:559–64.

43. Serruys PW, Morice MC, Kappetein AP, et al. Percutaneous coronary intervention versus coronary-artery bypass grafting for severe coronary artery disease. N Engl J Med 2009;360:961–72.

44. Head SJ, Davierwala PM, Serruys PW, et al. Coronary artery bypass grafting vs. percutaneous coronary intervention for patients with three-vessel disease: final five-year follow-up of the SYNTAX trial. Eur Heart J 2014;35:2821–30.

45. Girerd N, Magne J, Rabilloud M, et al. The impact of complete revascularization on long-term survival is strongly dependent on age. Ann Thorac Surg 2012;94:1166–72.

46. Ahn JM, Park DW, Lee CW, et al. Comparison of stenting versus bypass surgery according to the completeness of revascularization in severe coronary artery disease: patient-level pooled analysis of the SYNTAX, PRECOMBAT, and BEST Trials. JACC Cardiovasc Interv 2017;10:1415–24.

47. Farooq V, Serruys PW, Bourantas CV, et al. Quantification of incomplete revascularization and its association with five-year mortality in the synergy between percutaneous coronary intervention with taxus and cardiac surgery (SYNTAX) trial validation of the residual SYNTAX score. Circulation 2013; 128:141–51.

48. Boden WE, O'Rourke RA, Teo KK, et al. Optimal medical therapy with or without PCI for stable coronary disease. N Engl J Med 2007;356:1503–16.

49. Shaw LJ, Berman DS, Maron DJ, et al. Optimal medical therapy with or without percutaneous coronary intervention to reduce ischemic burden: results from the Clinical Outcomes Utilizing Revascularization and Aggressive Drug Evaluation (COURAGE) trial nuclear substudy. Circulation 2008;117: 1283–91.

50. Tonino PA, De Bruyne B, Pijls NH, et al. Fractional flow reserve versus angiography for guiding percutaneous coronary intervention. N Engl J Med 2009; 360:213–24.

51. Pijls NH, Fearon WF, Tonino PA, et al. Fractional flow reserve versus angiography for guiding percutaneous coronary intervention in patients with multivessel coronary artery disease: 2-year follow-up of the FAME (Fractional Flow Reserve versus Angiography for Multivessel Evaluation) study. J Am Coll Cardiol 2010;56:177–84.

52. Fearon WF, Bornschein B, Tonino PA, et al. Economic evaluation of fractional flow reserve-guided percutaneous coronary intervention in patients with multivessel disease. Circulation 2010;122:2545–50.

53. Fearon WF, Nishi T, De Bruyne B, et al. Clinical outcomes and cost-effectiveness of fractional flow reserve-guided percutaneous coronary intervention in patients with stable coronary artery disease: three-year follow-up of the FAME 2 trial (fractional flow reserve versus angiography for multivessel evaluation). Circulation 2018;137:480–7.

54. Xaplanteris P, Fournier S, Pijls NHJ, et al. Five-year outcomes with PCI guided by fractional flow reserve. N Engl J Med 2018;379:250–9.

55. Nam CW, Mangiacapra F, Entjes R, et al. Functional SYNTAX score for risk assessment in multivessel coronary artery disease. J Am Coll Cardiol 2011; 58:1211–8.

56. Kobayashi Y, Nam CW, Tonino PA, et al. The prognostic value of residual coronary stenoses after functionally complete revascularization. J Am Coll Cardiol 2016;67:1701–11.

57. Werner GS, Martin-Yuste V, Hildick-Smith D, et al. A randomized multicentre trial to compare revascularization with optimal medical therapy for the treatment of chronic total coronary occlusions. Eur Heart J 2018;39:2484–93.

58. Al-Lamee R, Thompson D, Dehbi HM, et al. Percutaneous coronary intervention in stable angina (ORBITA): a double-blind, randomised controlled trial. Lancet 2018;391:31–40.

59. Schueler R, Al-Lamee R, Mahfoud F, et al. Will ORBITA change my practice? ORBITA trial: objective Randomised Blinded Investigation with optimal medical Therapy of Angioplasty in stable angina. EuroIntervention 2018;14:951–4.

60. Maron DJ, Hochman JS, Reynolds HR, et al. Initial invasive or conservative strategy for stable coronary disease. N Engl J Med 2020;382:1395–407.

Patient Selection for Protected Percutaneous Coronary Intervention
Who Benefits the Most?

Seung-Hyun Kim, MD*, Stefan Baumann, MD, Michael Behnes, MD, Martin Borggrefe, MD, Ibrahim Akin, MD

KEYWORDS

- High-risk-PCI • Protected PCI • MCS devices • IABP • pLVAD • LAAD • VA-ECMO

KEY POINTS

- Definition of protected percutaneous coronary intervention (PCI) and hemodynamic impact of diverse mechanical circulatory support devices.
- Clinical criteria for patient selection for protected PCI.
- Procedure-related criteria for patient selection for protected PCI.
- Algorithm and scoring system for patient selection for protected PCI.

INTRODUCTION

A development of percutaneous coronary intervention (PCI) with device innovation, novel skills, and effective antiproliferative medications allows for addressing increasingly complex coronary artery disease (CAD).[1] However, simultaneously, patients are presenting nowadays with higher rates of comorbidities and more complex CAD, which may lead to a lower physiologic tolerance for complex PCI. This patient group would be poor candidates for coronary artery bypass grafting (CABG) because of the high risk of surgical morbidity and mortality.[2]

As an alternative approach, the concept of so-called "protected PCI" has been developed, in which mechanical circulatory support (MCS) is used for the PCI in this high-risk patient group. The purpose of MCS is to provide hemodynamic support for complex PCI, and concurrently to reduce left ventricular systolic work and myocardial oxygen demand while maintaining systemic and coronary perfusion.[3] Currently, the following devices are available for MCS: intra-aortic balloon pump (IABP), percutaneous left ventricular assist devices (pLVAD), left atrial to aorta assist devices (LAAD), and veno-arterial extracorporeal membrane oxygenation (VA-ECMO). Using MCS devices in combination with an optimal selection of patients and devices would potentially improve the success rate of interventional procedures and clinical outcomes in these high-risk patients.[4,5]

However, since multiple treatment modalities are available and the precise definition of "high-risk patients" has not yet been established, it is still not clearly determined who benefits the most from protected PCI and which MCS device offers the best result in each clinical scenario. Hence, this review aims to provide practical approaches for the appropriate selection of patients and MCS device types by outlining current clinical data that assess utility of diverse MCS devices in high-risk patients undergoing protected PCI.

First Department of Medicine, University Medical Centre Mannheim (UMM), Faculty of Medicine Mannheim, University of Heidelberg, European Center for AngioScience (ECAS), and DZHK (German Center for Cardiovascular Research) Partner Site Heidelberg/Mannheim, Theodor-Kutzer-Ufer 1-3, Mannheim 68167, Germany
* Corresponding author.
E-mail address: seung-hyun.kim@umm.de

0733-8651/20/© 2020 Elsevier Inc. All rights reserved.

cardiology.theclinics.com

DEFINITION OF PROTECTED PERCUTANEOUS CORONARY INTERVENTION

The evolution of PCI techniques has enhanced the number of patients eligible for PCI of complex coronary lesions, for example, unprotected left main coronary stenosis, heavily calcified stenosis, and chronic total occlusion.[6] Nevertheless, each aspect of PCI, beginning from guide catheter engagement and ending with balloon inflation and stent deployment, is associated with potential risk of vascular damage and impairment of myocardial perfusion. Especially, patients with more complex CAD evaluated by higher SYNTAX (Synergy between Percutaneous Coronary Intervention with Taxus and Cardiac Surgery) score and concurrent higher surgical mortality assessed by higher STS (the Society of Thoracic Surgeons) score would not be suitable for either PCI[7] or for CABG.[8] Specifically, the PCI in patients with reduced coronary perfusion gradients between coronary arterioles and venules could cause a severe myocardial ischemia and consequently ischemia-triggered cardiac arrhythmias or further depression of an already impaired left ventricular ejection fraction (LVEF), leading to circulatory collapse and cardiac arrest.[9,10] Furthermore, complete or sufficient revascularization could not be guaranteed due to hemodynamic instability during the procedures. To avoid this fatal consequence, so-called protected PCI using MCS device as an alternative strategy for safely achieving complete revascularization has been used for more than 25 years.[11] The purpose of MCS is to decrease myocardial oxygen demand by reducing left ventricular volume (preload) and pressure (afterload) during high-risk PCI.[12] Another goal of MCS is to achieve sufficient cardiac output to maintain myocardial, cerebral, renal, mesenteric, and peripheral tissue perfusion, thereby preventing systemic shock syndrome. In addition, the use of appropriate MCS devices can provide sufficient time to safely perform high-risk PCI with optimal results in this patient group who would not otherwise tolerate complete revascularization.[13]

HEMODYNAMIC IMPACT OF MECHANICAL CIRCULATORY SUPPORT DEVICES

Currently, diverse types of percutaneous MCS with different characteristics and hemodynamic impact are available for high-risk PCI.[14] First, IABP supports hemodynamic circulation by inflating and deflating the balloon based on an electrocardiogram (ECG) or pressure triggers.[15] The balloon inflating occurs with the onset of diastole timed to the middle of the T-wave on ECG.

Thereafter, the balloon deflates rapidly at the beginning of left ventricular systole corresponding to the pear of the R-wave on ECG. The IABP decreases myocardial oxygen demand by reducing left ventricular afterload, and increases coronary artery perfusion by enhancing diastolic blood pressure. However, there are some functional limitations of IABP. Whereas mean arterial pressure and coronary blood flow are increased by using IABP, it offers only modest left ventricular unloading defined by reducing left ventricular volume and pressure (**Fig. 1**A). A stable electrical rhythm is also a prerequisite for the optimal hemodynamic effect from IABP, because IABP works depending on the surface ECG. The further limitations of IABP are dependence on native left ventricular function, balloon capacity, and accurate timing of balloon inflation and deflation.[16]

Second, the pLVAD is a continuous nonpulsatile microaxial screw pump deployed into the left ventricle across the aortic valve to pump blood from the left ventricle to the ascending aorta.[17] In this way, the pLVAD increases forward flow to the ascending aorta and mean arterial pressure. At the same time, it reduces myocardial oxygen demand and pulmonary capillary wedge pressure.[18] In contrast to IABP, the hemodynamic support from pLVAD is dependent neither on the native left ventricular function of patients nor on electrical stability due to its direct continuous propelling of blood from the left ventricle to the ascending aorta. The pLVAD leads to a remarkable unloading of the left ventricle by reducing left ventricular systolic and diastolic pressures, left ventricular volumes, and stroke volume (**Fig. 1**B). In case of biventricular failure or unstable ventricular arrhythmias, concomitantly using a right ventricular assist device should be considered to maintain left ventricular preload and optimal hemodynamic support from pLVAD.

The LAAD is one of the MCS devices that extracorporeally pumps blood from the left atrium via a transseptally placed left atrial cannula to the iliofemoral arterial system, thereby bypassing the left ventricle.[17] The bypass of blood from the left atrium induces indirectly optimal left ventricular unload at a similar level to pLVAD that enables direct unloading of the left ventricle (see **Fig. 1**B). By this means, the LAAD reduces wall stress and myocardial oxygen demand.[19] However, the need for a transseptal puncture is an important obstacle for clinical use of LAAD.

Finally, VA-ECMO provides both oxygenation and circulation. A venous cannula drains deoxygenated blood into a membrane oxygenator for gas exchange, and oxygenated blood is subsequently infused into the patient via an arterial

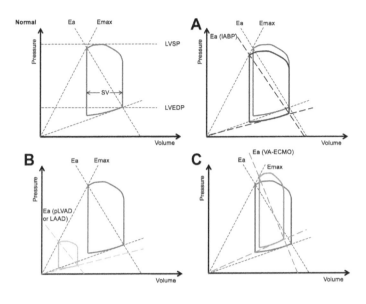

Fig. 1. Hemodynamic imbalance in acute myocardial infarction and cardiogenic shock, and hemodynamic impact of various MCS devices are illustrated by the pressure-volume loop. The normal pressure-volume loop is shown in blue. Emax representing a load-independent left ventricular contractility is defined as the maximal slope of the end-systolic pressure-volume point under various loading conditions, known as the end-systolic pressure-volume relationship. Effective arterial elastance (Ea) is a component of left ventricular afterload and is defined as the ratio of left ventricular systolic pressure (LVSP) and stroke volume (SV). (*A*) Pressure-volume loop in using IABP demonstrates a mildly decreased left ventricular end-diastolic pressure (LVEDP) and LVSP, leading to decreased an Ea. (*B*) Pressure-volume loop with pLVAD and LAAD shows a substantially decreased LVEDP, LVSP, and SV. The net effect is a pronounced reduction of left ventricular preload and afterload. (*C*) Pressure-volume loop with VA-ECMO without left ventricular venting indicates a decreased SV, whereas LVEDP und LVSP are significantly increased with a net effect of substantial increase of left ventricular afterload. (*Adapted from* Rihal CS, Naidu SS, Givertz MM, et al. 2015 SCAI/ACC/HFSA/STS Clinical Expert Consensus Statement on the Use of Percutaneous Mechanical Circulatory Support Devices in Cardiovascular Care: Endorsed by the American Heart Assocation, the Cardiological Society of India, and Sociedad Latino Americana de Cardiologia Intervencion; Affirmation of Value by the Canadian Association of Interventional Cardiology-Association Canadienne de Cardiologie d'intervention. J Am Coll Cardiol. 2015;65(19): e7-e26.)

cannula. VA-ECMO provides systemic circulatory support with flows sometimes exceeding 6 L/min depending on cannula sizes. However, it can significantly increase afterload on the left ventricle (**Fig. 1**C), thereby potentially reducing left ventricular stroke volume, increasing myocardial oxygen demand, and necessitating "venting" of the left ventricle by concomitant IABP or pLVAD.[20,21] In contrast to conventional VA-ECMO, the novel pulsatile ECMO triggered by ECG provides a more sufficient coronary perfusion with less increase in afterload.

CLINICAL CRITERIA FOR PATIENT SELECTION FOR PROTECTED PERCUTANEOUS CORONARY INTERVENTION

Recently, the clinical practice guidelines recommend consideration of the use of these devices in the setting of high-risk PCI.[3] To avoid underutilization or overutilization of MCS devices during high-risk PCI and to minimize the associated risk, however, a proper patient selection is paramount. Based on patient inclusion criteria adopted in prior various studies assessing utility of protected PCI, the following factors are generally considered as major criteria in patient selection for protected

PCI[22] (**Table 1**). First, one of these factors is the lesion characteristic that determines the complexity of PCI reflecting the technical perspectives and the potential risk of complications. It includes unprotected left main coronary stenosis, distal left main bifurcation stenosis, multivessel disease with high SYNTAX score ($\geq$33), myocardial jeopardy score ($\geq$8/12), last remaining coronary conduit, heavily calcified lesions (type C lesion), and chronic total occlusions. Shamekhi and colleagues[23] revealed that patients undergoing protected PCI with pLVAD achieved more often a complete revascularization without the occurrence of cardiac death at 30 days of follow-up compared with patients undergoing unprotected PCI despite a higher SYNTAX score (45% vs 36%, *P* = .07) and more often complex left main bifurcation lesions (71% vs 29%). Moreover, a similar major adverse cardiac event rate (MACE) at 1 year of follow-up between both groups was shown despite severe basic characteristics of the protected PCI group. These are consistent with results of another study, in which patients undergoing protected PCI with pLVAD had also a decreased rate of residual stenosis and increased rate of procedural success compared with patients with unprotected PCI. The short-term and

Table 1
Clinical criteria for patient selection for protected PCI

Lesion characteristic	Unprotected left main coronary stenosis
	Distal left main bifurcation stenosis
	Multivessel disease with higher SYNTAX score ($\geq$33) or myocardial jeopardy ($\geq$8/12)
	Last remaining coronary conduit
	Heavily calcified lesions (type C lesion)
	Chronic total occlusions
Severe decompensated heart failure	LVEF ($\leq$30–40%)
	NYHA classification III-IV
	Killip classification II-IV
	Electrical instability (eg, ventricular tachycardia)
Patient comorbidities with higher STS-score or EuroSCORE	Increased age (>75 y)
	Chronic obstructive lung disease
	Chronic kidney disease
	Peripheral vascular disease
	Diabetes mellitus
Hemodynamic parameters	Cardiac index (<2.2 L/min per m^2)
	Pulmonary capillary wedge pressure (>15 mm Hg)
	Mean pulmonary artery pressure (>30 mm Hg)

Abbreviations: LVEF, left ventricular ejection fraction; NYHA, New York Heart Association; PCI, percutaneous coronary intervention; STS, Society of Thoracic Surgeons; SYNTAX, synergy between percutaneous coronary intervention with taxus and cardiac surgery.

long-term outcomes in terms of MACE were also similar despite the significantly higher SYNTAX score in the protected PCI group (33% vs 24%, *P*<.01).[24] The extended randomized BCIS-1 trial (Balloon Pump-Assisted Coronary Intervention Study) demonstrated that protected PCI using IABP reduced relatively a long-term all-cause mortality in patients with higher myocardial jeopardy score ($\geq$8) compared with the unprotected PCI group.[25]

Second, protected PCI might be proper for patients with severe decompensated heart failure with reduced LVEF ($\leq$30–40%), New York Heart Association (NYHA) classification III-IV, Killip classification II–IV, or electrical instability (eg, ventricular tachycardia). Ameloot and colleagues[5] showed that patients with severely reduced LVEF (median 24%) and concomitant higher SYNTAX score (median 33) have benefited from protected PCI using pLVAD in terms of survival rate. In a registry trial involving patients with decreased LVEF (mean 31%) and higher SYNTAX score (median 37), it was shown that protected PCI with pLVAD significantly improved LVEF and NYHA class of these high-risk patients.[26] In the PROTECT II trial (Prospective Randomized Clinical Trial of Hemodynamic Support with Impella 2.5 vs Intra-Aortic Balloon Pump in Patients undergoing High-Risk Percutaneous Coronary Intervention) involving patients with reduced LVEF (<30%–35%) and concurrent unprotected left main stenosis or 3-

vessel disease, patients undergoing protected PCI with pLVAD have achieved a more hemodynamic stabilization.[27] Thereby, the frequent occurrence of complete revascularization and the associated reduction of MACE in the protected PCI group might be explained.

Third, patient comorbidities, including increased age (>75 years), chronic obstructive lung disease, chronic kidney disease, peripheral arterial disease, and diabetes mellitus, should be evaluated by STS-score or EuroSCORE when selecting patients for protected PCI. Patients with higher comorbidities assessed by higher STS-score or EuroSCORE could not be suitable for surgical revascularization due to the underlying increased expected risk of mortality and morbidity,.[28–30] In a multicenter registry study, it was shown that protected PCI using pLVAD might be a safe and effective alternative approach to revascularize coronary lesions in patients with higher SYNTAX score (median 32) and concurrent higher logistic EuroSCORE (median 14.7).[31] Another study demonstrated also the safety of both pLVAD and LAAD for protected PCI, especially in patients with complex coronary anatomy and reduced LVEF (median 31%) who were rejected for CABG because of higher mortality risk (median STS-score of 4.2%).[32] Recently, Baumann and colleagues[33] demonstrated in a multicenter registry study that patients undergoing protected PCI with pLVAD due to both higher SYNTAX score (median 33) and higher

EuroSCORE II (median 7.2%) had acceptable clinical results at 180 days of follow-up regarding MACE (22%) and all-cause mortality (18%).

Finally, hemodynamic parameters are also regarded as key factors, especially reduced cardiac index (<2.2 L/min per m^2), increased pulmonary capillary wedge pressure (>15 mm Hg), and mean pulmonary artery pressure (>30 mm Hg). The safety and efficacy of IABP and LAAD for protected PCI could be demonstrated in a randomized study including patients with a cardiac index less than 2.1 L/min per m^2 indicating an onset of cardiogenic shock.[34] In contrast, however, no study could clearly demonstrate the mortality advantage of MCS devices in patients with already manifested severe cardiogenic shock despite improvement in hemodynamic and metabolic parameters by using MCS devices.[35–38]

PROCEDURE-RELATED CRITERIA FOR PATIENT SELECTION FOR PROTECTED PERCUTANEOUS CORONARY INTERVENTION

In addition to the previously mentioned clinical criteria, procedure-related factors also should be considered in patient selection for protected PCI to reduce procedure-related complications and thus to improve clinical outcomes (**Table 2**). These depend basically on the selection of MCS devices due to the different implantation techniques and operating mechanisms.[39] The factor that is independent of types of MCS devices is a pathologic peripheral vessel condition, such as tortuosity and/or peripheral arterial disease. This factor does not actually represent an absolute contraindication for the implantation of MCS devices of all types.[3] However, it is associated with increased risk of limb ischemia or mechanical malfunction of MCS devices.[40] Especially in patients with known peripheral arterial disease, severity of disease should be assessed by imaging diagnostics, such as duplex ultrasonography or even computed tomography angiography to determine the appropriate access vessel for insertion of the device's sheath. In this regard, for example, patients with severe peripheral arterial disease or tortuosity in iliofemoral vessels could benefit more from pLVAD with an axillary access than from other devices.[22]

In addition, the indication of protected PCI should be carefully evaluated in patients with aortic valve disease (ie, aortic regurgitation or aortic stenosis).[41] Even with mild aortic regurgitation, all types of MCS devices could increase significantly the volume of regurgitation due to increased aortic pressure, leading to further dilatation of aorta and left ventricle and consequently

severe decompensating hemodynamics.[42,43] Specifically, in case of pLVAD in patients with aortic regurgitation, an optimal forward flow mediated by pLVAD could be not guaranteed due to the lack of a competent valve separating between the left ventricle and aorta.[44] Moreover, patients with an aortic stenosis will be also poorly served by pLVAD because of difficult placement caused by the aortic stenosis and an increased risk of thromboembolism as well as rupture. Therefore, assessment of aortic valve using transthoracic (TTE) or transesophageal echocardiography (TEE) before protected PCI is recommended.

The presence of thrombus is also one of criteria that should be excluded by TTE or TEE before the planed protected PCI using particularly pLVAD or LAAD.[44] An ingestion of left ventricular clot in pLVAD commonly leads to shutdown of the device. The likelihood of clot ingestion resulting in embolization is extremely unlikely; however, a mobile thrombus represents a risk for systemic embolization with any left ventricular catheter placement. When using LAAD, thrombus in the left atrium could lead to the shutdown of the LAAD or/and a systemic embolization, such as an ischemic stroke, mesenteric ischemia, and renal infarction. Hence, preprocedural visualization of the left ventricle and atrium excluding the presence of thrombus is advisable.

In protected PCI with pLVAD, LAAD, or VA-ECMO, an adequate anticoagulation is indispensable to prevent thrombus formation that leads to malfunctions of devices and systemic thromboembolism.[45] In this context, patients with hemorrhagic diathesis, for example, thrombocytopenia, liver synthesis disorder, von Willebrand disease, or disseminated intravascular coagulation, might benefit rather from protected PCI using IABP instead of pLVAD, LAAD or VA-ECMO.

ALGORITHM AND SCORING SYSTEM FOR PATIENT SELECTION FOR PROTECTED PERCUTANEOUS CORONARY INTERVENTION

According to recommendations of European Society of Cardiology 2017, IABP insertion should be considered in patients with hemodynamic instability or cardiogenic shock due to mechanical complications (Class IIa), whereas no other devices are recommended.[46] In patients with acute myocardial infarction complicated by cardiogenic shock, short-term MCS may be considered regardless of device types (Class IIb). According to the guidelines of American College of Cardiology/American Heart Association/Society for Cardiovascular Angiography and Interventions, elective insertion of an appropriate MCS device

Table 2
Procedure-related criteria for selection of patients and MCS devices for protected PCI

	Criterium	Available MCS Devices
Peripheral vessel condition assessed by duplex ultrasonography or CTA	Iliofemoral tortuosity Iliofemoral peripheral arterial disease	Axillary pLVAD, IABP
Aortic valve disease assessed by TTE or TEE	Aortic regurgitation Aortic stenosis	No devices recommended IABP, LAAD, VA-ECMO
Presence of thrombus assessed by TTE or TEE	Thrombus in left ventricle Thrombus in left atrium	IABP, LAAD, VA-ECMO IABP, VA-ECMO
Contraindication for anticoagulation	Thrombocytopenia Liver synthesis disorder von Willebrand disease Disseminated intravascular coagulation	IABP

Abbreviations: CTA, computed tomography angiography; IABP, intra-aortic balloon pump; LAAD, left atrial to aorta assist devices; MCS, mechanical circulatory support; PCI, percutaneous coronary intervention; pLVAD, percutaneous left ventricular assist devices; TEE, transesophageal echocardiography; TTE, transthoracic echocardiography; VA-ECMO, veno-arterial extracorporeal membrane oxygenation.

as an adjunct to PCI has been recommended in carefully selected high-risk patients who have a vessel subtending a large territory on a background of severely depressed left ventricular function, unprotected left main, or last remaining conduit (Class IIa).[47]

So far, however, no established algorithm or scoring system reflecting all clinical and procedure-related criteria has been developed that can be generally used in patient selection for protected PCI to prevent underestimating or overestimating. Werner and colleagues[48] suggested in their expert consensus an algorithm for patient selection for protected PCI based on coronary complexity, LVEF, cardiac index, and comorbidities; however, herewith also no procedure-related criteria were considered when selecting patients for protected PCI. In the algorithm suggested by Atkinson and colleagues,[22] an evaluation of femoral vessel was reflected to determine

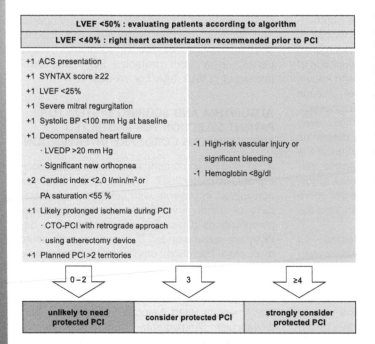

Fig. 2. Proposed scoring system based on clinical factors for optimal patient selection for protected PCI. ACS, acute coronary syndrome; BP, blood pressure; CI, cardiac index; CTO, chronic total occlusion; LVEF, left ventricular end-diastolic pressure; PA, pulmonary artery. (*Adapted from* McCabe JM. Hemodynamic support for CTO PCI: who, when & how. Presented at Transcatheter Cardiovascular Therapeutics (TCT). September 21-25, 2018, San Diego, California.)

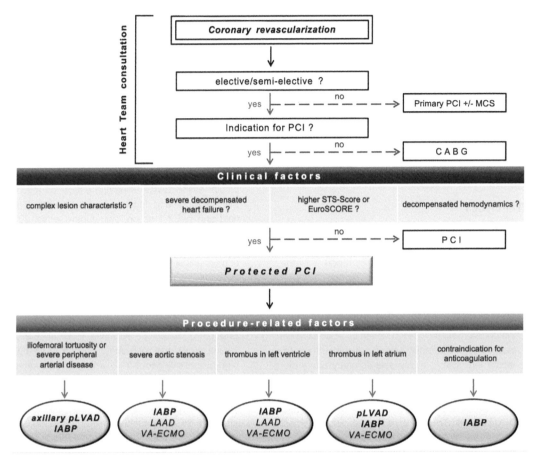

Fig. 3. Proposed practical approach for patient selection for protected PCI depending on the clinical and procedure-related factors. IABP or pLVAD should be preferred for protected PCI if there are no negative procedure-related factors for their use.

the access vessel for inserting MCS devices, but no other procedure-related factors were described in detail. A single-center registry by McCabe[49] evaluating a proposed scoring system to guide patient selection for protected PCI is ongoing, and findings regarding the adequacy of these characteristics to predict efficacy and safety of upfront protected PCI are still pending (**Fig. 2**). Based on the previously proposed algorithms, **Fig. 3** suggests a practical approach for patient selection for protected PCI depending on the clinical and technical aspects. To improve efficacy and safety of protected PCI in these high-risk patients exhibiting higher mortality, further clinical studies should be conducted to develop a universal reliable algorithm to select appropriate patients for protected PCI.

to maintain sufficient cardiac output and reduce myocardial oxygen demand in high-risk patients who would not otherwise tolerate complete revascularization of complex coronary lesions. However, a precise selection of patients for protected PCI based on various clinical criteria is imperative to achieve hemodynamic and prognostic benefit in this patient group with higher morbidity and mortality burden. Moreover, the use of MCS devices for protected PCI should be also strictly individualized based on procedure-related factors to prevent device-associated complications. Further registry and randomized trials should be conducted to establish an evidence-based algorithm and scoring system that enables more careful selection of patients for protected PCI to improve clinical outcomes.

SUMMARY

Protected PCI represents one of the most advanced PCI types using several MCS devices

ACKNOWLEDGMENTS

This review was supported by the Deutsches Zentrum fuer Herz-Kreislauf-Forschung - German

Centre for Cardiovascular Research (DZHK). The authors thank Hyoin Bai for her excellent technical assistance.

DISCLOSURE

The authors have nothing to disclose.

CONFLICT OF INTEREST

The authors declare that they have no potential conflict of interest.

REFERENCES

1. Venkitachalam L, Kip KE, Selzer F, et al. Twenty-year evolution of percutaneous coronary intervention and its impact on clinical outcomes: a report from the National Heart, Lung, and Blood Institute-sponsored, multicenter 1985-1986 PTCA and 1997-2006 Dynamic Registries. Circ Cardiovasc Interv 2009;2(1):6–13.

2. Waldo SW, Secemsky EA, O'Brien C, et al. Surgical ineligibility and mortality among patients with unprotected left main or multivessel coronary artery disease undergoing percutaneous coronary intervention. Circulation 2014;130(25):2295–301.

3. Rihal CS, Naidu SS, Givertz MM, et al. 2015 SCAI/ACC/HFSA/STS clinical expert consensus Statement on the Use of percutaneous mechanical circulatory support devices in Cardiovascular Care: Endorsed by the American Heart Assocation, the Cardiological Society of India, and Sociedad Latino Americana de Cardiologia Intervencion; Affirmation of Value by the Canadian Association of Interventional Cardiology-Association Canadienne de Cardiologie d'intervention. J Am Coll Cardiol 2015;65(19):e7–26.

4. Basir MB, Kapur NK, Patel K, et al. Improved outcomes associated with the use of shock protocols: updates from the national cardiogenic shock initiative. Catheter Cardiovasc Interv 2019;93(7):1173–83.

5. Ameloot K, Bastos MB, Daemen J, et al. New-generation mechanical circulatory support during high-risk PCI: a cross-sectional analysis. EuroIntervention 2019;15(5):427–33.

6. Mennuni MG, Pagnotta PA, Stefanini GG. Coronary stents: the impact of technological advances on clinical outcomes. Ann Biomed Eng 2016;44(2):488–96.

7. Vetrovec GW. Hemodynamic support devices for shock and high-risk PCI: when and which one. Curr Cardiol Rep 2017;19(10):100.

8. Velazquez EJ, Lee KL, Jones RH, et al. Coronary-artery bypass surgery in patients with ischemic cardiomyopathy. N Engl J Med 2016;374(16):1511–20.

9. Nayyar M, Donovan KM, Khouzam RN. When more is not better-appropriately excluding patients from mechanical circulatory support therapy. Ann Transl Med 2018;6(1):9.

10. Nellis SH, Liedtke AJ, Whitesell L. Small coronary vessel pressure and diameter in an intact beating rabbit heart using fixed-position and free-motion techniques. Circ Res 1981;49(2):342–53.

11. Ait Ichou J, Larivee N, Eisenberg MJ, et al. The effectiveness and safety of the Impella ventricular assist device for high-risk percutaneous coronary interventions: a systematic review. Catheter Cardiovasc Interv 2018;91(7):1250–60.

12. Drakos SG, Kfoury AG, Selzman CH, et al. Left ventricular assist device unloading effects on myocardial structure and function: current status of the field and call for action. Curr Opin Cardiol 2011;26(3):245–55.

13. Burkhoff D, Sayer G, Doshi D, et al. Hemodynamics of mechanical circulatory support. J Am Coll Cardiol 2015;66(23):2663–74.

14. Csepe TA, Kilic A. Advancements in mechanical circulatory support for patients in acute and chronic heart failure. J Thorac Dis 2017;9(10):4070–83.

15. Briguori C, Sarais C, Pagnotta P, et al. Elective versus provisional intra-aortic balloon pumping in high-risk percutaneous transluminal coronary angioplasty. Am Heart J 2003;145(4):700–7.

16. Papaioannou TG, Stefanadis C. Basic principles of the intraaortic balloon pump and mechanisms affecting its performance. ASAIO J 2005;51(3):296–300.

17. Basra SS, Loyalka P, Kar B. Current status of percutaneous ventricular assist devices for cardiogenic shock. Curr Opin Cardiol 2011;26(6):548–54.

18. Raess DH, Weber DM. Impella 2.5. J Cardiovasc Transl Res 2009;2(2):168–72.

19. Kapur NK, Paruchuri V, Urbano-Morales JA, et al. Mechanically unloading the left ventricle before coronary reperfusion reduces left ventricular wall stress and myocardial infarct size. Circulation 2013;128(4):328–36.

20. Koeckert MS, Jorde UP, Naka Y, et al. 5 for left ventricular unloading during venoarterial extracorporeal membrane oxygenation support. J Card Surg 2011;26(6):666–8.

21. Bavaria JE, Ratcliffe MB, Gupta KB, et al. Changes in left ventricular systolic wall stress during biventricular circulatory assistance. Ann Thorac Surg 1988;45(5):526–32.

22. Atkinson TM, Ohman EM, O'Neill WW, et al, Interventional Scientific Council of the American College of Cardiology. A practical approach to mechanical circulatory support in patients undergoing percutaneous coronary intervention: an interventional perspective. JACC Cardiovasc Interv 2016;9(9):871–83.

23. Shamekhi J, Putz A, Zimmer S, et al. Impact of hemodynamic support on outcome in patients

undergoing high-risk percutaneous intervention. Am J Cardiol 2019;124(1):20–30.

24. Becher T, Eder F, Baumann S, et al. Unprotected versus protected high-risk percutaneous coronary intervention with the Impella 2.5 in patients with multivessel disease and severely reduced left ventricular function. Medicine (Baltimore) 2018;97(43): e12665.

25. Perera D, Stables R, Clayton T, et al. Long-term mortality data from the balloon pump-assisted coronary intervention study (BCIS-1): a randomized, controlled trial of elective balloon counterpulsation during high-risk percutaneous coronary intervention. Circulation 2013;127(2):207–12.

26. Maini B, Naidu SS, Mulukutla S, et al. Real-world use of the Impella 2.5 circulatory support system in complex high-risk percutaneous coronary intervention: the USpella Registry. Catheter Cardiovasc Interv 2012;80(5):717–25.

27. O'Neill WW, Kleiman NS, Moses J, et al. A prospective, randomized clinical trial of hemodynamic support with Impella 2.5 versus intra-aortic balloon pump in patients undergoing high-risk percutaneous coronary intervention: the PROTECT II study. Circulation 2012;126(14):1717–27.

28. Roques F, Nashef SA, Michel P, et al. Risk factors and outcome in European cardiac surgery: analysis of the EuroSCORE multinational database of 19030 patients. Eur J Cardiothorac Surg 1999;15(6): 816–22 [discussion: 822–3].

29. Shahian DM, Jacobs JP, Badhwar V, et al. The Society of Thoracic Surgeons 2018 adult cardiac surgery risk models: part 1-background, design considerations, and model development. Ann Thorac Surg 2018;105(5):1411–8.

30. O'Brien SM, Feng L, He X, et al. The Society of Thoracic Surgeons 2018 adult cardiac surgery risk models: part 2-statistical methods and results. Ann Thorac Surg 2018;105(5):1419–28.

31. Baumann S, Werner N, Ibrahim K, et al. Indication and short-term clinical outcomes of high-risk percutaneous coronary intervention with microaxial Impella(R) pump: results from the German Impella(R) registry. Clin Res Cardiol 2018;107(8):653–7.

32. Kovacic JC, Nguyen HT, Karajgikar R, et al. The Impella Recover 2.5 and TandemHeart ventricular assist devices are safe and associated with equivalent clinical outcomes in patients undergoing high-risk percutaneous coronary intervention. Catheter Cardiovasc Interv 2013;82(1):E28–37.

33. Baumann S, Werner N, Al-Rashid F, et al. Six months follow-up of protected high-risk percutaneous coronary intervention with the microaxial Impella pump: results from the German Impella registry. Coron Artery Dis 2020;31(3):237–42.

34. Thiele H, Sick P, Boudriot E, et al. Randomized comparison of intra-aortic balloon support with a percutaneous left ventricular assist device in patients with revascularized acute myocardial infarction complicated by cardiogenic shock. Eur Heart J 2005;26(13):1276–83.

35. Lauten A, Engstrom AE, Jung C, et al. Percutaneous left-ventricular support with the Impella-2.5-assist device in acute cardiogenic shock: results of the Impella-EUROSHOCK-registry. Circ Heart Fail 2013; 6(1):23–30.

36. Thiele H, Zeymer U, Neumann FJ, et al. Intraaortic balloon support for myocardial infarction with cardiogenic shock. N Engl J Med 2012;367(14):1287–96.

37. Thiele H, Zeymer U, Neumann FJ, et al. Intra-aortic balloon counterpulsation in acute myocardial infarction complicated by cardiogenic shock (IABP-SHOCK II): final 12 month results of a randomised, open-label trial. Lancet 2013;382(9905): 1638–45.

38. Thiele H, Zeymer U, Thelemann N, et al. Intraaortic balloon pump in cardiogenic shock complicating acute myocardial infarction: long-term 6-year outcome of the randomized IABP-SHOCK II Trial. Circulation 2018. https://doi.org/10.1161/CIRCULATIONAHA. 118.038201.

39. Myat A, Patel N, Tehrani S, et al. Percutaneous circulatory assist devices for high-risk coronary intervention. JACC Cardiovasc Interv 2015;8(2):229–44.

40. Rastan AJ, Tillmann E, Subramanian S, et al. Visceral arterial compromise during intra-aortic balloon counterpulsation therapy. Circulation 2010; 122(11 Suppl):S92–9.

41. Asleh R, Resar JR. Utilization of percutaneous mechanical circulatory support devices in cardiogenic shock complicating acute myocardial infarction and high-risk percutaneous coronary interventions. J Clin Med 2019;8(8):1209.

42. Kar B, Basra SS, Shah NR, et al. Percutaneous circulatory support in cardiogenic shock: interventional bridge to recovery. Circulation 2012;125(14):1809–17.

43. Pham DT, Al-Quthami A, Kapur NK. Percutaneous left ventricular support in cardiogenic shock and severe aortic regurgitation. Catheter Cardiovasc Interv 2013;81(2):399–401.

44. Burzotta F, Trani C, Doshi SN, et al. Impella ventricular support in clinical practice: collaborative viewpoint from a European expert user group. Int J Cardiol 2015;201:684–91.

45. Pieri M, Agracheva N, Bonaveglio E, et al. Bivalirudin versus heparin as an anticoagulant during extracorporeal membrane oxygenation: a case-control study. J Cardiothorac Vasc Anesth 2013; 27(1):30–4.

46. Ibanez B, James S, Agewall S, et al. 2017 ESC guidelines for the management of acute myocardial infarction in patients presenting with ST-segment elevation. Rev Esp Cardiol (Engl Ed) 2017;70(12): 1082.

47. Levine GN, Bates ER, Blankenship JC, et al. 2011 ACCF/AHA/SCAI guideline for percutaneous coronary intervention. A report of the American College of Cardiology Foundation/American Heart Association Task Force on practice guidelines and the Society for Cardiovascular Angiography and Interventions. J Am Coll Cardiol 2011;58(24): e44–122.

48. Werner N, Akin I, Al-Rashid F, et al. Expertenkonsensus zum praktischen Einsatz von Herzkreislaufunterstützungssystemen bei Hochrisiko-Koronarinterventionen. Kardiologe 2017;11:460–72.

49. McCabe JM. Hemodynamic support for CTO PCI: who, when & how. Presented at Transcatheter Cardiovascular Therapeutics (TCT). San Diego, CA, September 21–25, 2018.

Echocardiographic Strain Imaging in Coronary Artery Disease
The Added Value of a Quantitative Approach

Alessandro Malagoli, MD[a,1], Diego Fanti, MD[b,1], Alessandro Albini, MD[c], Andrea Rossi, MD[b], Flavio L. Ribichini, MD, PhD[b], Giovanni Benfari, MD[b,*]

KEYWORDS

- Ischemic cardiomyopathy • Coronary artery disease • Speckle tracking echocardiography
- Global longitudinal strain • Left atrium • Right ventricular infarction

KEY POINTS

- Longitudinal left ventricular function by speckle tracking echocardiography provides incremental diagnostic and prognostic information in patients with subclinical and overt coronary artery disease. This technique may be on his way to an ultimate introduction in the clinical practice.
- Longitudinal strain-derived indexes (early systolic lengthening and postsystolic shortening) are further expanding and refining the applications of speckle tracking echocardiography, particularly in patients with coronary artery disease.
- Right ventricular and left atrial function by speckle tracking echocardiography are emerging prognosticators in ischemic cardiomyopathy, deserving great attention in the research field.

INTRODUCTION

Cardiovascular disease remains a leading and partially preventable cause of death worldwide; therefore, the early detection of incipient myocardial ischemia has always been a challenge for the clinicians. Echocardiography is part of the first-line patient assessment tools and may provide crucial incremental information to guide patients' management.[1]

The assessment of regional myocardial function is the cornerstone for the detection of myocardial ischemia by echocardiography. However, it is grounded on visual assessment and requires considerable expertise. Similarly, the quantification of damage after myocardial infarction (MI) relies on left ventricular ejection fraction (LVEF) calculation, which is based on ventricular volumes measurements, known to hold unsatisfactory intra- and interobserver variability, particularly in the context of distorted LV geometry or wall motion abnormalities.[2,3]

Assessment of LV function through strain imaging is currently increasing as an alternative method to identify early myocardial dysfunction before an

[a] Division of Cardiology, Nephro-Cardiovascular Department, "S. Agostino-Estense" Public Hospital, University of Modena and Reggio Emilia, Via Pietro Giardini N. 1355, Modena 41126, Italy; [b] Section of Cardiology, University of Verona, Piazzale A. Stefani 1, Verona 37126, Italy; [c] Division of Cardiology, Nephro-Cardiovascular Department, Policlinico University Hospital of Modena, University of Modena and Reggio Emilia, Largo del Pozzo N. 71, Modena 41125, Italy
[1] The authors equally contributed to the article.
* Corresponding author.
E-mail address: giovanni.benfari@gmail.com

Cardiol Clin 38 (2020) 517–526
https://doi.org/10.1016/j.ccl.2020.06.005

overt reduction in LVEF, thus revealing the so-called subclinical LV dysfunction.[4]

Furthermore, when applied to other cardiac chambers, as the right ventricle (RV) or the left atrium (LA), strain imaging has expanded the quantitative echocardiographic approach and has allowed the detection of myocardial dynamics to a level unreachable before.

The present review focuses mostly on speckle tracking echocardiography (STE) and its application on patients with coronary artery disease (CAD) to improve diagnosis and prognostic risk stratification; the analysis and the technical differences between STE and tissue Doppler methods are beyond the scope of this dissertation.

The analysis of myocardial strain by STE results, after an appropriate learning curve, is feasible and can provide a quantification of the active myocardial deformation.[5]

Strain indicates the tissue deformation (expressed in percentage) during the cardiac cycle, assuming positive strain values for elongation and negative strain values for shortening; strain-rate indicates the speed at which the deformation occurs.

Two-dimensional (2D) strain is progressively being introduced in the clinical practice; 3D-based strain has been proposed as a less time-consuming alternative, but it is not yet implemented in many laboratories and requires further validation as well as the definition of normal reference values.[6]

In particular, global longitudinal strain (GLS) is calculated as the average longitudinal strain from all segments made in standard apical 2-, 3-, and 4-chamber views,[7] with normal value reported between −18% and −25% in healthy individuals[8,9] (**Fig. 1**), whereas circumferential and radial strains are determined from short-axis views.

Although promising and appealing, 2D STE does not come without limitation at the current state. Indeed, strain normal range depends on multiple factors as age, gender, and weight[8]; furthermore, the systolic strain is not entirely independent from loading conditions.[9]

Strain calculation requires good imaging quality and according to the current guidelines its calculation should be avoided if more than 2 myocardial segments are not adequately visualized in a single view.[2] Lastly, intersoftware and intervendor variability must also be kept in mind, especially when assessing segmental strains.[7]

LEFT VENTRICULAR STRAIN AND MYOCARDIAL ISCHEMIC PROCESS

Three layers form the myocardial wall: the inner and the outer layers with oblique fibers and the middle layer with circular fibers. GLS, global circumferential strain, and global radial strain, as measured by STE, reflect the main shortening vectors of these fibers.[10]

Ischemic changes primarily affect the subendocardial layer, where longitudinal myocardial fibers are more represented.[11] Consequently, CAD and myocardial ischemia are more frequently associated with reduced strain values in the endocardium than in the epicardium. However, in current practice, STE is mostly used to evaluate the entire myocardial wall dynamic (see **Fig. 1**), as the applicability of layer-specific strain is not yet validated and further studies are needed.[12]

Speckle Tracking Echocardiography to Detect Subclinical Myocardial Damage

In terms of diagnostic accuracy improvement for patients with suspected CAD, STE analysis has been proposed as a feasible and reproducible method for the identification of myocardial ischemia during stress echocardiography recognizing functional defects before the development of regional wall motion abnormalities.[13,14]

A study investigated the role of strain imaging in dobutamine stress echocardiography on 102 patients with suspected CAD.[15] Longitudinal strain had similar diagnostic accuracy to wall motion score index; however, if combined with wall motion assessment by an expert reader its accuracy increased to 96% in the detection of regional ischemia.[15]

The routine adoption of speckle tracking during stress echocardiography is still a matter of debate,[16] as there are issues of applicability due to excessive myocardial motion at higher heart rates and the lack of definition of cutoff levels for each major coronary artery region. Joyce and colleagues[17] reported variable diagnostic accuracy using the same cutoff value for the strain parameter in different coronary perfusion regions. The adoption of cut-offs based on "sentinel segments" may be useful, but the heterogeneity of the perfusion territory distal to the stenosis makes it not always accurate.[16]

SPECKLE TRACKING ECHOCARDIOGRAPHY IN PATIENTS WITH STABLE ANGINA AND ACUTE CORONARY SYNDROME

Regional longitudinal peak systolic strain proved to be useful to diagnose CAD and identify the ischemic myocardial areas in patients with stable angina pectoris.[18] GLS may also be useful to identify high-risk patients with left main stem stenosis and 3-vessel CAD in the absence of regional wall motion abnormalities.[19]

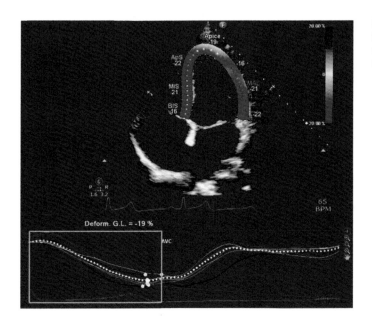

Fig. 1. Example of LV longitudinal strain measurement from the apical 4-chamber view. AVC, aortic valve closure; G.L., global longitudinal strain.

In the chronic phase of ischemic cardiomyopathy, GLS has shown to provide important prognostic information, being independently related to all-cause mortality and combined endpoint in a large cohort of 1060 patients.[20]

Regarding acute coronary syndrome, in the early phase of acute MI, reduced GLS may predict the occurrence of complications.[21] Performed right after the coronary revascularization, GLS seemed useful in distinguishing patients more prone to early recovery and reverse remodeling from those who acutely would merit more intensive monitoring and closer follow-up even after a successful percutaneous coronary intervention.[22] Indeed, GLS correlates with the final infarct size better than LVEF or wall motion score index and has a role in the prediction of major cardiovascular events and overall mortality.[23,24]

Strain parameters are also associated with the amount of myocardial fibrosis and might aid in discriminating transmural scarring from nontransmural to target further revascularization.[25,26] Lastly, although conflicting, some report indicates that GLS can identify stunned myocardium likely to recovery after an acute MI.[27]

Another important diagnostic application of myocardial strain is the identification of significant residual CAD after MI in the presence of existing concomitant wall motion abnormalities. A study investigated the role of dobutamine stress echocardiography in detecting residual ischemia in 105 patients at 3 months after first ST-elevation MI.[17] Not only patients with significant residual coronary disease demonstrated greater worsening in global peak longitudinal systolic strain from rest to peak-dose dobutamine but the authors found a significant drop of the peak longitudinal systolic strain in the segments with significant coronary artery using a sentinel segment approach, confirming the promising value of STE in this setting.[17]

EARLY SYSTOLIC LENGTHENING AND POSTSYSTOLIC SHORTENING OF LEFT VENTRICULAR SEGMENTS

Early systolic lengthening (ESL) is a novel predictor of cardiovascular events defined as the time from onset of the QRS complex to the peak positive systolic strain[28] (**Fig. 2**). ESL reflects a passive lengthening of an ischemic myocardial region before the beginning of systolic shortening, due to its reduced ability to generate an adequate active force during the pressure increase in the isovolumic contraction phase.

In patients with acute MI, ESL duration provides information about prognosis, infarct size, may identify patients with minimal myocardial damage, and may differentiate between occlusive and non-occlusive CAD.[28,29] It may represent a novel and complementary measure of ventricular damage and a predictor of long-term cardiovascular events in those patients who displayed good overall GLS after ST-elevation MI.[30]

Furthermore, ESL may discern between viable and nonviable segments, with akinetic segments displaying significantly higher ESL values.[30,31]

Postsystolic shortening (PSS) reflects a longitudinal shortening occurring after end-systole at

Global Longitudinal Strain

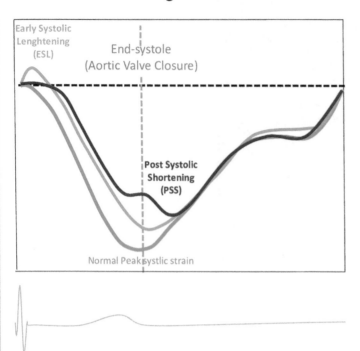

Fig. 2. Illustrative examples of longitudinal strain profile with postsystolic shortening (PSS) and end-systolic lengthening (ESL). PSS is considered myocardial contraction after the point of aortic valve closure, whereas ESL is a lengthening of a myocardial region before the beginning of systolic shortening.

aortic valve closure (see **Fig. 2**). PSS may be found in ischemic viable myocardium reflecting some degree of active contraction, whereas irreversibly injured myocardium remains passive after coronary occlusion.[32] PSS provides information about the ischemic burden[33] and is a predictor of major adverse cardiovascular events and death in patients with acute MI and [34] chronic CAD.[35]

In dobutamine stress echocardiography, diastolic dyssynchrony imaging is a good predictor of CAD,[36] as confirmed by a recent metanalysis.[37]

As a word of caution, PSS may not be ready to be adopted as a stand-alone to identify CAD, as it may be found in healthy individuals in up to one-third of myocardial segments.[38]

RIGHT VENTRICLE FUNCTION

RV involvement in patients with MI is associated with high in-hospital and late mortality, ventricular arrhythmias, advanced atrioventricular block, and mechanical complications.[39–41]

Because isolated RV infarction accounts for less than 3% of all cases of MI, concomitant RV involvement ranges from 14% to 84% of acute MI.[42] Clues of RV involvement in patients with not only inferior but also anterior LV infarcts have been provided by cardiac magnetic imaging studies.[43]

Multiple parameters based on monodimensional and 2D imaging, pulsed-wave (PW) Doppler, and tissue Doppler imaging (TDI) have been described to quantify RV function.[44] Although fully endorsed by the current guidelines, the efficacy of these parameters has been questioned by many investigators in recent years.

The recent application of newer myocardial deformation techniques to the RV could help in overcoming these limitations, allowing the detection of subtle RV dysfunction. RV strain by speckle tracking has proved to be a reliable and accurate tool for the evaluation of RV systolic function when validated against RV ejection fraction by cardiac magnetic resonance in different clinical settings.[45,46] In the latest recommendations for cardiac chamber quantification for the first time a clinical indication for RV strain is included.[2] RV speckle tracking strain is obtained from the apical 4-chamber view, and it could reflect the average value of the RV free wall strain alone or both the RV free wall and septal segments (**Fig. 3**). Currently, the use of RV free wall seems to have the largest body of evidence, but further investigations are needed to clarify this point. Interestingly, a group proposed an approach for a global assessment of RV function using 3 RV apical views, permitting a full reconstruction of the RV

A **B**

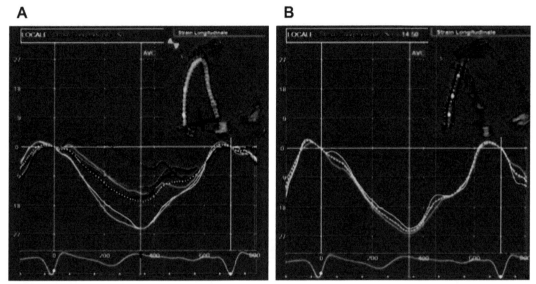

Fig. 3. Assessment of RV systolic function by 2D longitudinal strain from an apical 4-chamber view. Strain curves obtained automatically by tracing the endocardial margin of RV free wall and septal segments (*A*) or of the RV free wall alone (*B*). Each curve represents one RV segment. An average ventricular longitudinal strain along the cardiac cycle is depicted (*dashed curve*).

in an 18-segment model and a calculation of a "true" RV global longitudinal strain.[47] To date, wide agreement regarding normal values is lacking; a recent meta-analysis suggested −27 ± 2% as the normal range, but an RV free wall strain cutoff of −20% to −21% seems to be able to detect abnormal RV function.[48,49]

Few studies have investigated the relationship between RV speckle tracking strain and CAD. Among these investigations, acute MI has been discussed more than chronic ischemic heart disease. In patients with MI, RV strain has proved to be the best tool providing information about global and targeted regional function, with good feasibility and reproducibility.[50] Global longitudinal strain of the RV showed a better sensibility and specificity for prediction of major adverse cardiovascular events than standard RV function parameters.[51,52] It also provides important prognostic information about the arrhythmic risk and sudden cardiac death in patients with acute MI[39] due to interwoven scar tissue and viable myocardium constituting substrates for reentry arrhythmias. There is little evidence regarding outcomes associated with RV strain in chronic ischemic heart disease. In a study by Chang and colleagues[40] conducted on 208 patients with stable angina, impaired RV strain was significantly related to worse cardiovascular outcomes and new onset of arrhythmia. The same group successfully demonstrated the usefulness of RV strain for the detection of occult RV dysfunction in patients

with chronic right coronary artery stenosis.[41] Lastly, RV strain provides prognostic value also in stable outpatients with chronic heart failure. In a cohort of 171 consecutive patients with stable LV dysfunction (41% with ischemic cardiomyopathy), a lower magnitude of RV strain predicted adverse events after adjustment for age, cause of heart failure, and LVEF.[53] Although it has been accepted that RV dysfunction complicates and increases long-term mortality, whether RV strain is an independent predictor of adverse events in patients with CAD or a consequence of the progression of LV dysfunction still requires verification. Currently, preliminary results indicate that the RV itself plays a pivotal role in maintaining hemodynamic and rhythmic stability, but further prospective studies are needed.

LEFT ATRIAL FUNCTION

In recent years, the role of LA mechanical function has emerged to be of clinical value in several clinical settings including the ischemic heart disease.[54–57] LA function, in close interdependence with LV function, plays a crucial role in maintaining optimal cardiac performance. LA modulates LV filling through its 3 phases: reservoir, conduit, and booster pump. The reservoir function corresponds to the LV systole; the conduit function results from the blood transiting from the LA to the LV during early diastole (passive emptying); and finally the booster pump function in late diastolic phase corresponds to the LA contraction. The contribution of LA phasic function to LV filling depends on LV diastolic properties. With abnormal relaxation, the relative contribution of LA contractile function to LV filling increases, whereas the conduit function decreases. As LV filling pressures progressively increase, the limits of atrial preload reserve are reached, and the LA serves predominantly as a conduit.[58]

The estimation of LA function can be obtained by several methods, including the assessment of changes in LA volume during the cardiac cycle, analysis of transmitral flow by PW Doppler, and evaluation of LA myocardial velocities by TDI.

Despite these methods, the quantification of LA function remains a challenging issue because their application requires a skillful acquisition technique and calculations that are not routinely performed. To date, direct evaluation of LA function is also feasible with STE. This technique permits assessment of longitudinal myocardial LA deformation, which provides additive value concerning LA function when compared with conventional echocardiographic measurements and seems easier to apply.[59] In line with the current American Society of Echocardiography/European Association of Echocardiography consensus,[60] the LA endocardial border is manually traced in the 4- and 2-

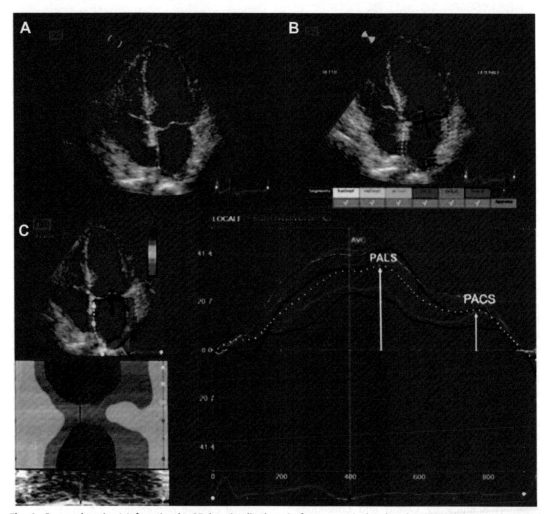

Fig. 4. Comprehensive LA function by 2D longitudinal strain from an apical 4-chamber view. (*A*) LA endocardial region of interest tracing. (*B*) The LA is divided into 6 segments: basal septal (basSept; *yellow*), midseptal (midSept; *light blue*), apical septal (apSept; *green*), apical lateral (apLat; lilac), mid lateral (midLat; *blue*), and basal lateral (basLat; *red*). (*C*) Strain curves during a cardiac cycle using the onset of the QRS complex as the starting point. Each curve represents one LA segment. An average atrial longitudinal strain along the cardiac cycle is depicted (*dashed curve*). AVC, aortic valve closure; PACS, peak atrial contraction strain; PALS, peak atrial longitudinal strain.

chamber views, thus delineating a region of interest composed by 6 segments. Then, after segmental tracking quality analysis and eventual manual adjustment of the region of interest, longitudinal strain curves are generated by the software for each atrial segment. Peak atrial longitudinal strain (PALS) is measured at the end of the reservoir phase, and peak atrial contraction strain (PACS) is measured just before the start of the active atrial contractile phase (**Fig. 4**).

There is increasing evidence demonstrating the value of PALS in acute and chronic ischemic heart disease. In patients with acute MI treated with primary percutaneous coronary intervention, PALS provides additional prognostic value beyond baseline risk factors and LA maximal volume.[61] Because of increased LV chamber stiffness and LV filling pressures occurring in acute LV ischemia, LA pressure may be increased. To maintain adequate LV filling, a preserved LA reservoir function is crucial. In contrast, in patients with noncompliant LA and reduced reservoir function, LV filling may be significantly impaired, increasing the risk of worse prognosis. LA reservoir function by STE was also related to adverse outcomes in stable outpatients with chronic heart failure and reduced left ventricular ejection fraction (HFrEF). In a cohort of 286 consecutive patients with stable HFrEF (64% with ischemic cardiomyopathy), patients with lower PALS showed worse event-free survival than those with higher PALS.[62] Mechanism linking LA function with outcome in this clinical setting is not fully understood. Chronic exposure to high LV filling pressures will cause an increase in LA volume, and it may be hypothesized that a decreased LA function is just a marker of a sicker LV.[63]

Because LA reservoir and conduit function reflect underlying LV function, there is some skepticism about the utility of LA strain compared with other markers of LV strain. The reciprocating changes in LV and LA volumes within the nearly constant total cardiac volume suggest that any measure of LA function will be highly influenced by LV longitudinal function. Thus, any longitudinal elongation of the atrium must correspond to the deformation of the ventricle.[64–66] This phenomenon has been reported by Ersbøll and colleagues,[67] who demonstrated that PALS provides a composite measure of LV longitudinal systolic function and maximum LA volume before mitral valve opening and as such, contains no added information when these readily obtained measures are known.

In contrast, PACS is less dependent on LV function, and changes to atrial pump function do not depend primarily on changes to the LV but may be due to the development of an underlying "atriopathy."[68] Currently, data about the prognostic role of PACS in the ischemic cardiomyopathy are lacking. Further research will allow us to understand this relationship better.

SUMMARY

Echocardiographic strain imaging is useful for the evaluation of acute and chronic ischemic heart disease. It may soon affect the guideline-based management of patients with ischemic heart disease. GLS of the LV holds both a diagnostic and prognostic value in patients with stable angina, acute coronary syndrome, and subclinical CAD; ESL and PSS of LV segments are innovative and not entirely validated markers of ischemia. Left atrium PALS reflects LV diastolic dysfunction and has a prognostic value in ischemic cardiomyopathy. Although less validated than the left counterpart, RV strain measures are useful for the diagnosis and risk stratification of patients with RV ischemic involvement. Even though we are getting closer, further accumulation of evidence is needed for the definitive introduction of strain parameters in clinical practice and guidelines for patients with ischemic heart disease.

DISCLOSURE

The authors declare that they have no competing financial interests or personal relationships that could have appeared to influence the work reported in this paper.

REFERENCES

1. Benfari G, Rossi A, Geremia G, et al. Optimizing the role of transthoracic echocardiography to improve the cardiovascular risk stratification: the dream of subclinical coronary artery disease detection. Minerva Med 2018;109:31–40.
2. Lang RM, Badano LP, Mor-Avi V, et al. Recommendations for cardiac chamber quantification by echocardiography in adults: an update from the American Society of Echocardiography and the European Association of Cardiovascular Imaging. J Am Soc Echocardiogr 2015;28:1–39.e14.
3. Salvo GD, Pergola V, Fadel B, et al. Strain echocardiography and myocardial mechanics: from basics to clinical applications. J Cardiovasc Echogr 2015; 25:1–8.
4. Shimoni S, Gendelman G, Ayzenberg O, et al. Differential effects of coronary artery stenosis on myocardial function: the value of myocardial strain analysis for the detection of coronary artery disease. J Am Soc Echocardiogr 2011;24:748–57.

5. Chan J, Shiino K, Obonyo NG, et al. Left ventricular global strain analysis by two-dimensional speckle-tracking echocardiography: the learning curve. J Am Soc Echocardiogr 2017;30:1081–90.

6. Truong VT, Phan HT, Pham KNP, et al. Normal ranges of left ventricular strain by three-dimensional speckle-tracking echocardiography in adults: a systematic review and meta-analysis. J Am Soc Echocardiogr 2019;32:1586–97.e5.

7. Voigt JU, Pedrizzetti G, Lysyansky P, et al. Definitions for a common standard for 2D speckle tracking echocardiography: consensus document of the EACVI/ASE/Industry Task Force to standardize deformation imaging. Eur Heart J Cardiovasc Imaging 2015;16:1–11.

8. Sugimoto T, Dulgheru R, Bernard A, et al. Echocardiographic reference ranges for normal left ventricular 2D strain: results from the EACVI NORRE study. Eur Heart J Cardiovasc Imaging 2017;18:833–40.

9. Yingchoncharoen T, Agarwal S, Popovic ZB, et al. Normal ranges of left ventricular strain: a meta-analysis. J Am Soc Echocardiogr 2013;26:185–91.

10. Gilbert SH, Benson AP, Li P, et al. Regional localisation of left ventricular sheet structure: integration with current models of cardiac fibre, sheet and band structure. Eur J Cardiothorac Surg 2007;32:231–49.

11. Sarvari SI, Haugaa KH, Zahid W, et al. Layer-specific quantification of myocardial deformation by strain echocardiography may reveal significant CAD in patients with non-ST-segment elevation acute coronary syndrome. JACC Cardiovasc Imaging 2013;6:535–44.

12. Hagemann CA, Hoffmann S, Hagemann RA, et al. Usefulness of layer-specific strain in diagnosis of coronary artery disease in patients with stable angina pectoris. Int J Cardiovasc Imaging 2019;35:1989–99.

13. Uusitalo V, Luotolahti M, Pietila M, et al. Two-Dimensional speckle-tracking during dobutamine stress echocardiography in the detection of myocardial ischemia in patients with suspected coronary artery disease. J Am Soc Echocardiogr 2016;29:470–9.e3.

14. Aggeli C, Lagoudakou S, Felekos I, et al. Two-dimensional speckle tracking for the assessment of cornary artery disease during dobutamine stress echo: clinical tool or merely research method. Cardiovasc Ultrasound 2015;13:43.

15. Ng AC, Sitges M, Pham PN, et al. Incremental value of 2-dimensional speckle tracking strain imaging to wall motion analysis for detection of coronary artery disease in patients undergoing dobutamine stress echocardiography. Am Heart J 2009;158:836–44.

16. Hanekom L, Cho GY, Leano R, et al. Comparison of two-dimensional speckle and tissue Doppler strain measurement during dobutamine stress echocardiography: an angiographic correlation. Eur Heart J 2007;28:1765–72.

17. Joyce E, Hoogslag GE, Al Amri I, et al. Quantitative dobutamine stress echocardiography using speckle-tracking analysis versus conventional visual analysis for detection of significant coronary artery disease after ST-segment elevation myocardial infarction. J Am Soc Echocardiogr 2015;28:1379–89.e1.

18. Biering-Sorensen T, Hoffmann S, Mogelvang R, et al. Myocardial strain analysis by 2-dimensional speckle tracking echocardiography improves diagnostics of coronary artery stenosis in stable angina pectoris. Circ Cardiovasc Imaging 2014;7:58–65.

19. Choi JO, Cho SW, Song YB, et al. Longitudinal 2D strain at rest predicts the presence of left main and three vessel coronary artery disease in patients without regional wall motion abnormality. Eur J Echocardiogr 2009;10:695–701.

20. Bertini M, Ng AC, Antoni ML, et al. Global longitudinal strain predicts long-term survival in patients with chronic ischemic cardiomyopathy. Circ Cardiovasc Imaging 2012;5:383–91.

21. Woo JS, Kim WS, Yu TK, et al. Prognostic value of serial global longitudinal strain measured by two-dimensional speckle tracking echocardiography in patients with ST-segment elevation myocardial infarction. Am J Cardiol 2011;108:340–7.

22. Meimoun P, Abouth S, Clerc J, et al. Usefulness of two-dimensional longitudinal strain pattern to predict left ventricular recovery and in-hospital complications after acute anterior myocardial infarction treated successfully by primary angioplasty. J Am Soc Echocardiogr 2015;28:1366–75.

23. Antoni ML, Mollema SA, Delgado V, et al. Prognostic importance of strain and strain rate after acute myocardial infarction. Eur Heart J 2010;31:1640–7.

24. Munk K, Andersen NH, Terkelsen CJ, et al. Global left ventricular longitudinal systolic strain for early risk assessment in patients with acute myocardial infarction treated with primary percutaneous intervention. J Am Soc Echocardiogr 2012;25:644–51.

25. Tarascio M, Leo LA, Klersy C, et al. Speckle-tracking layer-specific analysis of myocardial deformation and evaluation of scar transmurality in chronic ischemic heart disease. J Am Soc Echocardiogr 2017;30:667–75.

26. Becker M, Ocklenburg C, Altiok E, et al. Impact of infarct transmurality on layer-specific impairment of myocardial function: a myocardial deformation imaging study. Eur Heart J 2009;30:1467–76.

27. Mollema SA, Delgado V, Bertini M, et al. Viability assessment with global left ventricular longitudinal strain predicts recovery of left ventricular function after acute myocardial infarction. Circ Cardiovasc Imaging 2010;3:15–23.

28. Smedsrud MK, Sarvari S, Haugaa KH, et al. Duration of myocardial early systolic lengthening predicts the

presence of significant coronary artery disease. J Am Coll Cardiol 2012;60:1086–93.

29. Zahid W, Eek CH, Remme EW, et al. Early systolic lengthening may identify minimal myocardial damage in patients with non-ST-elevation acute coronary syndrome. Eur Heart J Cardiovasc Imaging 2014;15: 1152–60.

30. Vartdal T, Pettersen E, Helle-Valle T, et al. Identification of viable myocardium in acute anterior infarction using duration of systolic lengthening by tissue Doppler strain: a preliminary study. J Am Soc Echocardiogr 2012;25:718–25.

31. Brainin P, Haahr-Pedersen S, Olsen FJ, et al. Early systolic lengthening in patients with ST-segment-elevation myocardial infarction: a novel predictor of cardiovascular events. J Am Heart Assoc 2020;9: e013835.

32. Lyseggen E, Skulstad H, Helle-Valle T, et al. Myocardial strain analysis in acute coronary occlusion: a tool to assess myocardial viability and reperfusion. Circulation 2005;112:3901–10.

33. Brainin P, Hoffmann S, Fritz-Hansen T, et al. Usefulness of postsystolic shortening to diagnose coronary artery disease and predict future cardiovascular events in stable Angina pectoris. J Am Soc Echocardiogr 2018;31:870–879 e3.

34. Eek C, Grenne B, Brunvand H, et al. Strain echocardiography and wall motion score index predicts final infarct size in patients with non-ST-segment-elevation myocardial infarction. Circ Cardiovasc Imaging 2010;3:187–94.

35. Brainin P, Skaarup KG, Iversen AZ, et al. Post-systolic shortening predicts heart failure following acute coronary syndrome. Int J Cardiol 2019;276:191–7.

36. Onishi T, Uematsu M, Watanabe T, et al. Objective interpretation of dobutamine stress echocardiography by diastolic dyssynchrony imaging: a practical approach. J Am Soc Echocardiogr 2010;23:1103–8.

37. Agarwal R, Gosain P, Kirkpatrick JN, et al. Tissue Doppler imaging for diagnosis of coronary artery disease: a systematic review and meta-analysis. Cardiovasc Ultrasound 2012;10:47.

38. Voigt JU, Lindenmeier G, Exner B, et al. Incidence and characteristics of segmental postsystolic longitudinal shortening in normal, acutely ischemic, and scarred myocardium. J Am Soc Echocardiogr 2003;16:415–23.

39. Risum N, Valeur N, Sogaard P, et al. Right ventricular function assessed by 2D strain analysis predicts ventricular arrhythmias and sudden cardiac death in patients after acute myocardial infarction. Eur Heart J Cardiovasc Imaging 2018;19:800–7.

40. Chang WT, Liu YW, Liu PY, et al. Association of decreased right ventricular strain with worse survival in non-acute coronary syndrome angina. J Am Soc Echocardiogr 2016;29:350–8.e4.

41. Chang WT, Tsai WC, Liu YW, et al. Changes in right ventricular free wall strain in patients with coronary artery disease involving the right coronary artery. J Am Soc Echocardiogr 2014;27:230–8.

42. Kinch JW, Ryan TJ. Right ventricular infarction. N Engl J Med 1994;330:1211–7.

43. Masci PG, Francone M, Desmet W, et al. Right ventricular ischemic injury in patients with acute ST-segment elevation myocardial infarction: characterization with cardiovascular magnetic resonance. Circulation 2010;122:1405–12.

44. Surkova E, Muraru D, Iliceto S, et al. The use of multimodality cardiovascular imaging to assess right ventricular size and function. Int J Cardiol 2016; 214:54–69.

45. Longobardo L, Suma V, Jain R, et al. Role of two-dimensional speckle-tracking echocardiography strain in the assessment of right ventricular systolic function and comparison with conventional parameters. J Am Soc Echocardiogr 2017;30:937–46.e6.

46. Mondillo S, Galderisi M, Mele D, et al, Echocardiography Study Group Of The Italian Society Of Cardiology (Rome, Italy). Speckle-tracking echocardiography: a new technique for assessing myocardial function. J Ultrasound Med 2011;30: 71–83.

47. Forsha D, Risum N, Kropf PA, et al. Right ventricular mechanics using a novel comprehensive three-view echocardiographic strain analysis in a normal population. J Am Soc Echocardiogr 2014;27:413–22.

48. Fine NM, Chen L, Bastiansen PM, et al. Reference values for right ventricular strain in patients without cardiopulmonary disease: a prospective evaluation and meta-analysis. Echocardiography 2015;32: 787–96.

49. Fine NM, Shah AA, Han IY, et al. Left and right ventricular strain and strain rate measurement in normal adults using velocity vector imaging: an assessment of reference values and intersystem agreement. Int J Cardiovasc Imaging 2013;29:571–80.

50. Lemarie J, Huttin O, Girerd N, et al. Usefulness of speckle-tracking imaging for right ventricular assessment after acute myocardial infarction: a magnetic resonance imaging/echocardiographic comparison within the relation between aldosterone and cardiac remodeling after myocardial infarction study. J Am Soc Echocardiogr 2015;28:818–27.e4.

51. Park SJ, Park JH, Lee HS, et al. Impaired RV global longitudinal strain is associated with poor long-term clinical outcomes in patients with acute inferior STEMI. JACC Cardiovasc Imaging 2015;8:161–9.

52. Antoni ML, Scherptong RW, Atary JZ, et al. Prognostic value of right ventricular function in patients after acute myocardial infarction treated with primary percutaneous coronary intervention. Circ Cardiovasc Imaging 2010;3:264–71.

53. Motoki H, Borowski AG, Shrestha K, et al. Right ventricular global longitudinal strain provides prognostic value incremental to left ventricular ejection fraction in patients with heart failure. J Am Soc Echocardiogr 2014;27:726–32.

54. Benfari G, Noni M, Onorati F, et al. Effects of aortic valve replacement on left ventricular diastolic function in patients with aortic valve stenosis. Am J Cardiol 2019;124:409–15.

55. Cameli M, Mandoli GE, Loiacono F, et al. Left atrial strain: a new parameter for assessment of left ventricular filling pressure. Heart Fail Rev 2016;21: 65–76.

56. Sargento L, Vicente Simoes A, Longo S, et al. Left atrial function index predicts long-term survival in stable outpatients with systolic heart failure. Eur Heart J Cardiovasc Imaging 2017;18:119–27.

57. Cameli M, Mandoli GE, Loiacono F, et al. Left atrial strain: a useful index in atrial fibrillation. Int J Cardiol 2016;220:208–13.

58. Rosca M, Lancellotti P, Popescu BA, et al. Left atrial function: pathophysiology, echocardiographic assessment, and clinical applications. Heart 2011; 97:1982–9.

59. Cameli M, Caputo M, Mondillo S, et al. Feasibility and reference values of left atrial longitudinal strain imaging by two-dimensional speckle tracking. Cardiovasc Ultrasound 2009;7:6.

60. Mor-Avi V, Lang RM, Badano LP, et al. Current and evolving echocardiographic techniques for the quantitative evaluation of cardiac mechanics: ASE/EAE consensus statement on methodology and indications endorsed by the Japanese Society of Echocardiography. J Am Soc Echocardiogr 2011;24: 277–313.

61. Antoni ML, ten Brinke EA, Atary JZ, et al. Left atrial strain is related to adverse events in patients after acute myocardial infarction treated with primary percutaneous coronary intervention. Heart 2011;97: 1332–7.

62. Malagoli A, Rossi L, Bursi F, et al. Left atrial function predicts cardiovascular events in patients with chronic heart failure with reduced ejection fraction. J Am Soc Echocardiogr 2019;32:248–56.

63. Matsuda Y, Toma Y, Ogawa H, et al. Importance of left atrial function in patients with myocardial infarction. Circulation 1983;67:566–71.

64. Appleton CP, Kovacs SJ. The role of left atrial function in diastolic heart failure. Circ Cardiovasc Imaging 2009;2:6–9.

65. Bowman AW, Kovacs SJ. Assessment and consequences of the constant-volume attribute of the four-chambered heart. Am J Physiol Heart Circ Physiol 2003;285:H2027–33.

66. Bowman AW, Kovacs SJ. Left atrial conduit volume is generated by deviation from the constant-volume state of the left heart: a combined MRI-echocardiographic study. Am J Physiol Heart Circ Physiol 2004;286:H2416–24.

67. Ersbøll M, Andersen MJ, Valeur N, et al. The prognostic value of left atrial peak reservoir strain in acute myocardial infarction is dependent on left ventricular longitudinal function and left atrial size. Circ Cardiovasc Imaging 2013;6:26–33.

68. Ramkumar S, Yang H, Wang Y, et al. Association of the active and passive components of left atrial deformation with left ventricular function. J Am Soc Echocardiogr 2017;30:659–66.

Currently Available Options for Mechanical Circulatory Support for the Management of Cardiogenic Shock

Zachary K. Wegermann, MD*, Sunil V. Rao, MD

KEYWORDS

- Cardiogenic shock • Mechanical circulatory support • Myocardial infarction
- Advanced heart failure

KEY POINTS

- Multiple mechanical circulatory support (MCS) devices exist for management of cardiogenic shock (CS) refractory to vasoactive medications.
- MCS devices differ based on their mechanics, level of cardiac support provided, contraindications, and potential complications.
- Insufficient data exist to guide clinical device selection and the optimal timing for implantation for each patient.
- Shock teams and protocols can provide timely expert advice for CS management with MCS devices, tailored to local expertise.

INTRODUCTION

Cardiogenic shock (CS) is a complex condition of end-organ hypoperfusion driven by insufficient cardiac output.[1] This can occur both acutely, as with an acute myocardial infarction (AMI), or insidiously due to progressive chronic heart failure leading to end-stage heart failure.[2] A number of factors have been described as potential causes of acute CS beyond ischemic heart disease.[3,4] CS is most commonly driven by left ventricular (LV) systolic failure, but can result from right ventricular (RV) or biventricular dysfunction. As CS develops, multiple pathophysiologic pathways are affected, leading to upregulation of the neurohormonal cascade and triggering a Systemic Inflammatory Response Syndrome. These compound the effects of pump failure and lead to worsening shock.[1,3] The complexity of the pathophysiologic mechanisms of CS remain poorly understood with insufficient therapeutic targets, and as a result, morbidity and mortality remain high.[3] This has been compounded by the lack of a consensus definition of CS across multiple studies.[3]

CS is increasingly thought of as a condition occurring on a spectrum of escalating severity as opposed to a dichotomous condition. The recent Society for Cardiovascular Angiography and Interventions (SCAI) consensus statement on the classification of CS[5] laid out a framework for defining this spectrum of disease severity with 5 stages of

Division of Cardiology, Duke University Medical Center, Duke Clinical Research Institute, 200 Morris Street, Durham, NC 27710, USA
* Corresponding author.
E-mail address: zachary.wegermann@duke.edu

Table 1
Stages and definitions of cardiogenic shock from the Society for Coronary Angiography and Intervention expert consensus statement

A ⟷	B ⟷	C ⟷	D ⟷	E
At Risk for Cardiogenic Shock	Beginning of Cardiogenic Shock	Classic Cardiogenic Shock	Deteriorating Cardiogenic Shock	Extremis
Broad group of patients with risk factors for developing shock, but without active signs or symptoms	Relative vital sign instability from baseline (hypotension/ tachycardia) without overt evidence of end organ dysfunction.	Vital sign instability and overt tissue hypoperfusion requiring intervention (inotropes, pressors, mechanical circulatory support)	Worsening cardiogenic shock despite initial interventions, requiring more aggressive support measures.	Patients with active circulatory collapse despite maximal resuscitation and multiple active support measures.

shock, defined as A to E (**Table 1**). This definition shows how a patient could progress from stage A (at risk) to stage C (classic CS) to stage E (extremis). In many cases, CS remains refractory to medical management with vasopressors or inotropes, requiring a higher level of support to prevent progression to stage D or E shock. To stem the progression of shock, mechanical circulatory support (MCS) devices were developed to improve cardiac output and myocardial perfusion.

MCS devices can be divided into different categories related to their method of implantation, intended duration of use, and the supported ventricle.[6] Percutaneous MCS devices are generally a temporary support, implanted at the bedside, in a cardiac catheterization laboratory (CCL), or in an operating room, to halt the progression of shock. Durable MCS devices are surgically implanted in patients with end-stage disease. MCS devices are also classified as a bridging therapy versus a destination therapy. Percutaneous MCS devices are always a bridging therapy. They can be deployed as a short-term bridge to recovery, a bridge to stabilization before a destination therapy (durable MCS or transplant), or a bridge to a bridge (a durable MCS bridge to destination therapy). Finally, MCS devices are categorized by the ventricle they support: LV support, RV support, or biventricular support.

A number of MCS devices exist in current practice. This review describes commercially available devices, compares and contrasts their ability to support patients with CS, and reviews the currently available evidence supporting the use of each percutaneous MCS device. In so doing, it will also highlight areas where research is lacking, both in use of MCS and the treatment of shock.

FORMS OF PERCUTANEOUS MECHANICAL CIRCULATORY SUPPORT FOR LEFT VENTRICULAR SUPPORT

There are currently 4 commercially available forms of percutaneous MCS for left-sided support in CS: the intra-aortic balloon pump (IABP), the intravascular microaxial Impella pump family of devices (Abiomed, Danvers, MA), the TandemHeart percutaneous ventricular assist device (LivaNova, London, UK), and peripherally cannulated extracorporeal membrane oxygenation (ECMO). Each form varies in its route of placement, mechanics, and level of support (**Table 2**). Similarly, each form of MCS has different indications/contraindications, potential complications, and amount of evidence supporting its use.

Intra-aortic Balloon Pump

IABPs are counterpulsation devices used commonly in practice for CS due to the ease of insertion, low complexity, and favorable safety profile (see **Table 2**). The technology was initially developed in the 1960s but did not become widespread until the 2000s. An IABP is inserted percutaneously through an 8-Fr sheath via the femoral or axillary artery (**Fig. 1**A).

Theoretically, an IABP targets multiple pathways in CS. First, it improves coronary artery perfusion

Table 2
Characteristics of commercially available left ventricular, right ventricular, and biventricular mechanical circulatory support devices

	IABP	Impella 2.5	Impella CP	Impella 5.0	Impella 5.5	TandemHeart pVAD	VA ECMO	Impella RP	Percutaneous RVAD
Device Mechanics	Pneumatic Counter-pulsation	Axial pump	Axial pump	Axial pump	Axial pump	Centrifugal pump	Centrifugal pump	Axial pump	Centrifugal pump
Ventricular support	LV pressure unloading	LV volume and pressure unloading	LV volume and pressure unloading	LV volume and pressure unloading	LV volume and pressure unloading	LV volume unloading	Biventricular volume and pressure unloading	RV volume and pressure unloading	RV volume unloading
Cardiac output augmentation	0.5–1.0 L/min	2.5 L/min	2.5–3.7 L/min	5.0 L/min	6.2 L/min	4 L/min	2–6 L/min	2–4 L/min	2–4 L/min
Arterial cannula size and site	8 Fr Femoral artery	13 Fr Femoral artery	14 Fr Femoral artery	22 Fr Femoral artery	23 Fr Femoral artery	15–17 Fr Femoral artery	15–22 Fr Femoral artery	-	-
Venous cannula size and site	-	-	-	-	-	21 Fr Femoral vein	18–21 Fr Femoral vein	22 Fr Femoral vein	29–31 Fr Internal jugular vein (Protek Duo)
Alternative Access Sites	Axillary artery	Axillary artery	Axillary artery	Axillary artery	Axillary artery	-	Axillary artery and internal jugular vein or centrally cannulated	-	Centrally cannulated

(continued on next page)

Table 2
(continued)

	IABP	Impella 2.5	Impella CP	Impella 5.0	Impella 5.5	TandemHeart pVAD	VA ECMO	Impella RP	Percutaneous RVAD
Anticoagulation requirement	Recommended, particularly when augmentation is <1:1	Required	Required	Required	Required	Required	Required	Required	Required
Implantation times	Very short	Short	Short	Medium	Medium	Long	Long	Short	Medium
Monitoring complexity and requirements	Low complexity ICU level monitoring	Moderate complexity Specialized ICU monitoring	Moderate complexity Specialized ICU monitoring	Moderate complexity Specialized ICU monitoring	Moderate complexity Specialized ICU monitoring	High complexity Specialized ICU monitoring	High complexity Perfusionist supervision required Specialized ICU monitoring	Moderate complexity Specialized ICU monitoring	High complexity Specialized ICU monitoring
Complication rates	Very low	Low	Low	Low	Low	Moderate	High	Low	Low-Moderate

Contraindications	Moderate-severe aortic insufficiency High tachyarrhythmia burden	LV thrombus Peripheral arterial disease Moderate-severe aortic regurgitation or stenosis Mechanical aortic valves	LV thrombus Peripheral arterial disease Moderate-severe aortic regurgitation or stenosis Mechanical aortic valves	LV thrombus Peripheral arterial disease Moderate-severe aortic regurgitation or stenosis Mechanical aortic valves	LV thrombus Peripheral arterial disease Moderate-severe aortic regurgitation or stenosis Mechanical aortic valves	Peripheral arterial disease Ventricular septal defects RV failure	Peripheral arterial disease	Contraindication to anticoagulation Significant pulmonic or tricuspid stenosis or regurgitation	Contraindication to anticoagulation Venous stenosis Significant Pulmonic or Tricuspid Stenosis or Regurgitation

Abbreviations: IABP, intra-aortic balloon pump; ICU, intensive care unit; LV, left ventricular; pVAD, percutaneous left ventricular assist device; RV, right ventricular; VA ECMO, venous-arterial extracorporeal membrane oxygenation.

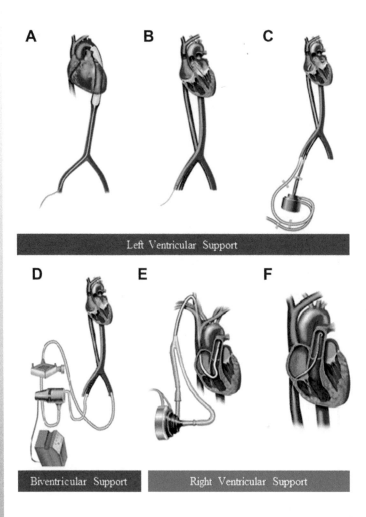

Fig. 1. Representative illustrations of the types of commercially available LV, RV, and biventricular mechanical circulatory support at the standard cannulation position. (*A*) Intra-aortic balloon pump, (*B*) Impella family of devices for LV support (Impella 2.5, CP, 5.0, and 5.5), (*C*) TandemHeart pVAD, (*D*) VA ECMO, (*E*) Percutaneous RVAD using a Protek Duo double lumen catheter and TandemHeart centrifugal pump, and (*F*) Impella RP. (*Adapted from* Mandawat A, Rao SV. Percutaneous mechanical circulatory support devices in cardiogenic shock. Circulation: Cardiovascular Interventions. 2017;10(5):e004337. Available at: https://www.ahajournals.org/doi/10.1161/CIRCINTERVENTIONS.116.004 337?url_ver=Z39.88-2003&rfr_id=ori %3Arid%3Acrossref.org&rfr_dat=cr_ pub++0pubmed&; with permission.)

by rapid inflation in diastole. Second, via rapid deflation in presystole, it reduces afterload. This LV pressure unloading improves CO, reducing myocardial workload and oxygen consumption.

IABP use is typically associated with a 0.5 to 1.0 L improvement in CO.[6] Most evidence for IABP use addresses CS associated with acute myocardial infarctions (AMI-CS); however, there is a growing body of evidence for IABP use in advanced heart failure for support and stabilization before either a durable bridge therapy or a destination therapy. There is a small amount of evidence for the use of IABP for other indications.

Intra-aortic Balloon Pump Use in Cardiogenic Shock Associated with Acute Myocardial Infarction

Although most data initially supporting IABP use were drawn from observational studies and meta-analyses, a number of clinical trials have subsequently evaluated the technology. Early observational studies suggested an association between IABP and improved survival from AMI-CS.[7–13] This led to IABP having a class I indication for treatment of AMI-CS in prior iterations of clinical practice guidelines. However, these findings have not been substantiated in prospective clinical trials.

The TACTICS trial[14] compared IABP for 48 hours versus optimal medical therapy in patients with AMI-CS post fibrinolysis. The study did not show any significant differences in the primary endpoint (6-month all-cause mortality), secondary endpoints, or safety events. Critiques of this study include its small sample size, large cross over from the medical therapy to IABP group, higher-risk characteristics in the IABP arm, lack of a strict definition of shock, and inclusion of patients with heart failure who did not truly have CS. Only 57 patients were enrolled in the study, with 9 patients in the optimal medical therapy arm deteriorating to the point they required IABP insertion. Although the trial was aimed at assessing IABP support in AMI-CS, nearly half of patients had Killip class I-II symptoms. Given the heterogeneity of the patient population and the other issues raised, this was not a definitive study. Other small trials have demonstrated similar results in a primary percutaneous coronary intervention (PCI) population.

The IABP-SHOCK II study[15] examined the use of IABP in addition to early revascularization and optimal medical therapy in a 600-patient, multicenter randomized controlled trial. The study assessed 30-day mortality and secondary endpoints including time to hemodynamic stabilization, intensive care unit (ICU) length of stay, serum lactate, and renal function. In addition, important safety endpoints were evaluated, including major bleeding, sepsis, peripheral ischemic complications, and stroke. There were no significant differences in primary or secondary endpoints, and safety profiles were similar between the 2 groups. As a result of this study, MCS with IABP was downgraded in subsequent iterations of international guidelines. The 2013 American Heart Association (AHA)/American College of Cardiology (ACC) ST-segment elevation myocardial infarction (STEMI) guidelines gave a IIa (level of evidence B) recommendation for IABP in patients with CS following STEMI who do not rapidly improve with pharmacologic therapy.[16] The 2017 European Society of Cardiology (ESC) STEMI guidelines gave a IIa recommendation for IABP therapy only in patients with mechanical complications leading to CS and a IIb recommendation for a short-duration MCS of any type in cases of refractory shock.[17] However, the ESC guidelines clearly recommended against routine use of IABP for AMI-CS, giving it a class III recommendation. Interestingly, the current AHA/ACC non-STEMI management guidelines do not discuss MCS use[18] and there are no dedicated practice guidelines for the management of CS by any large international guideline committees.

Intra-aortic Balloon Pump Use in Advanced Heart Failure

IABP use as a bridge to stabilization, a bridge to LV assist device (LVAD), and as a bridge to transplant has been reported in CS associated with progressive chronic systolic heart failure.[18–21] Early studies of IABP use in a progressive chronic heart failure population suggest it is relatively safe with low complication rates despite prolonged use. Gjesdal and colleagues[21] reported an average IABP duration of 21 days as a bridge to definitive therapy, with relatively low 30-day mortality (6.2%). Although 6 patients experienced IABP complications, this equated to approximately 0.05 complications per week of IABP use. Additional studies have shown IABP can be inserted through the axillary artery for patients needing IABP support before transplantation, allowing patients to maintain physical conditioning before transplantation.[22]

IMPELLA

The Impella device is a nonpulsatile, continuous axial flow device that provides support via LV volume unloading. It was initially developed as a bridging device to more definitive therapy in shock. The Archemedes screw device is placed across the aortic valve with an inflow cannula positioned in the LV and an outflow cannula crossing the aortic valve and ejecting blood into the ascending aorta (**Fig. 1**B). Currently, 4 types of Impella device are commercially available for LV support and vary based on the amount of support provided and caliber of the device (see **Table 2**). The Impella 2.5 provides approximately 2.5 L/min of increased CO support, whereas the Impella CP provides up to 3.7 L/min, the Impella 5.0 delivers up to 5.0 L/min, and the Impella 5.5 delivers up to 6.2 L/min. The Impella 2.5 and CP models can be inserted percutaneously through a 12 to 14-Fr sheath, but the Impella 5.0 and 5.5 generally require a surgical cut down to safely place the 22 to 23 Fr sheaths.

Impella for Cardiogenic Shock Associated with Acute Myocardial Infarction

Published data regarding the efficacy of Impella for AMI-CS are limited to observational studies and clinical trials with limited sample sizes and short-term, often surrogate outcomes. The first randomized trial of the effectiveness of Impella in treating AMI-CS was the ISAR-SHOCK trial.[23] It evaluated improvement in cardiac index (CI) at 30 minutes post insertion in 26 patients treated with Impella 2.5 versus IABP. There was a statistically greater change in CI from baseline to 30 minutes in the Impella group compared with the IABP group; However, by 4 hours, the CIs in both groups were equivalent (2.23 ± 0.58 L/min/m^2 Impella vs 2.25 ± 0.92 L/min/m^2 IABP). There were no significant differences in secondary endpoints (vasopressor dose, vasopressor treatment time, mechanical ventilation time, serum lactate) between the 2 groups. Safety endpoints, such as transfusion requirements, were worse in the Impella group compared with IABP. In addition, there was a trend toward longer implant times in the Impella group, but this difference did not reach statistical significance.

Other trials evaluating mortality with Impella versus IABP have shown no differences between the 2 modalities. The IMPRESS trial[24] showed no differences in 30-day and 6-month mortality between patients with AMI-CS treated with either modality. However, this was a small exploratory trial with only 48 patients enrolled (24 Impella, 24 IABP), all of whom were mechanically ventilated. Similar results noted in an observational study by Schrage and colleagues[25] appear to confirm the lack of a mortality difference between Impella and IABP for AMI-CS. In this study, 237 patients with Impella placed for AMI-CS were matched to 237 patients from the IABP-SHOCK II trial. Although no difference in 30-day mortality was present between Impella and IABP groups, there was a significantly higher rate of severe bleeding and peripheral vascular complications in the Impella group.

Recent observational analyses have shown similar outcomes for patients with AMI-CS treated with Impella versus IABP. In a propensity-matched analysis of 28,304 patients with AMI-CS included in the National Cardiovascular Data Registry Chest Pain-MI and CathPCI registries, Dhruva and colleagues[26] demonstrated higher in-hospital mortality (45.0% vs 34.1%, $P<.001$) and high bleeding rates (31.3 vs 16.0%, $P<.001$) for patients treated with Impella versus IABP. Although this analysis is limited by its observational design, it is consistent with prior randomized trial findings, and involves the largest population studied on the topic to date. This observation supports a prior analysis by Amin and colleagues[27] evaluating trends of Impella use and outcomes for Impella-assisted PCI using a commercial claims database. This analysis showed that although Impella use increased since Food and Drug Administration approval in 2008, its use was associated with worsening mortality, higher rates of bleeding, and greater risk of stroke. Given the lack of data for any benefit from Impella, and the worsening safety profile compared with IABP, there are no specific indications for Impella in international guidelines for treating AMI-CS. Both AHA/ACC and ESC STEMI guidelines allow for LV support devices in the setting of refractory shock.[16,17] However, neither specifically recommend Impella.

Impella for Advanced Heart Failure

Observational studies have described the use of Impella devices for short-term treatment of acute decompensated heart failure. A single-center case series reported the use of the Impella 5.0 as a bridge to destination therapy with either LVAD or heart transplantation.[28] Hall and colleagues[29] expanded this in reporting the use of Impella 5.0 across 5 centers for stabilization in hemodynamically unstable advanced heart failure, serving as a short-term bridge to destination therapy or decision making. Yet, there are no randomized trials evaluating the use of Impella as a bridging therapy in advanced heart failure and there is insufficient comparative evidence between Impella and other forms of MCS in this setting.

Impella for Intraprocedural Prevention of Cardiogenic Shock and Other Indications

Impella devices have been used for temporary support in the recovery from other etiologies of shock and for prevention of intraprocedural shock. Case series and feasibility studies have demonstrated the utility of Impella for recovery from postcardiotomy shock.[30] However, no comparative effectiveness trials currently exist comparing Impella with other forms of temporary MCS for postcardiotomy shock. Case series of Impella use for support during ventricular tachycardia (VT) ablation show this is a feasible form of MCS.[31] The PROTECT II trial[32] compared Impella with IABP for patients undergoing high-risk PCI. Although the primary endpoint of 30-day major adverse cardiac events was no different between the 2 groups, there was a trend toward decreased events at 90 days in the Impella-supported group. Although observational research has shown Impella use for protected PCI has significantly increased over time, a wide variation in use exists. In addition, increased costs and worse outcomes have been associated with its use despite increased volume of utilization.[27]

TandemHeart

The TandemHeart device (LivaNova, London, UK) is a continuous flow, centrifugal pump that draws oxygenated blood from the left atrium and expels it into the aorta (**Fig. 1**C). The device is placed percutaneously into the left atrium via a transvenous and transseptal puncture with a 21-Fr cannula. Separately, a 15 to 17-Fr cannula is placed transarterially (see **Table 2**). Facility with a transseptal puncture technique is essential for timely and safe placement of the device, and may be a limitation to its use with some operators.

TandemHeart Use in Cardiogenic Shock Associated with Acute Myocardial Infarction

Early studies of TandemHeart device use focused on the feasibility of implantation and effects on hemodynamic and metabolic parameters of CS. Thiele and colleagues[33] demonstrated the feasibility of TandemHeart percutaneous LVAD (pVAD) insertion in a study of 18 patients. This study also showed TandemHeart device insertion lead to a significant increase in CI and mean arterial blood pressure, with a coinciding significant reduction in pulmonary capillary wedge pressure (PCWP) and pulmonary artery (PA) pressure. However, 30-day mortality was 44% in this cohort of patients.

Comparative studies of TandemHeart pVAD and IABP in AMI-CS showed that pVAD use was associated with improved hemodynamic performance, but longer implantation times, higher complication rates, and no improvement in mortality.[34] In a study of 41 patients randomized to pVAD (n = 21) and IABP (n = 20), improvement in cardiac power was significantly higher for the pVAD compared with IABP (0.15 vs 0.06, $P = .004$).[34] There were also significant improvements in PCWP, PA pressure, serum lactate and urine output in the pVAD group compared with the IABP cohort. However, pVAD was associated with significantly higher complication rates including major bleeding (19 vs 8, $P = .002$), limb ischemia (7 vs 0, $P = .009$), disseminated intravascular coagulation (13 vs 3), and transfusion requirements. Implantation times for pVADs were more than double that of IABP (25 min vs 11.5 min, $P<.001$). Despite these differences, there was no difference in mortality between the 2 groups (43% pVAD vs 45% IABP, $P = .86$).

A subsequent randomized controlled trial of TandemHeart pVAD versus IABP was undertaken to test whether pVAD placement was associated with greater hemodynamic support than IABP. This study enrolled 42 patients in total, 70% of who had AMI-CS with the remaining population presenting with decompensated heart failure. This study demonstrated significantly increased CI and MAP, and decreased PCWP in patients with pVAD compared with IABP. Interestingly, overall mortality and adverse events were no different between the 2 groups.[35]

TandemHeart Use in Advanced Heart Failure

Percutaneous LVAD systems have been reported as successful bridge therapy in patients with shock related to progressive systolic heart failure. This includes reports, case series, and observational studies of TandemHeart pVAD use as a bridge to recovery,[36] short-term bridge to a durable bridge therapy (bridge to a bridge),[36,37] and a bridge to cardiac transplantation.[38] Trials using pVAD support have included patients with CS related to progressive systolic heart failure from nonischemic cardiomyopathy,[35,39] with similar mortality rates noted between patients with nonischemic cardiomyopathy and those with ischemic cardiomyopathy.

TandemHeart Use in Severe Refractory Shock

Given the study data showing improved hemodynamic performance with pVAD compared with IABP,[35] TandemHeart pVAD were studied in shock refractory to standard treatments with IABP and/or vasopressors. In a cohort of 117 patients (80 ischemic, 37 nonischemic cardiomyopathy) with CS refractory to standard treatment, Kar and colleagues[39] demonstrated pVAD use was associated with improvement in hemodynamic, metabolic, and examination parameters of shock. Patients included in this group were by critically ill, with 56 (47.9%) of the 117 patients having undergone cardiopulmonary resuscitation (CPR) immediately before or during implantation of the pVAD. Hemodynamic improvements were similar to previously reported studies, with significant improvements in CI and systolic blood pressure, and a significant decreased in PCWP. Metabolic parameters also improved following pVAD placement with decreases in serum lactate (24.5 mg/dL to 11 mg/dL, $P<.001$), improved serum creatinine (1.5 mg/dL to 1.2 mg/dL, $P = .009$), and increased mixed venous oxygen saturation (75 mm Hg to 100 mm Hg, $P<.001$). In addition, urine output significantly improved (70.7 mL/d prior vs 1200 mL/d after placement, $P<.001$). However, 30-day and 6-month mortality rates remained very high (40.2% and 45.3%, respectively), in line with prior studies.

PERIPHERALLY CANNULATED EXTRACORPOREAL MEMBRANE OXYGENATION

Venous-arterial extracorporeal membrane oxygenation (VA ECMO) provides biventricular support by drawing deoxygenated blood from the central venous system through a centrifugal pump and oxygenator, and expelling oxygenated blood into the systemic central arterial system (**Fig. 1**D). It can be deployed percutaneously as well as centrally. When deployed percutaneously, it is typically placed in the femoral vasculature via an 18 to 21-Fr venous inflow cannula in the femoral vein and a 15 to 22-Fr outflow cannula in the femoral artery. VA ECMO can also be deployed via the internal jugular vein and axillary artery to allow patients the use of their legs (see **Table 2**). This potentially allows for physical therapy while VA ECMO is in place, but at the cost of increased deployment times. VA ECMO provides the greatest hemodynamic support of all MCS, providing effectively complete cardiopulmonary bypass.

One important physiologic consideration in use of VA ECMO is the extent of blood return to the left-sided cardiac chambers while the patient is effectively on cardiopulmonary bypass. This leads to progressive LV and left atrial (LA) dilation, with stagnant blood pooling and pulmonary edema. Although oxygenation issues can be overcome with the oxygenator, ventilation is still required to exchange CO_2, and stagnant blood flow can lead to LA and LV clots that can have devastating consequences for patients. The concept of LV venting overcomes this physiologic limitation, by pressure and volume unloading the LV or LA. Potential strategies include concomitant IABP or Impella placement, atrial septostomy, or a surgically placed LV vent. There are no data suggesting improved outcomes with any of these adjunct therapies; however, data do suggest improved PA pressures and LV dimensions with IABP and Impella use.[40,41]

An additional physiologic challenge with peripherally cannulated VA ECMO is ensuring that adequate oxygenated blood flow supplies all 3 arch vessels to adequately feed the cerebral vasculature and both upper extremities. One way to monitor for this is to sample right upper extremity arterial blood gas samples. However, there is no way to definitively ensure cerebral vasculature is receiving oxygenated blood.

Venous-Arterial Extracorporeal Membrane Oxygenation in Cardiogenic Shock Associated with Acute Myocardial Infarction

VA ECMO can be used in cases of severe refractory shock secondary to AMI-CS as well as in cases of refractory cardiac arrest or severe refractory shock in the early stages following cardiac arrest. In these cases, it is referred to as extracorporeal CPR (eCPR). Small observational studies have examined VA ECMO use in severe refractory AMI-CS.[42–45] In-hospital mortality for cohorts receiving VA ECMO for refractory AMI-CS remains high, greater than 50% in some studies, but with small sample sizes contributing to large variability in reported mortality rates.[42,44–46]

Given the extremely high mortality rate and resource utilization associated with VA ECMO use, studies have attempted to identify predictors of mortality and survival. The ENCOURAGE score was developed in a cohort of patients with AMI-CS treated in 2 ICUs in France. It incorporated 7 predeployment patient predictors of mortality (age, sex, body mass index, Glasgow coma scale, creatinine, lactate, and prothrombin activity). Although the score performed well in the development data set with an area under the receiver operating characteristic curve of 0.84, it was not validated as part of the study[42] and remains to be validated in an external AMI-CS population.

When examined in a post cardiac surgery population on VA ECMO, the prediction score did not perform well (c-statistic of 0.55 and 0.56 for 30-day and long-term mortality, respectively).[47] However, no other existing scores performed well enough to be considered reliable predictors of mortality.

Another limitation to the current understanding of the role of VA ECMO in treating AMI-CS is the lack of randomized data or large comparative registry analyses. Analyses from administrative datasets have attempted to overcome this limitation. A recent analysis of National Inpatient Sample data compared outcomes for patients with AMI-CS treated with VA ECMO versus Impella.[48] The propensity score matched analysis of 5730 patients receiving Impella and 560 treated with VA EMCO in a nonelective setting for AMI-CS showed rates of in-hospital mortality, respiratory failure, and vascular complications were lower in patients treated with Impella. In addition, costs were lower and hospital length of stay was shorter among Impella treated patients. Although this analysis attempts to use existing real-world data to compare VA ECMO and Impella, it is limited by its observational design and inability to completely control for differences between patients and factors that may have influenced the selection of one support apparatus over the other.

Venous-Arterial Extracorporeal Membrane Oxygenation in Extracorporeal Cardiopulmonary Resuscitation

Although most studies of eCPR have reported a benefit compared with standard CPR for both in and out of hospital cardiac arrest, there have been conflicting results.[49–55] Meta-analyses of eCPR have suggested a benefit from eCPR,[56] but with one systematic review suggesting the overall quality of evidence remained poor with significant bias from confounding.[57] Extracorporeal CPR programs for out of hospital refractory VT/ventricular fibrillation cardiac arrest have been successfully established and facilitate rapid transport for patients meeting criteria directly from the field to cardiac catheterization laboratories for VA ECMO deployment, coronary angiography, and PCI.[58] When compared with historical control cohorts, eCPR programs are associated with improved outcomes.[59] However, studies of eCPR have been limited by small sample size studies and randomized, multicenter data are still needed to assess the efficacy of eCPR programs compared with existing systems of care.[60]

Venous-Arterial Extracorporeal Membrane Oxygenation in Advanced Heart Failure and Other Indications

VA ECMO can serve as a bridge to recovery, bridge to a bridge, and as a bridge to transplant for patients with refractory shock.[44,61–63] Its use has been reported for cases of fulminant myocarditis, rejection, primary graft dysfunction, postcardiotomy shock, and refractory shock from progressive chronic systolic heart failure.[44,63,64] A meta-analysis by Khorsandi and colleagues[64] of studies evaluating VA ECMO for postcardiotomy shock showed an in-hospital mortality rate of nearly 69.2%. This is higher than reported with other studies examining a cohort of mixed etiologies for refractory CS, with in-hospital mortality reported at nearly 60%.[44,65] Although prior studies suggest age older than 70 and long-term ECMO support are the most common predictors of adverse outcomes with ECMO,[65,66] this was not substantiated in a meta-analysis.[64] In-hospital mortality for patients with myocarditis supported by VA ECMO is reported to be more favorable, with one study reporting an in-hospital survival rate of 71.9%.[67] Limited data exist comparing outcomes for patients with refractory shock secondary to progressive chronic systolic heart failure, particularly among cases of ischemic and nonischemic cardiomyopathy.

PERCUTANEOUS MECHANICAL CIRCULATORY SUPPORT FOR RIGHT VENTRICULAR SUPPORT

Isolated RV failure as an etiology of CS is much less common than LV dysfunction or biventricular failure. However, it can occur in isolation with RV infarction and commonly with pulmonary embolism. In cases refractory to medical management, there are forms of RV support that are discussed briefly.

Percutaneous Right Ventricular Assist Device

Percutaneous VAD devices have been adapted to provide RV support. Kapur and colleagues[68] described a cohort of 46 patients with RV failure treated with a TandemHeart centrifugal pVAD adapted to provide RV support. Similar to experiences with pVAD use for LV failure, patients had significant improvement in hemodynamic parameters, but in-hospital mortality remained high at 57%.

The ProtekDuo cannula (LivaNova, London, UK) was developed to provide a dual-lumen cannula for percutaneous right ventricular assist devices (pRVADs),[69] in combination with a TandemHeart centrifugal pump (**Fig. 1**E). The 29 to 31-Fr catheter is delivered via the internal jugular vein, drawing blood from the RA and expelling it into the PA (see **Table 2**). Small observational data suggest this is associated with a low complication rate and leads to improved hemodynamic support following implantation.[70] However, limited data exist reporting long-term outcomes and comparing this modality with other forms of RV support.

Impella RP

The Impella RP device was developed for isolated RV support. It functions by drawing blood from the RV and expelling it into the PA (**Fig. 1**F). The RECOVER RIGHT study[71] examined the use of Impella RP in 30 patients across 15 centers with refractory RV failure following LVAD placement, postcardiotomy shock, or MI. The device was successfully delivered in 29 of 30 patients. There was a significant improvement in patients' hemodynamics following insertion, and 30-day survival was 73.3%.

Case studies have demonstrated the Impella RP can be combined with left-sided Impella placement for biventricular support, with observational data showing improved cardiac output[72]; however, evidence for this is very limited and there is no evidence comparing this with other MCS therapies, including other forms of biventricular support.

SELECTING THE APPROPRIATE MECHANICAL CIRCULATORY SUPPORT DEVICE

A dilemma commonly faced by clinicians is how to select the ideal MCS device for a given patient. This problem does not have a one-size-fits-all answer. Instead, it should be dependent on individualized patient factors, the level of hemodynamic support needed, and operator and institutional experience with particular MCS devices. Key patient factors important to device selection include the etiology of CS, the expected treatment course, patient comorbidities and other end-organ function, invasive hemodynamic measurements, and echocardiographic features including ventricular function, chamber size, and valvular pathology. Given the complexities of managing patients with any mechanical circulatory device in place, institutional experience is a key factor in successful use of each device. Unique perspectives from all members of a multidisciplinary shock team should be incorporated into treatment decisions. Furthermore, shock protocols have been adopted with success across institutions to ensure patients receive timely and appropriate care, including selection of appropriate MCS.

MULTIDISCIPLINARY SHOCK TEAMS AND SHOCK PROTOCOLS
Cardiogenic Shock Teams

Given the incredibly high in-hospital mortality associated with CS, timely recognition and initiation of appropriate therapy is critical to improving survival. As the complexity of MCS continues to increase, multidisciplinary teams are needed to coordinate the rapid and appropriate care of patients with CS. Building off of the lessons learned with code teams for cardiac arrest,[73] as well as coordinated systems of care of MI,[74] stroke,[75] and trauma,[76] the concept of multidisciplinary shock teams seems attractive. Such teams are generally composed of specialists across multiple disciplines, including interventional cardiology, advanced heart failure cardiologists, critical care medicine, cardiothoracic surgery, and cardiac anesthesiology.

Although schema for developing shock teams within hospitals have been published,[3,77] shock teams need not all look the same and should be tailored to the strengths and needs of local hospital systems. The structure and function of the shock team should be to rapidly assess and deploy the appropriate treatment of shock for each patient based on local expert consensus. Experiences of health systems in developing shock teams have been well documented, notably within the INOVA health system.[78–80] Given the potential differences in shock teams at the local level, a randomized trial of shock teams is unlikely to be feasible. However, observational data should be rigorously collected by sites creating shock teams to allow systems of care to continually reassess performance and refine the way care is delivered for shock patients.

Cardiogenic Shock Protocols

Not only should sites work to establish multidisciplinary shock teams, but they should also nest them within clear protocols for the delivery of shock care. There are multiple examples of protocol-driven medicine improving patient outcomes, and given the exceedingly poor outcomes for patients with shock, protocol-driven care may improve outcomes. Demonstrations of shock protocols to improve outcomes include the Detroit Shock Initiative[81] and the University of Minnesota eCPR program.[58] Protocols should clearly delineate guidelines for inclusion and exclusion in care pathways, and data required for timely decisions affecting management. Care protocols should also make efforts to define futility criteria where appropriate.

MECHANICAL CIRCULATORY SUPPORT DEVICES IN DEVELOPMENT

There are multiple MCS devices currently at various stages of development and across a spectrum of indications. These include the NuPulse device (NuPulseCV, Raleigh, NC), Aortix device (Procyrion, Houston, TX), HeartMate Percutaneous Heart Pump (Abbott Laboratories, Abbott Park, IL), Reitan Catheter Pump (Cardiobridge, Hechingen, Germany), iVAC2L pVAD (Terumo Interventional Systems, Tokyo, Japan), Impella ECP (Abiomed, Danvers, MA), CSI hemodynamic support for complex PCI (CSI, St. Paul, MN), and Perkat pulsatile RV support device (NovaPump, Jena, Germany). Advances in technology include expandable-collapsible axial pump platforms (Impella ECP, HeartMate Percutaneous Heart Pump)[82,83] for smaller-caliber vascular access and indwelling counterpulsation devices that can be used in the outpatient setting (NuPulse device).

SUMMARY

Although the use of MCS devices for treatment of CS continues to increase, the evidence base supporting their use has not kept pace. Limited data exist to guide clinicians on the selection of the appropriate device for a given patient and the ideal time at which it should be implanted. Furthermore, insufficient comparative evidence exists among different MCS devices. This is particularly problematic for devices used for severe refractory shock in patients already treated with vasopressors and an IABP where equipoise may not exist.

Most of the current evidence for use of particular MCS devices has been generated from limited observational studies and clinical trials with small sample sizes. Problems with the current evidence that should be urgently addressed are a lack of large observational datasets with the ability to compare clinical endpoints in the treatment of CS across device types, a lack of clinical trials examining MCS device use with clinical endpoints rather than surrogate hemodynamic endpoints, and a lack of multicenter studies with large study populations. Although any randomized trial involving CS faces challenges with randomization, well-crafted studies remain essential in determining the optimal MCS treatment strategy for patients with shock refractory to vasoactive medications.

Another problem that has hampered research in CS is a lack of a consistent definition for it in trials and observational datasets.[84] CS is not a binary state, and the spectrum of shock has not been well captured in prior studies. Although the recent SCAI shock classification[5] has helped shed light on how to define and categorize patients with varying levels of CS, its use in guiding MCS device selection and utilization is not well established.

Further research in CS should focus on rapid early detection of shock and the optimal timing of MCS device use. As shock remains a multifaceted clinical diagnosis that is often based on clinical assessment before invasive measurements can be obtained, studies examining diagnostic approaches to CS are greatly needed. Although studies demonstrate that the use of MCS after the development of significant end-organ dysfunction is associated with worse outcomes, and that early use of MCS is associated with improved outcomes, the optimal timing of implantation remains unclear. Current data are insufficient for clinicians to be able to adequately counsel patients on the risks and benefits of an early invasive strategy with MCS devices in CS. Due to the myriad unanswered questions in this field, additional research is urgently needed to guide clinical decision making and improve outcomes in CS.

DISCLOSURE

Z.K. Wegermann and S.V. Rao report no relevant disclosures.

REFERENCES

1. Reynolds HR, Hochman JS. Cardiogenic shock: current concepts and improving outcomes. Circulation 2008;117(5):686–97.
2. Patel CB, Alexander KM, Rogers JG. Mechanical circulatory support for advanced heart failure. Curr Treat Options Cardiovasc Med 2010;12(6):549–65.
3. van Diepen S, Katz JN, Albert NM, et al. Contemporary management of cardiogenic shock: a scientific statement from the American Heart Association. Circulation 2017;136(16):e232–68.
4. Reyentovich A, Barghash MH, Hochman JS. Management of refractory cardiogenic shock. Nat Rev Cardiol 2016;13(8):481–92.
5. Baran DA, Grines CL, Bailey S, et al. SCAI clinical expert consensus statement on the classification of cardiogenic shock: this document was endorsed by the American College of Cardiology (ACC), the American Heart Association (AHA), the Society of Critical Care Medicine (SCCM), and the Society of Thoracic Surgeons (STS) in April 2019. Catheter Cardiovasc Interv 2019;94(1):29–37.
6. Rihal CS, Naidu SS, Givertz MM, et al. 2015 SCAI/ACC/HFSA/STS clinical expert consensus statement on the use of percutaneous mechanical circulatory support devices in cardiovascular care: endorsed by the American Heart Association, the Cardiological Society of India, and Sociedad Latino Americana de Cardiologia Intervencion; affirmation of value by the Canadian Association of Interventional Cardiology-Association Canadienne de Cardiologie d'intervention. J Am Coll Cardiol 2015;65(19):e7–26.
7. Moulopoulos S, Stamatelopoulos S, Petrou P. Intra-aortic balloon assistance in intractable cardiogenic shock. Eur Heart J 1986;7(5):396–403.
8. Waksman R, Weiss AT, Gotsman MS, et al. Intra-aortic balloon counterpulsation improves survival in cardiogenic shock complicating acute myocardial infarction. Eur Heart J 1993;14(1):71–4.
9. Anderson RD, Ohman EM, Holmes DR Jr, et al. Use of intraaortic balloon counterpulsation in patients presenting with cardiogenic shock: observations from the GUSTO-I Study. Global Utilization of Streptokinase and TPA for Occluded Coronary Arteries. J Am Coll Cardiol 1997;30(3):708–15.
10. Kovack PJ, Rasak MA, Bates ER, et al. Thrombolysis plus aortic counterpulsation: improved survival in patients who present to community hospitals with cardiogenic shock. J Am Coll Cardiol 1997;29(7):1454–8.
11. Sanborn TA, Sleeper LA, Bates ER, et al. Impact of thrombolysis, intra-aortic balloon pump counterpulsation, and their combination in cardiogenic shock complicating acute myocardial infarction: a report from the SHOCK Trial Registry. SHould we emergently revascularize Occluded Coronaries for cardiogenic shocK? J Am Coll Cardiol 2000;36(3 Suppl A):1123–9.
12. Barron HV, Every NR, Parsons LS, et al. The use of intra-aortic balloon counterpulsation in patients with cardiogenic shock complicating acute myocardial infarction: data from the National Registry of Myocardial Infarction 2. Am Heart J 2001;141(6): 933–9.
13. Gu J, Hu W, Xiao H, et al. Intra-aortic balloon pump improves clinical prognosis and attenuates C-reactive protein level in acute STEMI complicated by cardiogenic shock. Cardiology 2010;117(1):75–80.
14. Ohman EM, Nanas J, Stomel RJ, et al. Thrombolysis and counterpulsation to improve survival in myocardial infarction complicated by hypotension and suspected cardiogenic shock or heart failure: results of the TACTICS Trial. J Thromb Thrombolysis 2005; 19(1):33–9.
15. Thiele H, Zeymer U, Neumann FJ, et al. Intraaortic balloon support for myocardial infarction with cardiogenic shock. N Engl J Med 2012;367(14): 1287–96.
16. O'Gara PT, Kushner FG, Ascheim DD, et al. 2013 ACCF/AHA guideline for the management of ST-elevation myocardial infarction: a report of the American College of Cardiology Foundation/American

Heart Association Task Force on practice guidelines. J Am Coll Cardiol 2013;61(4):e78–140.

17. Ibanez B, James S, Agewall S, et al. 2017 ESC Guidelines for the management of acute myocardial infarction in patients presenting with ST-segment elevation: the Task Force for the management of acute myocardial infarction in patients presenting with ST-segment elevation of the European Society of Cardiology (ESC). Eur Heart J 2018;39(2):119–77.

18. Amsterdam EA, Wenger NK, Brindis RG, et al. 2014 AHA/ACC guideline for the management of patients with non-ST-elevation acute coronary syndromes: a report of the American College of Cardiology/American Heart Association Task Force on practice guidelines. J Am Coll Cardiol 2014;64(24): e139–228.

19. Bezerra CG, Adam EL, Baptista ML, et al. Aortic counterpulsation therapy in patients with advanced heart failure: analysis of the TBRIDGE registry. Arq Bras Cardiol 2016;106(1):26–32.

20. Sintek MA, Gdowski M, Lindman BR, et al. Intra-aortic balloon counterpulsation in patients with chronic heart failure and cardiogenic shock: clinical response and predictors of stabilization. J Card Fail 2015;21(11):868–76.

21. Gjesdal O, Gude E, Arora S, et al. Intra-aortic balloon counterpulsation as a bridge to heart transplantation does not impair long-term survival. Eur J Heart Fail 2009;11(7):709–14.

22. Estep JD, Cordero-Reyes AM, Bhimaraj A, et al. Percutaneous placement of an intra-aortic balloon pump in the left axillary/subclavian position provides safe, ambulatory long-term support as bridge to heart transplantation. JACC Heart Fail 2013;1(5): 382–8.

23. Seyfarth M, Sibbing D, Bauer I, et al. A randomized clinical trial to evaluate the safety and efficacy of a percutaneous left ventricular assist device versus intra-aortic balloon pumping for treatment of cardiogenic shock caused by myocardial infarction. J Am Coll Cardiol 2008;52(19):1584–8.

24. Ouweneel DM, Eriksen E, Sjauw KD, et al. Percutaneous mechanical circulatory support versus intra-aortic balloon pump in cardiogenic shock after acute myocardial infarction. J Am Coll Cardiol 2017;69(3):278–87.

25. Schrage B, Ibrahim K, Loehn T, et al. Impella support for acute myocardial infarction complicated by cardiogenic shock. Circulation 2019;139(10): 1249–58.

26. Dhruva SS, Ross JS, Mortazavi BJ, et al. Association of use of an intravascular microaxial left ventricular assist device vs intra-aortic balloon pump with in-hospital mortality and major bleeding among patients with acute myocardial infarction complicated by cardiogenic shock. JAMA 2020;323(8):734–45.

27. Amin AP, Spertus JA, Curtis JP, et al. The evolving landscape of Impella use in the United States among patients undergoing percutaneous coronary intervention with mechanical circulatory support. Circulation 2020;141(4):273–84.

28. Lima B, Kale P, Gonzalez-Stawinski GV, et al. Effectiveness and safety of the Impella 5.0 as a bridge to cardiac transplantation or durable left ventricular assist device. Am J Cardiol 2016;117(10):1622–8.

29. Hall SA, Uriel N, Carey SA, et al. Use of a percutaneous temporary circulatory support device as a bridge to decision during acute decompensation of advanced heart failure. J Heart Lung Transplant 2018;37(1):100–6.

30. Griffith BP, Anderson MB, Samuels LE, et al. The RECOVER I: a multicenter prospective study of Impella 5.0/LD for postcardiotomy circulatory support. J Thorac Cardiovasc Surg 2013;145(2):548–54.

31. Miller MA, Dukkipati SR, Chinitz JS, et al. Percutaneous hemodynamic support with Impella 2.5 during scar-related ventricular tachycardia ablation (PERMIT 1). Circ Arrhythm Electrophysiol 2013; 6(1):151–9.

32. O'Neill WW, Kleiman NS, Moses J, et al. A prospective, randomized clinical trial of hemodynamic support with Impella 2.5 versus intra-aortic balloon pump in patients undergoing high-risk percutaneous coronary intervention: the PROTECT II study. Circulation 2012;126(14):1717–27.

33. Thiele H, Lauer B, Hambrecht R, et al. Reversal of cardiogenic shock by percutaneous left atrial-to-femoral arterial bypass assistance. Circulation 2001;104(24):2917–22.

34. Thiele H, Sick P, Boudriot E, et al. Randomized comparison of intra-aortic balloon support with a percutaneous left ventricular assist device in patients with revascularized acute myocardial infarction complicated by cardiogenic shock. Eur Heart J 2005; 26(13):1276–83.

35. Burkhoff D, Cohen H, Brunckhorst C, et al. A randomized multicenter clinical study to evaluate the safety and efficacy of the TandemHeart percutaneous ventricular assist device versus conventional therapy with intraaortic balloon pumping for treatment of cardiogenic shock. Am Heart J 2006; 152(3):469.e1-8.

36. Smith L, Peters A, Mazimba S, et al. Outcomes of patients with cardiogenic shock treated with TandemHeart((R)) percutaneous ventricular assist device: Importance of support indication and definitive therapies as determinants of prognosis. Catheter Cardiovasc Interv 2018;92(6):1173–81.

37. Gregoric ID, Jacob LP, La Francesca S, et al. The TandemHeart as a bridge to a long-term axial-flow left ventricular assist device (bridge to bridge). Tex Heart Inst J 2008;35(2):125–9.

38. Bruckner BA, Jacob LP, Gregoric ID, et al. Clinical experience with the TandemHeart percutaneous ventricular assist device as a bridge to cardiac transplantation. Tex Heart Inst J 2008;35(4):447–50.

39. Kar B, Gregoric ID, Basra SS, et al. The percutaneous ventricular assist device in severe refractory cardiogenic shock. J Am Coll Cardiol 2011;57(6):688–96.

40. Petroni T, Harrois A, Amour J, et al. Intra-aortic balloon pump effects on macrocirculation and microcirculation in cardiogenic shock patients supported by venoarterial extracorporeal membrane oxygenation*. Crit Care Med 2014;42(9):2075–82.

41. Cheng A, Swartz MF, Massey HT. Impella to unload the left ventricle during peripheral extracorporeal membrane oxygenation. ASAIO J 2013;59(5):533–6.

42. Muller G, Flecher E, Lebreton G, et al. The ENCOURAGE mortality risk score and analysis of long-term outcomes after VA-ECMO for acute myocardial infarction with cardiogenic shock. Intensive Care Med 2016;42(3):370–8.

43. Sheu JJ, Tsai TH, Lee FY, et al. Early extracorporeal membrane oxygenator-assisted primary percutaneous coronary intervention improved 30-day clinical outcomes in patients with ST-segment elevation myocardial infarction complicated with profound cardiogenic shock. Crit Care Med 2010;38(9):1810–7.

44. Combes A, Leprince P, Luyt CE, et al. Outcomes and long-term quality-of-life of patients supported by extracorporeal membrane oxygenation for refractory cardiogenic shock. Crit Care Med 2008;36(5):1404–11.

45. Esper SA, Bermudez C, Dueweke EJ, et al. Extracorporeal membrane oxygenation support in acute coronary syndromes complicated by cardiogenic shock. Catheter Cardiovasc Interv 2015;86(Suppl 1):S45–50.

46. Sakamoto S, Taniguchi N, Nakajima S, et al. Extracorporeal life support for cardiogenic shock or cardiac arrest due to acute coronary syndrome. Ann Thorac Surg 2012;94(1):1–7.

47. Schrutka L, Rohmann F, Binder C, et al. Discriminatory power of scoring systems for outcome prediction in patients with extracorporeal membrane oxygenation following cardiovascular surgery. Eur J Cardiothorac Surg 2019;56(3):534–40.

48. Lemor A, Dehkordi SHH, Basir MB, et al. Impella versus extracorporeal membrane oxygenation for acute myocardial infarction cardiogenic shock. Cardiovasc Revasc Med 2020 [Epub ahead of print].

49. Thiagarajan RR, Brogan TV, Scheurer MA, et al. Extracorporeal membrane oxygenation to support cardiopulmonary resuscitation in adults. Ann Thorac Surg 2009;87(3):778–85.

50. Kagawa E, Dote K, Kato M, et al. Should we emergently revascularize occluded coronaries for cardiac arrest?: rapid-response extracorporeal membrane oxygenation and intra-arrest percutaneous coronary intervention. Circulation 2012;126(13):1605–13.

51. Chen Z, Liu C, Huang J, et al. Clinical efficacy of extracorporeal cardiopulmonary resuscitation for adults with cardiac arrest: meta-analysis with trial sequential analysis. Biomed Res Int 2019;2019:6414673.

52. Blumenstein J, Leick J, Liebetrau C, et al. Extracorporeal life support in cardiovascular patients with observed refractory in-hospital cardiac arrest is associated with favourable short and long-term outcomes: a propensity-matched analysis. Eur Heart J Acute Cardiovasc Care 2016;5(7):13–22.

53. Kim SJ, Jung JS, Park JH, et al. An optimal transition time to extracorporeal cardiopulmonary resuscitation for predicting good neurological outcome in patients with out-of-hospital cardiac arrest: a propensity-matched study. Crit Care 2014;18(5):535.

54. Shin TG, Jo IJ, Sim MS, et al. Two-year survival and neurological outcome of in-hospital cardiac arrest patients rescued by extracorporeal cardiopulmonary resuscitation. Int J Cardiol 2013;168(4):3424–30.

55. Chen YS, Lin JW, Yu HY, et al. Cardiopulmonary resuscitation with assisted extracorporeal life-support versus conventional cardiopulmonary resuscitation in adults with in-hospital cardiac arrest: an observational study and propensity analysis. Lancet 2008;372(9638):554–61.

56. Ouweneel DM, Schotborgh JV, Limpens J, et al. Extracorporeal life support during cardiac arrest and cardiogenic shock: a systematic review and meta-analysis. Intensive Care Med 2016;42(12):1922–34.

57. Holmberg MJ, Geri G, Wiberg S, et al. Extracorporeal cardiopulmonary resuscitation for cardiac arrest: a systematic review. Resuscitation 2018;131:91–100.

58. Yannopoulos D, Bartos JA, Martin C, et al. Minnesota Resuscitation Consortium's advanced perfusion and reperfusion cardiac life support strategy for out-of-hospital refractory ventricular fibrillation. J Am Heart Assoc 2016;5(6).

59. Yannopoulos D, Bartos JA, Raveendran G, et al. Coronary artery disease in patients with out-of-hospital refractory ventricular fibrillation cardiac arrest. J Am Coll Cardiol 2017;70(9):1109–17.

60. Bol ME, Suverein MM, Lorusso R, et al. Early initiation of extracorporeal life support in refractory out-of-hospital cardiac arrest: design and rationale of the INCEPTION trial. Am Heart J 2019;210:58–68.

61. Sun T, Guy A, Sidhu A, et al. Veno-arterial extracorporeal membrane oxygenation (VA-ECMO) for emergency cardiac support. J Crit Care 2018;44:31–8.

62. Schwarz B, Mair P, Margreiter J, et al. Experience with percutaneous venoarterial cardiopulmonary bypass for emergency circulatory support. Crit Care Med 2003;31(3):758–64.

63. Pagani FD, Lynch W, Swaniker F, et al. Extracorporeal life support to left ventricular assist device bridge to heart transplant: a strategy to optimize survival and resource utilization. Circulation 1999; 100(19 Suppl):II206–10.

64. Khorsandi M, Dougherty S, Bouamra O, et al. Extracorporeal membrane oxygenation for refractory cardiogenic shock after adult cardiac surgery: a systematic review and meta-analysis. J Cardiothorac Surg 2017;12(1):55.

65. Smith M, Vukomanovic A, Brodie D, et al. Duration of veno-arterial extracorporeal life support (VA ECMO) and outcome: an analysis of the Extracorporeal Life Support Organization (ELSO) registry. Crit Care 2017;21(1):45.

66. Rastan AJ, Dege A, Mohr M, et al. Early and late outcomes of 517 consecutive adult patients treated with extracorporeal membrane oxygenation for refractory postcardiotomy cardiogenic shock. J Thorac Cardiovasc Surg 2010;139(2):302–11, 311.e1.

67. Lorusso R, Centofanti P, Gelsomino S, et al. Venoarterial extracorporeal membrane oxygenation for acute fulminant myocarditis in adult patients: a 5-year multi-institutional experience. Ann Thorac Surg 2016;101(3):919–26.

68. Kapur NK, Paruchuri V, Jagannathan A, et al. Mechanical circulatory support for right ventricular failure. JACC Heart Fail 2013;1(2):127–34.

69. Wang D, Jones C, Ballard-Croft C, et al. Development of a double-lumen cannula for a percutaneous RVAD. ASAIO J 2015;61(4):397–402.

70. Schmack B, Farag M, Kremer J, et al. Results of concomitant groin-free percutaneous temporary RVAD support using a centrifugal pump with a double-lumen jugular venous cannula in LVAD patients. J Thorac Dis 2019;11(Suppl 6):S913–20.

71. Anderson MB, Goldstein J, Milano C, et al. Benefits of a novel percutaneous ventricular assist device for right heart failure: the prospective RECOVER RIGHT study of the Impella RP device. J Heart Lung Transplant 2015;34(12):1549–60.

72. Kuchibhotla S, Esposito ML, Breton C, et al. Acute biventricular mechanical circulatory support for cardiogenic shock. J Am Heart Assoc 2017;6(10): e006670.

73. Morrison LJ, Neumar RW, Zimmerman JL, et al. Strategies for improving survival after in-hospital cardiac arrest in the United States: 2013 consensus recommendations: a consensus statement from the American Heart Association. Circulation 2013;127(14): 1538–63.

74. Jollis JG, Al-Khalidi HR, Roettig ML, et al. Impact of regionalization of ST-segment-elevation myocardial infarction care on treatment times and outcomes for emergency medical services-transported patients presenting to hospitals with percutaneous coronary intervention: mission: lifeline accelerator-2. Circulation 2018;137(4):376–87.

75. Adeoye O, Nystrom KV, Yavagal DR, et al. Recommendations for the establishment of stroke systems of care: a 2019 update. Stroke 2019;50(7): e187–210.

76. Celso B, Tepas J, Langland-Orban B, et al. A systematic review and meta-analysis comparing outcome of severely injured patients treated in trauma centers following the establishment of trauma systems. J Trauma 2006;60(2):371–8 [discussion: 378].

77. Doll JA, Ohman EM, Patel MR, et al. A team-based approach to patients in cardiogenic shock. Catheter Cardiovasc Interv 2016;88(3):424–33.

78. Truesdell AG, Tehrani B, Singh R, et al. 'Combat' approach to cardiogenic shock. Interv Cardiol 2018;13(2):81–6.

79. Tehrani BN, Truesdell AG, Sherwood MW, et al. Standardized team-based care for cardiogenic shock. J Am Coll Cardiol 2019;73(13):1659–69.

80. Tehrani B, Truesdell A, Singh R, et al. Implementation of a cardiogenic shock team and clinical outcomes (INOVA-SHOCK registry): observational and retrospective study. JMIR Res Protoc 2018;7(6):e160.

81. Basir MB, Schreiber T, Dixon S, et al. Feasibility of early mechanical circulatory support in acute myocardial infarction complicated by cardiogenic shock: the Detroit cardiogenic shock initiative. Catheter Cardiovasc Interv 2018;91(3):454–61.

82. Van Mieghem NM, Daemen J, den Uil C, et al. Design and principle of operation of the HeartMate PHP (percutaneous heart pump). EuroIntervention 2018;13(14):1662–6.

83. Dudek D, Ebner A, Sobczynski R, et al. Efficacy and safety of the HeartMate percutaneous heart pump during high-risk percutaneous coronary intervention (from the SHIELD I trial). Am J Cardiol 2018;121(12): 1524–9.

84. Samsky M, Krucoff M, Althouse AD, et al. Clinical and regulatory landscape for cardiogenic shock: a report from the Cardiac Safety Research Consortium ThinkTank on cardiogenic shock. Am Heart J 2020; 219:1–8.

Noninvasive Imaging Risk Stratification with Computed Tomography Angiography for Coronary Artery Disease

Monica Verdoia, MD, PhD[a,b,*], Rocco Gioscia, MD[b],
Marco Marcolongo, MD[a], Giuseppe De Luca, MD, PhD[b]

KEYWORDS

- Coronary stenosis • Coronary imaging • Computed tomography • Cardiovascular risk

KEY POINTS

- The role of Coronary Computed Tomography Angiography (CTA) for the diagnosis and prognosis assessment in coronary artery disease (CAD) still needs definition.
- CTA use is currently indicated for the exclusion of CAD in low-risk patients and in special settings, as coronary total occlusions and bypass grafts.
- Intermediate-risk patients may benefit of the assessment of the ischemic power of coronary lesions of the fusion of functional and anatomic data from CTA.
- Further definition of the impact of CTA as a gatekeeper test before invasive coronary angiography is still warranted.

BACKGROUND

In recent years, the evolution in imaging technology has improved the evaluation of coronary artery disease (CAD). Coronary computed tomography angiography (CTA) has emerged among imaging methods for its high accuracy in visualizing the lumen and wall of the coronary vessels, including a variety of examinations with different degrees of complexity and radiation exposure, from calcium score to the traditional contrast-mediated angiography and even allowing the fusion of anatomic and functional information in the assessment of obstructive coronary stenoses.[1–3]

Although invasive coronary angiography remains the gold standard for the diagnosis and treatment of CAD, previous large-scale registries have shown that almost two-thirds of patients undergoing invasive angiography appear to have normal or nonobstructive disease.[4]

Therefore, a stepwise strategy based on a noninvasive stratification of the patients according to the risk of CAD, and subsequent selective invasive approach in patients with documented ischemia, is currently suggested in guidelines,[5] being associated with similar effectiveness but increased safety, preventing the complications associated with the invasive angiography.

However, the definition of the most accurate diagnostic algorithms comprising CTA as a first-line strategy for ruling out CAD and the correct management of the patients according to the results of imaging tests is still debated,[6] requiring further dedicated studies.

a Cardiologia e Unità Coronarica, Ospedale degli Infermi, ASL Biella, Via dei Ponderanesi, Biella 13900, Italy;
b Division of Cardiology, Azienda Ospedaliera-Universitaria "Maggiore della Carità", Università del Piemonte Orientale, corso Mazzini, Novara 28100, Italy
* Corresponding author. Ospedale degli Infermi, ASL Biella, Università del Piemonte Orientale, Via dei Ponderanesi, Biella 13900, Italy.
E-mail address: monica.verdoia@aslbi.piemonte.it

Cardiol Clin 38 (2020) 543–550
https://doi.org/10.1016/j.ccl.2020.07.002
0733-8651/20/© 2020 Elsevier Inc. All rights reserved.

CURRENT INDICATIONS FOR CORONARY COMPUTED TOMOGRAPHY ANGIOGRAPHY: THE DEFINITION OF CLINICAL LIKELIHOOD

Clinical evaluation is still the initial diagnostic management of patients with suspected obstructive CAD, aiming at the identification of symptoms and at the definition of a pretest clinical risk of obstructive CAD.

This initial assessment, or clinical likelihood, according to guidelines, is generally based on patients' sex, age, and geographic region. However, the key point in the evaluation of patients with suspected coronary disease is the presence of symptoms that suggest angina.[7] The definition of pretest probability of CAD according to the most recent European Society of Cardiology guidelines is shown in **Fig. 1**.[5] In addition to this primary assessment, cardiovascular risk factors, which are often incorporated in several available scores,[8,9] should be considered in the global evaluation of the cardiovascular risk.

Thus, asymptomatic patients with low pretest probability of CAD (<15%) should generally not undergo further testing.[9] However, in specific settings, as in patients with several cardiovascular risk factors, the assessment of calcium score by coronary CTA has emerged as the most accurate imaging tool for ruling out CAD.[10] Coronary calcium is an early marker of atherosclerotic disease, and coronary calcifications are quickly and easily evaluated by computed tomography (CT) with low radiation exposure and no need for contrast agents.[11] The Agatston score is the most widely used calcium score, and an Agatston score of zero in asymptomatic patients is associated with an excellent prognosis.

Shaw and colleagues[12] showed that an Agatston score of 0 accurately predicted the 15-year overall mortality with an absolute events rate of 3%, and more recent studies found a low prevalence of obstructive CAD (<5%) and low risk of death or nonfatal MI (<1% annual risk) in the absence of coronary calcium. However, coronary calcium imaging does not exclude coronary stenosis caused by a noncalcified atherosclerotic lesion, and although the negative predictive value of a zero calcium score for excluding severe stenosis (on CTA) was 99.5%,[13] in patients with a marked increase of calcium score (>400), an abnormal myocardial perfusion single-photon emission CT (SPECT) was observed only in 31% to 46% of patients.[14–16] The identification of coronary calcium can influence the subsequent management of the patient, allowing a direct second-level complete CTA examination with contrast medium but also an earlier introduction of preventive measures, such as statin therapy and lifestyle modifications[17–19]

Nevertheless, this stepwise approach to CTA is considered but not recommended in guidelines[20] and the protocols for the management of the diagnostic process in asymptomatic patients with incidental detection of coronary calcium are still poorly defined.

In contrast, although patients with a high pretest probability of CAD are better to undergo directly invasive coronary angiography offering the possibility of treatment in the same procedure, further noninvasive testing represents the most appropriate strategy in presence of symptoms and an intermediate probability (15%–85%) of CAD.

CORONARY COMPUTED TOMOGRAPHY ANGIOGRAPHY IN SUSPECT OBSTRUCTIVE CORONARY ARTERY DISEASE

For patients with suspected angina and an intermediate pretest probability of CAD, guidelines[5] recommend the use of either a noninvasive functional test of ischemia or anatomic imaging. Debate is still open, attempting to define the strategy that offers the best risk stratification and prognostic benefit. In patients with known CAD, research in ischemia is needed, especially because patients with stents and prior coronary artery bypass grafts are not optimal candidates for CTA.

The recent publication of the data derived from 2 large multicenter randomized controlled trials[21,22] and 2 smaller randomized trials[23,24] significantly

Age (y)	Angina		Atypical/Dyspnea		Nonanginal	
	Men	Women	Men	Women	Men	Women
40–49	22%					
50–59	32%		17%/20%			
60–69	44%	16%	26%/27%		22%	
>=70	52%	27%	34%/32%	19%	24%	

Fig. 1. Pretest (PTP) of obstructive coronary artery disease according to age, sex, and the nature of symptoms. Only patients with PTP greater than or equal to 15% and potential indication to coronary CTA are shown.

favored the use of coronary CTA among other imaging modalities in patients with no history of CAD, leading to the present indication as the first-line strategy (class Ia) in symptomatic patients in whom obstructive CAD cannot be excluded by clinical assessment alone.

The PROMISE[23] (Prospective Multicenter Imaging Study for Evaluation of Chest Pain) trial randomly assigned more than 10,000 patients to an initial strategy of anatomic testing with the use of coronary CTA or to functional testing. Over a median follow-up of 2 years, there were similar outcomes in the coronary CTA and functional testing groups of patients.[25] More patients in the coronary CTA than in the functional group underwent coronary angiography early after testing (12.2 vs 8.1%) but also 50% of patients previously classified as having an intermediate likelihood of obstructive CAD were reclassified to a low (<15%) risk after CTA evaluation, pointing to a good negative predictive value and prognostic impact of coronary CTA.

The Scottish computed tomography of the heart (SCOT-HEART)[21] trial assessed the use of coronary CTA in a large population of more than 20,000 patients, randomized to standard care or standard care plus CT. At 5 years follow-up, the use of imaging significantly reduced the coronary mortality, without increasing the rate of coronary angiography or coronary revascularization.

Similar results were reported in a subsequent meta-analysis, including the PROMISE[22] and other 2 studies, but not the 5-year SCOT-HEART results,[25] where patients undergoing CTA had a significant reduction in the annual rate of myocardial infarction (P = .038) but no difference in all-cause mortality. Most acute ischemic events occur because of the complication of non–flow-limiting plaques,[26] which might be underestimated by the use of a functional test, because they do not induce ischemia, therefore delaying those pharmacologic measures that could prevent major cardiovascular events.[27] In SCOT-HEART, patients assigned to CTA were more likely than patients assigned to standard care alone to have commenced preventive and antianginal therapies and to have undergone earlier coronary revascularization, although only the overall differences in pharmacologic prescribing persisted over 5 years.[21,28] This finding could suggest that CTA can guide the early selection of appropriate patients for both invasive coronary angiography and revascularization and also that earlier onset of treatment in the CTA group prevented downstream longer-term disease progression, whereas the unrecognized disease in the standard care group underwent only more delayed management,

often after the occurrence of a major ischemic event.[29]

Therefore, although functional testing is very effective for risk prediction but is unable to exclude CAD, coronary CTA has shown a 94% to 99% sensitivity and a 64% to 83% specificity for the identification of coronary stenosis,[30] with a 97% to 99% negative predictive value to rule out anatomic CAD. Moreover, the exclusion of CAD by coronary CTA offers the unique opportunity to reassure the patients of presenting a very low risk of adverse cardiac events extending over the following 5 years, often referred to as a warranty period. Initial prognostic studies have estimated that the rate of myocardial infarction or cardiac death remains less than 1% per year for at least 8 years,[2] thus potentially avoiding unnecessary downstream hospital visits and investigations,[31] whereas the severity of CAD, as defined by coronary CTA, clearly affected the long-term outcomes, as shown in **Fig. 2**.[31]

However, the anatomic evaluation of coronary lesions presents some limitations, and mainly for nonthigh (50%–90%) stenoses. Coronary obstructions detected by visual inspection are not necessarily functionally significant, and assessing the ischemic power of a lesion represents a key point for establishing the indications for revascularization, even with invasive coronary angiography. In the Fractional Flow Reserve versus Angiography for Multivessel Evaluation (FAME-2) trial,[32] among patients with stable CAD, PCI was superior to medical therapy alone in the reduction of the primary composite end point at 5 years, when PCI was guided by fractional flow reserve (FFR) to assess the functional ischemic effect of a lesion. Similar conclusions were confirmed by Johnson and colleagues[33] in a subsequent patient-level meta-analysis.

However, the technical limitations of coronary CTA should be acknowledged.[34] For example, irregular heart rate and the presence of extensive coronary calcifications are associated with increased nondiagnostic quality of coronary CTA. To obtain good-quality scans, patients should be in sinus rhythm with a heart rate less than 65 beats per minute and should have good breath holding and collaboration capabilities. In addition, in patients with renal failure, CTA may not be an appropriate choice because of the contrast medium that is needed.[35]

The progressive evolution of CT imaging, allowing high-quality examinations to be obtained with lower radiation exposure and increased accuracy, has partially overcome these technical issues. In the SCOT-HEART trial, the positive results of CTA were confirmed despite the inclusion of those

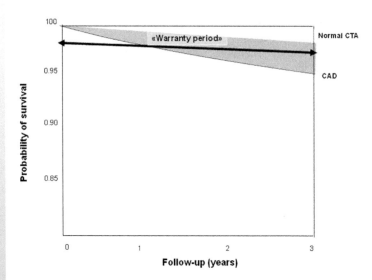

Fig. 2. Unadjusted all-cause 3-year Kaplan-Meier survival by the maximal per-patient presence of normal coronary arteries or obstructive CAD.

patients generally representing the pitfalls of CTA, such as those in atrial fibrillation, with higher body mass index or coronary calcium level.[28]

However, a more tailored approach should be considered in the selection of the noninvasive tests, accounting for the clinical characteristics of the patients and the features of the test, attempting to apply it in those settings where the usefulness of its application is maximal.[5,6] Combination strategies, with the use of multiple noninvasive tests, should be considered in equivocal cases, because both anatomic and functional information are generally required in order to proceed to coronary revascularization (**Fig. 3**).

CORONARY COMPUTED TOMOGRAPHY ANGIOGRAPHY IN SPECIAL SETTINGS

The pressing need for both anatomic and functional data for the assessment of coronary obstructions has led to the progressive development of hybrid technologies, combining the visualization of the coronary vessel by CTA with the evaluation of myocardial ischemia and perfusion. In particular, hybrid imaging with nuclear cardiology imaging (PET or SPECT) combines the high negative predictive value of coronary CTA with one of the most sensitive and specific functional tests.[36] Benz and colleagues[37] showed that a matched combination of a reversible perfusion defect on SPECT in a territory supplied by a coronary artery with CAD on CTA was independently associated with an improved outcome compared with medical therapy alone. In contrast, patients with unmatched findings did not benefit from early revascularization, irrespective of the presence or absence of high-risk CAD.

Another recent acquisition in CT technology is the noninvasive calculation of FFR noninvasively (FFRCT), based on the application of computational fluid dynamics to model and predict FFR from conventionally acquired CTA, without requiring further exposure to radiation or contrast media.[38] Three large multicenter studies (NXT, DISCOVER-FLOW [Diagnosis of Ischemia-Causing Stenoses Obtained Viat Noninvasive Fractional Flow Reserve], and DeFACTO,[39–41]) have compared the accuracy of FFRCT with invasive FFR measurements, and reported sensitivities of between 88% and 90% and specificities between 54% and 90%.[42,43] A meta-analysis of the 3 trials concluded that FFRCT has a pooled sensitivity similar to coronary CTA (0.89 vs 0.89 at per-patient analysis; 0.83 vs 0.86 at per-vessel analysis) but improved specificity (0.71 vs 0.35 at per-patient analysis; 0.78 vs 0.56 at per-vessel analysis),[44] leading to a reduction in the number of unnecessary invasive angiographies.[2]

Another unique opportunity that recently emerged for coronary CTA is the identification of high-risk plaques. An important advantage of coronary CTA is that, in addition to the identification of coronary artery stenosis, it can also assess plaque characteristics, which can be in the form of visual assessment, or more recently using software capable of semiautomated quantitative and qualitative assessment of the plaque.[45] More detailed visual assessment includes the identification of adverse features, including positive remodeling, low-attenuation plaque, spotty calcification, and the so-called napkin-ring sign. These features are associated with markers of histologic vulnerability[46] and with prognosis in several studies, being more frequently observed in patients experiencing

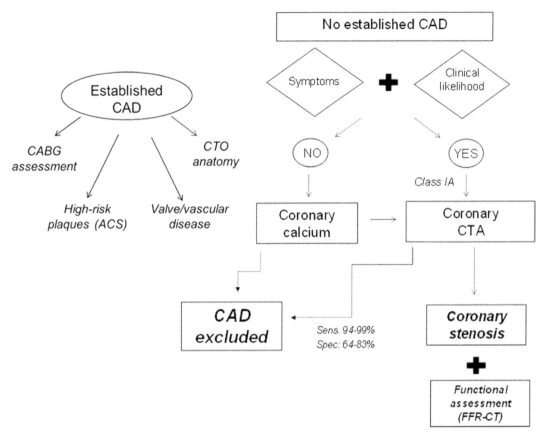

Fig. 3. Proposed tailored approach for CAD risk stratification using a stepwise approach. ACS, acute coronary syndrome; CABG, coronary artery bypass graft; CTO, chronic total occlusion.

a future acute coronary syndrome.[47,48] The largest study on this topic was reported by Motoyama and colleagues,[49] which included 3158 patients followed up for 4 years. They found that positive remodeling or low-attenuation plaque was associated with an increased likelihood of acute cardiovascular events. Similarly, in the PROMISE trial, high-risk plaques were associated with an increased risk of death, myocardial infarction, or hospitalization for unstable angina at 2 years.[50]

In effect, adverse plaques are frequently identified on coronary CTA, ranging from 15% of patients in the stable population of the PROMISE trial[50] to the 35% in the Multicenter Study to Rule Out Myocardial Infarction by Cardiac Computed Tomography (ROMICAT-II).[51] In the latter study, among 1000 patients admitted to the emergency department with symptoms suggestive of acute coronary syndromes, incorporating coronary CTA into a triage strategy improved the efficiency of clinical decision making, compared with a standard evaluation in the emergency department, allowing the time of hospitalization to be shortened, especially when combined with high-sensitivity troponin.

In addition, a special mention is needed about the role of coronary anatomy in certain special subsets of patients with established cardiovascular disease, where the tridimensional imaging offered by coronary CTA compared with invasive angiography can provide useful information for the assessment of CAD and planning of interventions.

In effect, the progressive increase of the indication to the percutaneous reopening of chronic coronary occlusions has led to the need to face more and more complex lesions, where the information provided by the coronary CTA can help in the procedural success.[52] Coronary CTA can feature the coronary course and connections with collaterals, the extent of calcification, vessel tortuosity, stump morphology, presence of multiple occlusions, and lesion length. Previous studies have suggested that the procedural success in chronic total occlusions was larger in patients in whom preprocedural CTA was performed.[53]

In addition, the progressive aging of the population has led to the increase of comorbidities, such as renal failure and aortic stenosis, where the possibility of performing multiple anatomic evaluations with a smaller amount of contrast medium can render CTA more advantageous compared with invasive angiography, especially among special subsets of patients, such as those who need aortic valve treatment[54] or patients with prior bypass grafting.[55] CTA of coronary bypass is more demanding from a technical point of view, because it requires a larger scan range (12.5–22.0 cm) and consequently a longer breath hold, and the nondynamic nature of CTA makes the assessment of competitive flow or vasospasm in the arterial graft difficult. Also, arterial grafts pose some limitations to CTA study, as does the presence of metallic clips in mammary artery and, particularly, in radial artery grafts, which interfere with the visualization of lesions.

In contrast, invasive evaluation of grafts can be challenging and exposes patients to large contrast volumes in addition to rare complications such as injury to the graft vessel during catheter engagement. In addition, coronary artery bypass grafts are more amenable to CTA imaging, because of their larger diameters and lower pulsatile movements along the cardiac cycle than native arteries and their relative freedom from calcification, therefore rendering noninvasive assessment a promising opportunity for these patients.

SUMMARY

The availability of imaging technologies for the assessment of CAD, both in elective settings and in emergency room departments, and the options to combine functional and anatomic information, allow clinicians to stratify cardiovascular risk by noninvasive methods. Coronary CTA has recently emerged as the most accurate and effective technique for the exclusion of CAD, whereas different tests could be more appropriate for specific subsets of patients. However, the contests where the different noninvasive tests could provide the greatest advantages still lack a unique definition. Therefore, future large randomized trials are needed in order to draw tailored diagnostic and therapeutic pathways, allowing the assessment of cardiovascular risk to be individualized and the outcome benefits maximized.

REFERENCES

1. Miller JM, Rochitte CE, Dewey M, et al. Diagnostic performance of coronary angiography by 64-row CT. N Engl J Med 2008;359(22):2324–36.
2. Andreini D, Pontone G, Mushtaq S, et al. A long-term prognostic value of coronary CT angiography in suspected coronary artery disease. JACC Cardiovasc Imaging 2012;5(7):690–701.
3. Williams MC, Newby DE, Nicol ED. Coronary atherosclerosis imaging by CT to improve clinical outcomes. J Cardiovasc Comput Tomogr 2019;13(5):281–7.
4. Patel MR, Peterson ED, Dai D, et al. Low diagnostic yield of elective coronary angiography. N Engl J Med 2010;362(10):886–95.
5. Knuuti J, Wijns W, Saraste A, et al, ESC Scientific Document Group. 2019 ESC Guidelines for the diagnosis and management of chronic coronary syndromes. Eur Heart J 2020;41(3):407–77.
6. Steurer J, Fischer JE, Bachmann LM, et al. Communicating accuracy of tests to general practitioners: a controlled study. BMJ 2002;324:824–6.
7. Diamond GA, Forrester JS. Analysis of probability as an aid in the clinical diagnosis of coronary-artery disease. N Engl J Med 1979;300:1350–8.
8. Genders TS, Steyerberg EW, Hunink MG, et al. Prediction model to estimate presence of coronary artery disease: retrospective pooled analysis of existing cohorts. BMJ 2012;344:3485.
9. Reeh J, Therming CB, Heitmann M, et al. Prediction of obstructive coronary artery disease and prognosis in patients with suspected stable angina. Eur Heart J 2018;40:1426–35.
10. Budoff MJ, Dowe D, Jollis JG, et al. Diagnostic performance of 64-multidetector row coronary computed tomographic angiography for evaluation of coronary artery stenosis in individuals without known coronary artery disease: results from the prospective multicenter ACCURACY (Assessment by Coronary Computed Tomographic Angiography of Individuals Undergoing Invasive Coronary Angiography) trial. J Am Coll Cardiol 2008;52(21):1724–32.
11. Gräni C, Vontobel J, Benz DC, et al. Ultra-low-dose coronary artery calcium scoring using novel scoring thresholds for low tube voltage protocols-a pilot study. Eur Heart J Cardiovasc Imaging 2018;19(12):1362–71.
12. Shaw LJ, Giambrone AE, Blaha MJ, et al. Long-term prognosis after coronary artery calcification testing in asymptomatic patients: a cohort study. Ann Intern Med 2015;163(1):14–21.
13. Hoff JA, Chomka EV, Krainik AJ, et al. Age and gender distributions of coronary artery calcium detected by electron beam tomography in 35,246 adults. Am J Cardiol 2001;87(12):1335–9.
14. Engbers EM, Timmer JR, Ottervanger JP, et al. Prognostic value of coronary artery calcium scoring in addition to single-photon emission computed tomographic myocardial perfusion imaging in symptomatic patients. Circ Cardiovasc Imaging 2016;9(5):e003966.
15. Chang SM, Nabi F, Xu J, et al. The coronary artery calcium score and stress myocardial perfusion

imaging provide independent and complementary prediction of cardiac risk. J Am Coll Cardiol 2009; 54(20):1872–82.

16. He ZX, Hedrick TD, Pratt CM, et al. Severity of coronary artery calcification by electron beam computed tomography predicts silent myocardial ischemia. Circulation 2000;101(3):244–51.

17. Kalia NK, Cespedes L, Youssef G, et al. Motivational effects of coronary artery calcium scores on statin adherence and weight loss. Coron Artery Dis 2015; 26(3):225–30.

18. Gupta A, Lau E, Varshney R, et al. The identification of calcified coronary plaque is associated with initiation and continuation of pharmacological and lifestyle preventive therapies: a systematic review and meta-analysis. JACC Cardiovasc Imaging 2017; 10(8):833–42.

19. Mamudu HM, Paul TK, Veeranki SP, et al. The effects of coronary artery calcium screening on behavioral modification, risk perception, and medication adherence among asymptomatic adults: a systematic review. Atherosclerosis 2014;236(2):338–50.

20. Assessing and diagnosing suspected stable angina (NICE pathways). 2018. Available at: http://pathwaysnice.org.uk/pathways/chest-pain.

21. SCOT-HEART investigators, Newby DE, Adamson PD, Berry C, et al. Coronary CT angiography and 5-year risk of myocardial infarction. N Engl J Med 2018;379(10):924–33.

22. Douglas PS, Hoffmann U, Lee KL, et al. PROspective Multicenter Imaging Study for Evaluation of chest pain: rationale and design of the PROMISE trial. Am Heart J 2014;167(6):796–803.

23. McKavanagh P, Lusk L, Ball PA, et al. A comparison of cardiac computerized tomography and exercise stress electrocardiogram test for the investigation of stable chest pain: the clinical results of the CAPP randomized prospective trial. Eur Heart J Cardiovasc Imaging 2015;16(4):441–8.

24. Min JK, Koduru S, Dunning AM, et al. Coronary CT angiography versus myocardial perfusion imaging for near-term quality of life, cost and radiation exposure: a prospective multicenter randomized pilot trial. J Cardiovasc Comput Tomogr 2012;6(4): 274–83.

25. Bittencourt MS, Hulten EA, Murthy VL, et al. Clinical outcomes after evaluation of stable chest pain by coronary computed tomographic angiography versus usual care: a meta-analysis. Circ Cardiovasc Imaging 2016;9(4):e004419.

26. Hoffmann U, Moselewski F, Nieman K, et al. Noninvasive assessment of plaque morphology and composition in culprit and stable lesions in acute coronary syndrome and stable lesions in stable angina by multidetector computed tomography. J Am Coll Cardiol 2006;47(8): 1655–62.

27. Hulten E, Bittencourt MS, Singh A, et al. Coronary artery disease detected by coronary computed tomographic angiography is associated with intensification of preventive medical therapy and lower low-density lipoprotein cholesterol. Circ Cardiovasc Imaging 2014;7(4):629–38.

28. SCOT-HEART investigators. CT coronary angiography in patients with suspected angina due to coronary heart disease (SCOT-HEART): an open-label, parallel-group, multicentre trial. Lancet 2015; 385(9985):2383–91.

29. Doris M, Newby DE. Coronary CT angiography as a diagnostic and prognostic tool: perspectives from the SCOT-HEART trial. Curr Cardiol Rep 2016; 18(2):18.

30. Meijboom WB, Meijs MF, Schuijf JD, et al. Diagnostic accuracy of 64-slice computed tomography coronary angiography: a prospective, multicenter, multivendor study. J Am Coll Cardiol 2008;52(25): 2135–44.

31. Min JK, Dunning A, Lin FY, et al. Age- and sex-related differences in all-cause mortality risk based on coronary computed tomography angiography findings results from the International Multicenter CONFIRM (Coronary CT Angiography Evaluation for Clinical Outcomes: an International Multicenter Registry) of 23,854 patients without known coronary artery disease. J Am Coll Cardiol 2011;58:849–60.

32. Xaplanteris P, Fournier S, Pijls NHJ, et al. Five-year outcomes with PCI guided by fractional flow reserve. N Engl J Med 2018;379(3):250–9.

33. Johnson NP, Toth GG, Lai D, et al. Prognostic value of fractional flow reserve: linking physiologic severity to clinical outcomes. J Am Coll Cardiol 2014;64: 16411654.

34. Schmermund A, Marwan M, Hausleiter J, et al. Declining radiation dose of coronary computed tomography angiography: German cardiac CT registry experience 2009-2014. Clin Res Cardiol 2017; 106(11):905–12.

35. Knuuti J, Bengel F, Bax JJ, et al. Risks and benefits of cardiac imaging: an analysis of risks related to imaging for coronary artery disease. Eur Heart J 2014; 35:633–8.

36. Rochitte CE, George RT, Chen MY, et al. Computed tomography angiography and perfusion to assess coronary artery stenosis causing perfusion defects by single photon emission computed tomography: the CORE320 study. Eur Heart J 2014;35:1120–30.

37. Benz DC, Gaemperli L, Gräni C, et al. Impact of cardiac hybrid imaging-guided patient management on clinical long-term outcome. Int J Cardiol 2018;261: 218–22.

38. Min JK, Taylor CA, Achenbach S, et al. Noninvasive fractional flow reserve derived from coronary CT angiography: clinical data and scientific principles. JACC Cardiovasc Imaging 2015;8:1209–22.

39. Koo BK, Erglis A, Doh JH, et al. Diagnosis of ischemia-causing coronary stenoses by noninvasive fractional flow reserve computed from coronary computed omographic angiograms. Results from the prospective multicentre DISCOVER-FLOW (Diagnosis of Ischemia-Causing Stenoses Obtained Via Noninvasive Fractional Flow Reserve) study. J Am Coll Cardiol 2011;58:1989–97.

40. Nakazato R, Park HB, Berman DS, et al. Noninvasive fractional flow reserve derived from computed tomography angiography for coronary lesions of intermediate stenosis severity: results from the DeFACTO study. Circ Cardiovasc Imaging 2013;6:881–9.

41. Nørgaard BL, Leipsic J, Gaur S, et al. Diagnostic performance of noninvasive fractional flow reserve derived from coronary computed tomography angiography in suspected coronary artery disease: the NXT trial (Analysis of Coronary Blood Flow Using CT Angiography: next Steps). J Am Coll Cardiol 2014;63:1145–55.

42. Morise AP, Diamond GA. Comparison of the sensitivity and specificity of exercise electrocardiography in biased and unbiased populations of men and women. Am Heart J 1995;130(4):741–7.

43. Nandalur KR, Dwamena BA, Choudhri AF, et al. Diagnostic performance of stress cardiac magnetic resonance imaging in the detection of coronary artery disease: a meta-analysis. J Am Coll Cardiol 2007;50(14):1343–53.

44. Schwitter J, Wacker CM, Wilke N, et al, MR-IMPACT Investigators. MR-IMPACT II: magnetic Resonance Imaging for Myocardial Perfusion Assessment in Coronary artery disease Trial: perfusion-cardiac magnetic resonance vs. single-photon emission computed tomography for the detection of coronary artery disease: a comparative multicentre, multivendor trial. Eur Heart J 2013;34(10):775–81.

45. Dey D, Schepis T, Marwan M, et al. Automated three-dimensional quantification of noncalcified coronary plaque from coronary CT angiography: comparison with intravascular US. Radiology 2010;257:516–22.

46. Obaid DR, Calvert PA, Brown A, et al. Coronary CT angiography features of ruptured and high-risk atherosclerotic plaques: correlation with intra-vascular ultrasound. J Cardiovasc Comput Tomogr 2017;11(6):455–61.

47. Schlett CL, Maurovich-Horvat P, Ferencik M, et al. Histogram analysis of lipid-core plaques in coronary computed tomographic angiography: ex vivo validation against histology. Invest Radiol 2013;48(9):646–53.

48. Narula J, Nakano M, Virmani R, et al. Histopathologic characteristics of atherosclerotic coronary disease and implications of the findings for the invasive and noninvasive detection of vulnerable plaques. J Am Coll Cardiol 2013;61(10):1041–51.

49. Motoyama S, Ito H, Sarai M, et al. Plaque characterization by coronary computed tomography angiography and the likelihood of acute coronary events in mid-term follow-up. J Am Coll Cardiol 2015;66(4):337–46.

50. Ferencik M, Mayrhofer T, Bittner DO, et al. Use of high-risk coronary atherosclerotic plaque detection for risk stratification of patients with stable chest pain: a secondary analysis of the PROMISE randomized clinical trial. JAMA Cardiol 2018;3(2):144–52.

51. Puchner SB, Liu T, Mayrhofer T, et al. High-risk plaque detected on coronary CT angiography predicts acute coronary syndromes independent of significant stenosis in acute chest pain: results from the ROMICAT-II trial. J Am Coll Cardiol 2014;64(7):684–92.

52. Rolf A, Werner GS, Schuhbäck A, et al. Preprocedural coronary CT angiography significantly improves success rates of PCI for chronic total occlusion. Int J Cardiovasc Imaging 2013;29(8):1819–27.

53. Opolski MP, Achenbach S. CT angiography for revascularization of CTO: crossing the borders of diagnosis and treatment. JACC Cardiovasc Imaging 2015;8(7):846–58.

54. Annoni AD, Andreini D, Pontone G, et al. CT angiography prior to TAVI procedure using third-generation scanner with wide volume coverage: feasibility, renal safety and diagnostic accuracy for coronary tree. Br J Radiol 2018;91(1090):20180196.

55. Chow BJ, Ahmed O, Small G, et al. Prognostic value of CT angiography in coronary bypass patients. JACC Cardiovasc Imaging 2011;4(5):496–502.

Antithrombotic Therapy in Patients with Atrial Fibrillation Undergoing Percutaneous Coronary Intervention

Anton Camaj, MD, MS, Michael S. Miller, MSc, Jonathan L. Halperin, MD, Gennaro Giustino, MD*

KEYWORDS

- Triple antithrombotic therapy • Dual antithrombotic therapy • Atrial fibrillation
- Percutaneous coronary intervention

KEY POINTS

- The antithrombotic strategy in patients with atrial fibrillation (AF) undergoing percutaneous coronary intervention (PCI) should be chosen after a thorough assessment of an individual patient's bleeding and ischemic risks.
- Dual antithrombotic therapy with a direct oral anticoagulant should be the default antithrombotic strategy in most patients with AF undergoing PCI.
- Monotherapy with an oral anticoagulant after 6 months or 1-year post-PCI should be favored over a dual antithrombotic strategy, combining an oral anticoagulant with an antiplatelet agent, especially in patients whose bleeding risk outweighs the ischemic risk.

INTRODUCTION

It is estimated that 20% to 40% of patients with atrial fibrillation (AF) have coronary artery disease (CAD) and approximately 10% of patients who undergo percutaneous coronary intervention (PCI) with drug-eluting stent (DES) implantation have AF.[1] AF is associated with increased risk of thromboembolic events, thus warranting prophylaxis with long-term oral anticoagulation (OAC).[1] In contrast, dual antiplatelet therapy (DAPT) with a combination of aspirin and an oral P2Y$_{12}$-receptor inhibitor is necessary to prevent coronary thrombotic events after PCI with DES.[2] Historically, triple antithrombotic therapy (TAT), combining OAC and DAPT, has been the default antithrombotic strategy for these patients. TAT is associated, however, with a high risk for bleeding complications, which are associated with morbidity and mortality.[3] Therefore, balancing the risk of cardiogenic embolism, coronary events, and major bleeding in this patient population poses a clinical dilemma. Evidence from randomized controlled trials (RCT)[4–9] has prompted the rapid evolution of recommendations surrounding optimal antithrombotic strategies for patients with AF after PCI.[10–16] The purpose of this review is to provide an update on the evidence, recommendations, and future directions in the field of antithrombotic therapy for patients with AF who undergo PCI.

The Zena and Michael A. Wiener Cardiovascular Institute, The Icahn School of Medicine at Mount Sinai, 1 Gustave L. Levy Place, New York, NY 10029, USA
* Corresponding author.
E-mail address: Gennaro.Giustino@mountsinai.org

Cardiol Clin 38 (2020) 551–561
https://doi.org/10.1016/j.ccl.2020.07.006

ANTITHROMBOTIC STRATEGIES IN PATIENTS UNDERGOING PERCUTANEOUS CORONARY INTERVENTION WITHOUT AN INDICATION FOR ORAL ANTICOAGULATION

The evidence informing antithrombotic strategies in patients undergoing PCI with stent implantation who do not have an indication for OAC favors DAPT over OAC with respect to both ischemic and bleeding events.[17–20] American and European guidelines both provide a class I recommendation for DAPT after PCI with stent implantation with the type of P2Y$_{12}$ inhibitor dependent on the clinical scenario.[14,21]

With respect to DAPT duration, prolonged DAPT reduces the risks of stent thrombosis and myocardial infarction (MI) but increases the risk of bleeding. Both the American and European guidelines strongly recommend a shorter course (eg, 6 months) of DAPT in patients with stable CAD undergoing PCI with implantation of a DES (American College of Cardiology [ACC]/American Heart Association [AHA]: class of recommendation [COR] I, level of evidence [LOE] B; European Society of Cardiology [ESC]: COR I, LOE A).[14,21] For patients with acute coronary syndrome (ACS) undergoing PCI with DES, the guidelines recommend a minimum of 12 months of DAPT (ACC/AHA: COR I, LOE B; ESC: COR I, LOE A) unless the patient is at high bleeding risk (HBR), when shorter therapy (eg, 6 months) should be considered (ACC/AHA: COR IIb, LOE C; ESC: COR IIa, LOE B).[14,21] After this period, in patients who have tolerated DAPT without adverse events and who are not at HBR, DAPT might be extended beyond 12 months (ACC/AHA COR: IIb, LOE A).

More recently, multiple randomized controlled trials (RCTs) compared the efficacy and safety of single antiplatelet therapy (SAPT) using a P2Y$_{12}$-receptor inhibitor monotherapy, instead of aspirin, versus DAPT after PCI with newer-generation DES.[22–25] None of these trials included patients with AF or another indication for chronic OAC. The Ticagrelor With Aspirin or Alone in High-Risk Patients After Coronary Intervention (TWILIGHT) study tested the hypothesis that after a 3-month course of DAPT using aspirin and ticagrelor, ticagrelor monotherapy would be superior to DAPT with respect to clinically significant bleeding without ischemic harm in a cohort of HBR and ischemic risk patients after PCI.[22] In this randomized, double-blind trial, the investigators found a significantly lower rate of Bleeding Academic Research Consortium (BARC) 2 to 5 bleeding (primary endpoint) in the experimental arm (hazard ratio [HR] 0.56; 95% CI, 0.45–0.68; P<.001) without

an increased risk of death, nonfatal MI or nonfatal stroke.[22]

ANTITHROMBOTIC THERAPIES IN PATIENTS UNDERGOING PERCUTANEOUS CORONARY INTERVENTION WITH AN INDICATION FOR ORAL ANTICOAGULATION
Vitamin K Antagonist Trials

The What Is the Optimal Antiplatelet and Anticoagulant Therapy in Patients With Oral Anticoagulation and Coronary Stenting (WOEST) trial was the first of a series of studies comparing double antithrombotic therapy (DAT) using a vitamin K antagonist (VKA) plus a P2Y$_{12}$-receptor inhibitor to TAT, using a VKA, a P2Y$_{12}$-receptor inhibitor, and aspirin in patients with an indication for chronic OAC following PCI.[6] WOEST was an open-label RCT that included 573 patients (69% of whom had AF) randomized to DAT (VKA plus clopidogrel) versus TAT (VKA plus clopidogrel plus aspirin) after PCI in order to test the hypothesis that SAPT with clopidogrel would reduce the risk of bleeding without increasing the risk of thrombotic events compared with DAPT. WOEST demonstrated that the early discontinuation of aspirin reduced the relative risk of any bleeding event by 64%, which was driven largely by Thrombolysis in Myocardial Infarction (TIMI) minor and Global Strategies for Opening Occluded Coronary Arteries (GUSTO) moderate bleeding.[6] Although underpowered, the DAT group did not show any increase in the risk of ischemic events and all-cause death was significantly lower in the DAT group.[6]

The Intracoronary Stenting and Antithrombotic Regimen–Testing of a 6-Week versus a 6-Month Clopidogrel Treatment Regimen in Patients With Concomitant Aspirin and Oral Anticoagulant Therapy Following Drug-Eluting Stenting (ISAR-TRIPLE) trial tested whether 6 weeks of DAPT was superior to 6 months of DAPT in patients with an indication for chronic OAC after PCI.[7] The study randomized 614 patients (83% AF or atrial flutter) and found no difference in its primary composite endpoint of death, MI, definite stent thrombosis, stroke, or TIMI major bleeding at 9 months between the 2 groups. Furthermore, the abbreviated strategy showed a lower risk of BARC types 2 to 5 bleeding in a post hoc landmark analysis of events between 6 weeks and 6 months.[7]

Direct Oral Anticoagulant Trials

Multiple trials have evaluated the safety and efficacy of a direct oral anticoagulant (DOAC)-based antithrombotic strategy after PCI in patients with AF requiring chronic OAC. These trials had varying designs and randomization schemes and were powered to demonstrate superiority for reduction in bleeding with a DOAC-based strategy versus a VKA-based strategy. Individually, they were underpowered to detect significant differences in major adverse cardiac events between antithrombotic strategies.

The Study Exploring Two Strategies of Rivaroxaban and One of Oral Vitamin K Antagonist in Patients With Atrial Fibrillation Who Undergo Percutaneous Coronary Intervention (PIONEER AF-PCI) study included 2124 patients who were stratified prior to randomization by DAPT duration (1 month, 6 months, or 12 months) and $P2Y_{12}$ inhibitor (clopidogrel, ticagrelor, or prasugrel) and then were randomized into 2 groups: (group 1) low-dose rivaroxaban (15 mg daily) plus SAPT with a $P2Y_{12}$ inhibitor; (group 2) very-low-dose rivaroxaban (2.5 mg twice daily) plus DAPT; and (group 3, control) VKA plus DAPT.[5] Only 22% of patients received TAT for 1 year. The rivaroxaban-based strategies led to a reduction in the primary safety endpoint of clinically significant bleeding driven by reduction in rates of bleeding requiring medical attention as opposed to TIMI major or minor bleeding without significant differences in rates of major adverse cardiovascular (CV) events between the 3 groups.[5]

In the Evaluation of Dual Therapy With Dabigatran versus Triple Therapy With Warfarin in Patients With AF That Undergo a PCI With Stenting (RE-DUAL PCI) trial, 2725 patients were randomized post-PCI to DAT consisting of dabigatran, 110 mg or 150 mg twice daily, plus a $P2Y_{12}$ inhibitor (86.6% clopidogrel, 12.4% ticagrelor) or TAT consisting of warfarin plus DAPT (90.3% clopidogrel, 7.8% ticagrelor).[8] Aspirin was discontinued 1 month after bare-metal stent implantation or 3 months after DES implantation in the TAT group. Although powered for noninferiority analysis, both DAT regimens proved superior to the TAT regimen with respect to the primary endpoint of major or clinically relevant nonmajor bleeding at 14 months irrespective of clinical presentation or $P2Y_{12}$ inhibitor selection.[8]

Although both PIONEER AF-PCI and RE-DUAL PCI support a DAT over a TAT strategy, neither was designed to delineate whether the reduction in bleeding was due to aspirin withdrawal, the doses of DOACs, or both. This was addressed in the an open-label, 2 × 2 factorial, randomized controlled trial to evaluate the safety of apixaban versus VKA and aspirin versus placebo in patients with AF and acute coronary syndrome and/or percutaneous coronary intervention (AUGUSTUS) trial.[4] AUGUSTUS randomized 4614 AF patients within 14 days after having an ACS or PCI in a

2 × 2 factorial design to apixaban, 5 mg twice daily, or VKA (open-label) and to aspirin or matching placebo (double-blind) for 6 months.[4] A $P2Y_{12}$ inhibitor was prescribed for all patients: 92.6% clopidogrel, 6.2% ticagrelor, or 1.1% prasugrel. The primary endpoint of major or clinically relevant nonmajor bleeding was lower in those receiving apixaban compared with a VKA (HR 0.69; 95% CI, 0.58–0.81; P<.001 for both noninferiority and superiority) and higher in those receiving aspirin compared with placebo (HR 1.89; 95% CI, 1.59–2.24; P<.001).[4] Additionally, the apixaban group had a lower incidence of death or hospitalization compared with the VKA group (HR 0.83; 95% CI, 0.74–0.93) without a significant difference in rates of ischemic events.[4] Although aspirin increased the risk of bleeding compared with placebo, there was no significant difference in the incidence of coronary ischemic events (eg, MI, CV death, stent thrombosis, and urgent revascularization).[4] The results from AUGUSTUS support a DAT strategy with DOACs over VKAs and early aspirin withdrawal, but the optimal duration of aspirin therapy remains uncertain and may vary based on a patient's thrombotic risk.

The recent Edoxaban Treatment versus Vitamin K Antagonist in Patients With Atrial Fibrillation Undergoing Percutaneous Coronary Intervention (ENTRUST-AF PCI) trial randomized 1506 AF patients after successful PCI (52% ACS) to a DAT strategy with edoxaban (60 mg daily) and a $P2Y_{12}$ inhibitor (92% clopidogrel) or a TAT strategy with a VKA.[9] DAT was noninferior to TAT with regards to the primary composite endpoint of major or clinically relevant nonmajor bleeding at 12 months. There was no significant difference in rates of ischemic events between groups. It is important to acknowledge the results from the landmark analysis at 14 days, when a higher risk of bleeding was observed with edoxaban and a high proportion of patients in the VKA group had an international normalized ratio less than 2 (69% in the first week and 42% in the second week). Beyond 14 days, edoxaban consistently was associated with less bleeding (HR 0.68; 95% CI, 0.53–0.88; $P_{interaction}$<0.0001).

A meta-analysis of these 4 DOAC-based trials comparing DAT versus TAT in 10,234 AF-PCI/ACS patients[26] found DAT associated with a reduction in major or clinically relevant nonmajor bleeding compared with TAT (risk ratio [RR] 0.66; 95% CI, 0.56 to 0.78) at the cost of an increase in stent thrombosis (RR 1.59; 95% CI, 1.01–2.50).[26] There were no significant differences in rates of MI, CV death, or all-cause death. There were 1715 major or clinically relevant nonmajor bleeding events (523 major bleeding events) versus 85 stent thrombosis events across the more than 10,000 patients with no between-group differences in CV death or major adverse clinical events.[26] Given that bleeding complications are numerically significantly more frequent than stent thrombosis and associated with substantial morbidity and mortality, these findings support the safety of a DAT strategy using a DOAC over a TAT strategy, whereas patients at very high risk of stent thrombosis may benefit from a brief course of TAT.

Summaries of the study designs and trial results of the VKA and DOAC trials are provided in **Figs. 1** and **2**, respectively.

ANTITHROMBOTIC MANAGEMENT OF PATIENTS WITH ATRIAL FIBRILLATION AFTER PERCUTANEOUS CORONARY INTERVENTION: GUIDELINE AND CONSENSUS RECOMMENDATIONS
Guideline and Consensus Recommended Strategies

Emerging RCT data largely have replaced expert consensus as the basis for international guidelines and consensus recommendations.[10–13] The

precepts underlying these recommendations as follows:

1. Assess individual patient thrombotic and bleeding risks.
2. Minimize TAT duration to mitigate bleeding.
3. DOAC preferred over a VKA unless contraindicated.
4. Clopidogrel is the $P2Y_{12}$ inhibitor of choice.
5. Beyond 1 year, OAC monotherapy preferred over DAT.

International guidelines and consensus documents, at present, do not incorporate results from AUGUSTUS or ENTRUST-AF PCI. Summaries of the American and European consensus document recommendations are provided in **Figs. 3** and **4**, respectively.

Assessment of Thrombotic and Bleeding Risks

Once the need for OAC has been established, risk stratification according to the individual risk of coronary thrombosis and major bleeding becomes critical, because this determines subsequent decisions surrounding TAT duration and antiplatelet selection. The most recent North American

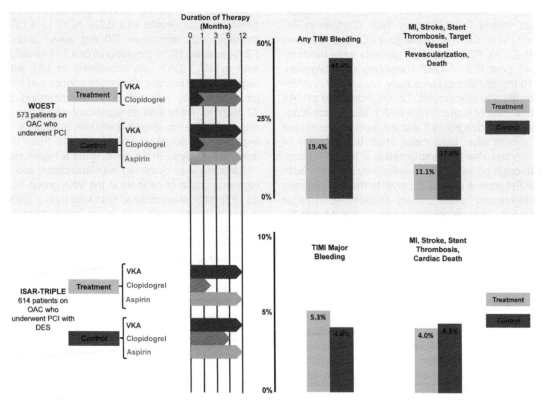

Fig. 1. Study design and outcomes of WOEST and ISAR-TRIPLE: patients with atrial fibrillation on VKAs undergoing PCI.

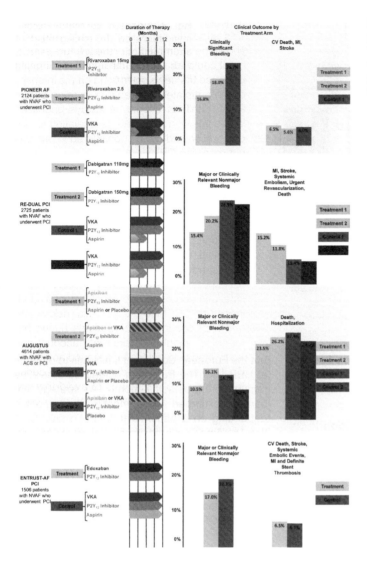

Fig. 2. Study design and outcomes of PIONEER AF, RE-DUAL PCI, AUGUSTUS, and ENTRUST-AF PCI: patients with atrial fibrillation DOACs undergoing PCI. NVAF, nonvalvular atrial fibrillation.

consensus document highlights multiple patient and complex procedural characteristics that may predispose to increased ischemic and thrombotic risks, including ACS presentation, age, prior MI, extent of CAD, diabetes mellitus, chronic kidney disease, older-generation stents, smaller stent diameter, longer stent length, and bifurcation stents, among others.[12] In a similar, qualitative fashion, the North American document cites a history of prior bleeding, OAC therapy, female sex, age, diabetes mellitus, chronic kidney disease, and anemia, among others, as bleeding risk factors.[12] The European counterpart emphasizes the use of risk scores to quantify ischemic and bleeding risk in addition to patient and procedural characteristics.[10] For ischemic risk assessment, the European document recommends the Synergy Between Percutaneous Coronary Intervention

With Taxus (SYNTAX) score in elective cases and the Global Registry of Acute Coronary Events (GRACE) score (>140) in patients with ACS, while accounting for other risk factors, including left main PCI, proximal left anterior descending artery, proximal bifurcation, recurrent MI, and a history of stent thrombosis.[10] For bleeding risk assessment, the European document recommends the Hypertension, Abnormal renal/liver function, Stroke, Bleeding history or predisposition, Labile international normalized ratio, Elderly (>65 years), Drugs/alcohol concomitantly (HAS-BLED) score.[10] A consensus document from the Academic Research Consortium (ARC) proposed 20 clinical criteria (14 major and 6 minor) to define patients at HBR undergoing PCI (ARC-HBR definition).[27] Although long-term OAC use is a major criterion, this definition may inform the estimation of

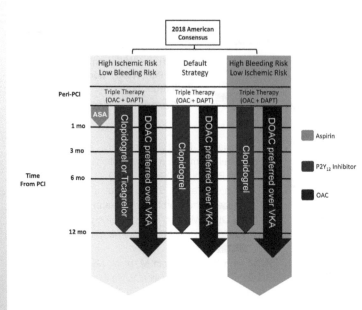

Fig. 3. American consensus recommendations on the management of antithrombotic therapy in patients with atrial fibrillation undergoing PCI. ASA, aspirin.

bleeding risk. The ARC-HBR definition has not been validated in an independent patient data set.[27]

Triple Antithrombotic Therapy Duration

The recommended duration of TAT differs slightly between the 2019 ACC/AHA/Heart Rhythm Society (HRS) guidelines for AF and the 2018 ESC guidelines for myocardial revascularization.[11,13] Both provide a COR IIa recommendation for DAT as an alternative to TAT to reduce bleeding, but the European document limits this to patients at HBR.[11,13] The European guidelines otherwise recommend a default 1-month TAT strategy that can be extended for 3 months to 6 months depending on a patient's thrombotic risk (COR IIa). The American guidelines, conversely, recommend a default DAT strategy, limiting aspirin to the periprocedural, in-hospital period.[11] Moreover, the American guidelines recommend 4 weeks to 6 weeks of TAT in patients at greatest risk of stent thrombosis, such as those with STEMI (COR IIb).[11]

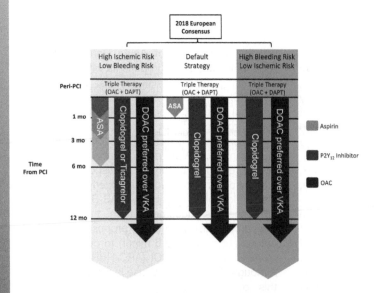

Fig. 4. European consensus recommendations on the management of antithrombotic therapy in patients with atrial fibrillation undergoing PCI. ASA, aspirin.

Oral Anticoagulation Selection and Dosage

Unless contraindicated, DOACs are favored over VKAs given their relative safety and ease of use.[10–13] Regarding dosing, the North American consensus document recommends DOACs as dosed in the AF-PCI trials. Because the 110-mg twice daily dose of dabigatran is not approved in the United States for stroke prevention, the 2018 AHA/ACC/HRS guidelines for AF recommend 150 mg twice daily (COR IIa, LOE B),[11] whereas the 2018 ESC guidelines on myocardial revascularization offer a COR IIa, LOE C recommendation for the 110-mg twice daily dose during TAT and a COR IIb, LOE B recommendation for the 150-mg twice daily dose during DAT.[13] The American and European guidelines also differ slightly in recommendations for rivaroxaban, 15 mg daily, with the 2019 ACC/AHA/HRS guidelines for AF providing a COR IIa, LOE B recommendation and the 2018 ESC guidelines for myocardial revascularization providing a COR IIb, LOE B recommendation.[11,13] When a decision is made to discontinue the $P2Y_{12}$ inhibitor (typically at 1 year), the North American and European consensus documents recommend increasing the OAC to its labeled dose.[10,12] Lastly, specific dosage recommendations for apixaban and edoxaban are not provided by either the guidelines or consensus documents, which were written prior to publication of the results from AUGUSTUS and ENTRUST-AF PCI. In both trials, the full recommended doses of DOACs were used, and it is likely that future guidelines and consensus documents will incorporate these options.[4,9]

Antiplatelet Regimen

The default $P2Y_{12}$ inhibitor per American and European guidelines and consensus documents should be clopidogrel.[10–13] The 2019 ACC/AHA/HRS guidelines for AF provide a COR IIa, LOE B recommendation for clopidogrel irrespective of TAT versus DAT strategy whereas the 2018 ESC guidelines for myocardial revascularization provide a COR IIa, LOE A recommendation for clopidogrel in DAT strategies and COR IIa, LOE B recommendation for clopidogrel during TAT treatment.[11,13] The 2018 ESC guidelines for myocardial revascularization caution against the use of more potent $P2Y_{12}$ inhibitors (ie, prasugrel or ticagrelor) in combination with OAC.[13] The North American consensus document also recommends against prasugrel, given the results from a small study that demonstrated a 4-fold increase in bleeding with prasugrel-based TAT[28] but recommends ticagrelor as a suitable option for patients at high

thrombotic and low bleeding risk who otherwise are not on triple therapy.[12]

Once the transition from TAT to DAT occurs, aspirin should be dropped in favor of continuing $P2Y_{12}$ inhibitor therapy.[10,12] A significant proportion of patients who undergo PCI might be hyporesponsive to clopidogrel.[29] High platelet reactivity on clopidogrel reflects inadequate platelet inhibition and has been associated with an increased risk of stent thrombosis.[29] Randomized trials comparing platelet function-guided antiplatelet therapy failed to show benefit,[30–32] but further research is needed to evaluate the use of platelet function testing to guide antiplatelet therapies in patients treated concurrently with OAC.

Long-Term Oral Anticoagulation

Upon completion of DAT therapy, patients should continue OAC monotherapy at the dose recommended for stroke prevention, accounting for renal function.[10,12] Because there appears to be little advantage to continuing SAPT plus OAC beyond 1 year,[33–35] these recommendations are aimed at reducing bleeding in patients with AF and stable CAD. Support for this recommendation comes from the Atrial Fibrillation and Ischemic Events With Rivaroxaban in Patients With Stable Coronary Artery Disease (AFIRE) trial.[36] The investigators randomized 2236 patients with stable CAD to rivaroxaban, 15 mg daily, or a DAT with rivaroxaban plus SAPT (70% aspirin vs. 27% P2Y12 inhibitor). When the trial was terminated because of increased mortality in the DAT group, rivaroxaban monotherapy was noninferior to DAT for the primary efficacy endpoint of all-cause mortality, MI, stroke, unstable angina requiring revascularization, or systemic embolism ($P<.001$) and superior to DAT for the primary safety endpoint of major bleeding.[36] Still, those at high thrombotic risk may benefit from a prolonged course of DAT. The ongoing French Assessment of Quitting versus Using Aspirin Therapy In Patients Treated With Oral Anticoagulation for Atrial Fibrillation and With Stabilized Coronary artery disease (AQUATIC) trial aims to study the superiority of DAT with aspirin plus OAC for 24 months to 48 months versus placebo plus OAC in high-risk, stable CAD-AF patients and will provide more data on this issue.

Additional Strategies and Future Directions

Other practices to incorporate in the routine care of AF-PCI patients include radial over femoral access, use of bivalirudin in HBR patients, use of newer-generation DES, use of proton pump inhibitors post-PCI for patients on DAPT or DAT/TAT,

Table 1
Ongoing trials evaluating antithrombotic strategies in patients with atrial fibrillation undergoing percutaneous coronary intervention

Trials	ClinicalTrials.gov Identifier	Target Population	Experimental Arm(s)	Control Arm	Endpoint(s)	Timeline	Anticipated Completion Date
APPROACH-ACS-AF (N = 400)	NCT02789917	ACS + NVAF or atrial flutter + successful PCI	Apixaban and clopidogrel for 6 mo	VKA, clopidogrel, and aspirin for 6 mo if HAS-BLED <3 VKA, clopidogrel, and aspirin for 1 mo followed by VKA and clopidogrel for 5 mo if HAS-BLED ≥3	Primary: major bleeding Secondary: combined death, MI, ST, STE	6 mo	TBD
COACH-AF-PCI (N = 1120)	NCT03536611	NVAF + successful PCI with DES	Dabigatran, aspirin, and clopidogrel for 1 mo followed by dabigatran and clopidogrel for 5 mo	Warfarin, aspirin and clopidogrel for 1 mo followed by Warfarin and Cclopidogrel for 5 mo	Primary: clinically relevant bleeding Secondary: death MI, STE, ischemia-induced revascularization	24 mo	June 2020
OPTIMAL-1/2 (N = 1550)	NCT03234114	ACS + NVAF + successful PCI with DES	OPTIMAL-1: warfarin, clopidogrel, and aspirin for 1 mo, then quit aspirin until 12 mo after PCI OPTIMAL-2: dabigatran with ticagrelor for 12 mo	OPTIMAL-1: warfarin, clopidogrel, and aspirin for 6 mo, then quit aspirin until 12 mo after PCI OPTIMAL-2: dabigatran with clopidogrel for 12 mo	OPTIMAL-1: combined death, MI, STE, unplanned revascularization OPTIMAL-2: major or clinically relevant bleeding	12 mo	December 2021
SAFE-A (N = 600)	N/A	NVAF + PCI with DES	Aspirin and apixaban for 12 mo with $P2Y_{12}$ inhibitor for 1 mo	Aspirin and apixaban for 12 mo with $P2Y_{12}$ inhibitor for 6 mo	Primary: all bleeding complications Secondary: combined death, MI, STE	12 mo	TBD

| MASTER-DAPT (N = 430) | NCT03023020 | HBR who underwent PCI | DAPT for 1 mo, then SAPT for 11 more months | DAPT for 6 mo, then aspirin for 6 more months | Combined death, MI, stroke, bleeding Major or clinically relevant bleeding | 12 mo | March 2021 |

Abbreviations: APPROACH-ACS-AF, APixaban Versus PhenpRoccoumon: Oral AntiCoagulation Plus Antiplatelet therapy in Patients With Acute Coronary Syndrome and Atrial Fibrillation; COACH-AF-PCI, Comparing Dabigatran Etexilate Versus Warfarin in Chinese Patients With Nonvalvular Atrial Fibrillation Who Undergo Percutaneous Coronary Intervention With Stenting (DES); MASTER-DAPT, Management of High Bleeding Risk Patients Post Bioresorbable Polymer Coated Stent Implantation With an Abbreviated Versus Prolonged DAPT Regimen; NVAF, nonvalvular atrial fibrillation; OPTIMAL-1/2, Optimal Antithrombotic Therapy for Acute Coronary Syndrome Patients Concomitant Atrial Fibrillation Undergoing New Generation Drug Eluting Stent Implantation; SAFE-A, SAFety and Effectiveness trial of Apixaban use in association with dual antiplatelet therapy in patients with AF undergoing percutaneous coronary intervention; STE, systemic thrombolic event; TBD, to be determined.

and avoidance of nonsteroidal anti-inflammatory drugs.[10,12] Finally, ongoing trials evaluating novel approaches to antithrombotic strategies using contemporary DES platforms will provide more data to inform clinical decision making (**Table 1**).

SUMMARY

PCI in the setting of AF necessitates concomitant antiplatelet and anticoagulant agents to prevent ischemic events. The totality of data supports use of a DOAC-based DAT strategy, combining OAC with a $P2Y_{12}$-receptor inhibitor for most patients requiring chronic OAC who undergo PCI. A TAT strategy should be considered in selected cases, when the thrombotic risk exceeds bleeding risk. In this setting, the optimal duration of aspirin, in combination with an OAC and a $P2Y_{12}$-receptor inhibitor, remains unclear and could vary from weeks to months. Finally, in patients who have completed an initial 6-month or 1-year course of DAT, withdrawal of the $P2Y_{12}$-receptor inhibitor and ongoing treatment with an OAC alone are recommended to reduce the risk of bleeding.

DISCLOSURE

Dr J.L. Halperin has received consulting fees from Boehringer Ingelheim, Bayer Healthcare, Ortho-McNeil-Janssen Pharmaceuticals, and Medtronic. Dr G. Giustino received consultation fees (Advisory Board) for Bristol-Myers Squibb/Pfizer. The other coauthors have no conflicts of interest to disclose.

REFERENCES

1. Baber U, Mastoris I, Mehran R. Balancing ischaemia and bleeding risks with novel oral anticoagulants. Nat Rev Cardiol 2015;12(2):66.
2. Mehta SR, Yusuf S, Peters RJ, et al. Effects of pretreatment with clopidogrel and aspirin followed by long-term therapy in patients undergoing percutaneous coronary intervention: the PCI-CURE study. Lancet 2001;358(9281):527–33.
3. van Rein N, Heide-Jorgensen U, Lijfering WM, et al. Major bleeding rates in atrial fibrillation patients on single, dual, or triple antithrombotic therapy. Circulation 2019;139(6):775–86.
4. Lopes RD, Heizer G, Aronson R, et al. Antithrombotic therapy after acute coronary syndrome or PCI in atrial fibrillation. N Engl J Med 2019;380(16):1509–24.
5. Gibson CM, Mehran R, Bode C, et al. Prevention of bleeding in patients with atrial fibrillation undergoing PCI. N Engl J Med 2016;375(25):2423–34.
6. Dewilde WJ, Oirbans T, Verheugt FW, et al. Use of clopidogrel with or without aspirin in patients taking oral anticoagulant therapy and undergoing percutaneous coronary intervention: an open-label, randomised, controlled trial. Lancet 2013;381(9872):1107–15.
7. Fiedler KA, Maeng M, Mehilli J, et al. Duration of triple therapy in patients requiring oral anticoagulation after drug-eluting stent implantation: the ISAR-TRIPLE trial. J Am Coll Cardiol 2015;65(16):1619–29.
8. Cannon CP, Bhatt DL, Oldgren J, et al. Dual antithrombotic therapy with dabigatran after PCI in atrial fibrillation. N Engl J Med 2017;377(16):1513–24.
9. Vranckx P, Valgimigli M, Eckardt L, et al. Edoxaban-based versus vitamin K antagonist-based antithrombotic regimen after successful coronary stenting in patients with atrial fibrillation (ENTRUST-AF PCI): a randomised, open-label, phase 3b trial. Lancet 2019;394(10206):1335–43.
10. Lip GYH, Collet JP, Haude M, et al. 2018 Joint European consensus document on the management of antithrombotic therapy in atrial fibrillation patients presenting with acute coronary syndrome and/or undergoing percutaneous cardiovascular interventions: a joint consensus document of the European Heart Rhythm association (EHRA), European Society of Cardiology Working Group on Thrombosis, European Association of Percutaneous Cardiovascular Interventions (EAPCI), and European Association of Acute Cardiac Care (ACCA) endorsed by the Heart Rhythm Society (HRS), Asia-Pacific Heart Rhythm Society (APHRS), Latin America Heart Rhythm Society (LAHRS), and Cardiac Arrhythmia Society of Southern Africa (CASSA). Europace 2019;21(2):192–3.
11. January CT, Wann LS, Calkins H, et al. 2019 AHA/ACC/HRS focused update of the 2014 AHA/ACC/HRS guideline for the management of patients with atrial fibrillation: a Report of the American College of Cardiology/American Heart association Task Force on clinical practice guidelines and the Heart Rhythm Society. J Am Coll Cardiol 2019;74(1):104–32.
12. Angiolillo DJ, Goodman SG, Bhatt DL, et al. Antithrombotic therapy in patients with atrial fibrillation treated with oral anticoagulation undergoing percutaneous coronary intervention. Circulation 2018;138(5):527–36.
13. Neumann FJ, Sousa-Uva M, Ahlsson A, et al. 2018 ESC/EACTS Guidelines on myocardial revascularization. Eur Heart J 2019;40(2):87–165.
14. Valgimigli M, Bueno H, Byrne RA, et al. 2017 ESC focused update on dual antiplatelet therapy in coronary artery disease developed in collaboration with EACTS: the Task Force for dual antiplatelet therapy in coronary artery disease of the European Society of Cardiology (ESC) and of the European

Association for Cardio-Thoracic Surgery (EACTS). Eur Heart J 2018;39(3):213–60.

15. Steffel J, Verhamme P, Potpara TS, et al. The 2018 European Heart Rhythm Association Practical Guide on the use of non-vitamin K antagonist oral anticoagulants in patients with atrial fibrillation. Eur Heart J 2018;39(16):1330–93.

16. Knuuti J, Wijns W, Saraste A, et al. 2019 ESC Guidelines for the diagnosis and management of chronic coronary syndromes. Eur Heart J 2020;41(3): 407–77.

17. Leon MB, Baim DS, Popma JJ, et al. A clinical trial comparing three antithrombotic-drug regimens after coronary-artery stenting. Stent Anticoagulation Restenosis Study Investigators. N Engl J Med 1998;339(23):1665–71.

18. Schomig A, Neumann FJ, Kastrati A, et al. A randomized comparison of antiplatelet and anticoagulant therapy after the placement of coronary-artery stents. N Engl J Med 1996;334(17):1084–9.

19. Bertrand ME, Legrand V, Boland J, et al. Randomized multicenter comparison of conventional anticoagulation versus antiplatelet therapy in unplanned and elective coronary stenting. The full anticoagulation versus aspirin and ticlopidine (fantastic) study. Circulation 1998;98(16):1597–603.

20. Urban P, Macaya C, Rupprecht HJ, et al. Randomized evaluation of anticoagulation versus antiplatelet therapy after coronary stent implantation in high-risk patients: the multicenter aspirin and ticlopidine trial after intracoronary stenting (MATTIS). Circulation 1998;98(20):2126–32.

21. Levine GN, Bates ER, Bittl JA, et al. 2016 ACC/AHA guideline focused update on duration of dual antiplatelet therapy in patients with coronary artery disease: a Report of the American College of Cardiology/American Heart association Task Force on clinical practice guidelines. J Am Coll Cardiol 2016;68(10):1082–115.

22. Mehran R, Baber U, Sharma SK, et al. Ticagrelor with or without aspirin in high-risk patients after PCI. N Engl J Med 2019;381(21):2032–42.

23. Hahn JY, Song YB, Oh JH, et al. Effect of P2Y12 inhibitor monotherapy vs dual antiplatelet therapy on cardiovascular events in patients undergoing percutaneous coronary intervention: the SMART-CHOICE randomized clinical trial. JAMA 2019;321(24): 2428–37.

24. Watanabe H, Domei T, Morimoto T, et al. Effect of 1-month dual antiplatelet therapy followed by clopidogrel vs 12-month dual antiplatelet therapy on cardiovascular and bleeding events in patients receiving PCI: the STOPDAPT-2 randomized clinical trial. JAMA 2019;321(24):2414–27.

25. Vranckx P, Valgimigli M, Juni P, et al. Ticagrelor plus aspirin for 1 month, followed by ticagrelor monotherapy for 23 months vs aspirin plus clopidogrel or ticagrelor for 12 months, followed by aspirin monotherapy for 12 months after implantation of a drug-eluting stent: a multicentre, open-label, randomised superiority trial. Lancet 2018;392(10151):940–9.

26. Gargiulo G, Goette A, Tijssen J, et al. Safety and efficacy outcomes of double vs. triple antithrombotic therapy in patients with atrial fibrillation following percutaneous coronary intervention: a systematic review and meta-analysis of non-vitamin K antagonist oral anticoagulant-based randomized clinical trials. Eur Heart J 2019;40(46):3757–67.

27. Urban P, Mehran R, Colleran R, et al. Defining high bleeding risk in patients undergoing percutaneous coronary intervention. Circulation 2019;140(3): 240–61.

28. Sarafoff N, Martischnig A, Wealer J, et al. Triple therapy with aspirin, prasugrel, and vitamin K antagonists in patients with drug-eluting stent implantation and an indication for oral anticoagulation. J Am Coll Cardiol 2013;61(20):2060–6.

29. Stone GW, Witzenbichler B, Weisz G, et al. Platelet reactivity and clinical outcomes after coronary artery implantation of drug-eluting stents (ADAPT-DES): a prospective multicentre registry study. Lancet 2013;382(9892):614–23.

30. Collet JP, Cuisset T, Range G, et al. Bedside monitoring to adjust antiplatelet therapy for coronary stenting. N Engl J Med 2012;367(22):2100–9.

31. Price MJ, Berger PB, Teirstein PS, et al. Standard- vs high-dose clopidogrel based on platelet function testing after percutaneous coronary intervention: the GRAVITAS randomized trial. JAMA 2011; 305(11):1097–105.

32. Cayla G, Cuisset T, Silvain J, et al. Platelet function monitoring to adjust antiplatelet therapy in elderly patients stented for an acute coronary syndrome (ANTARCTIC): an open-label, blinded-endpoint, randomised controlled superiority trial. Lancet 2016;388(10055):2015–22.

33. Lamberts M, Gislason GH, Lip GY, et al. Antiplatelet therapy for stable coronary artery disease in atrial fibrillation patients taking an oral anticoagulant: a nationwide cohort study. Circulation 2014;129(15): 1577–85.

34. Hamon M, Lemesle G, Tricot O, et al. Incidence, source, determinants, and prognostic impact of major bleeding in outpatients with stable coronary artery disease. J Am Coll Cardiol 2014;64(14):1430–6.

35. Alexander JH, Lopes RD, Thomas L, et al. Apixaban vs. warfarin with concomitant aspirin in patients with atrial fibrillation: insights from the ARISTOTLE trial. Eur Heart J 2014;35(4):224–32.

36. Yasuda S, Kaikita K, Akao M, et al. Antithrombotic therapy for atrial fibrillation with stable coronary disease. N Engl J Med 2019;381(12):1103–13.

State of the Art
No-Reflow Phenomenon

Gianluca Caiazzo, MD, PhD[a], Rita Leonarda Musci, MD[b], Lara Frediani, MD[c],
Julia Umińska, MD, PhD[d], Wojciech Wanha, MD, PhD[e], Krzysztof J. Filipiak, MD, PhD[f],
Jacek Kubica, MD, PhD[d], Eliano Pio Navarese, MD, PhD[d,g],*

KEYWORDS

• No-reflow • Primary PCI • Microvascular obstruction

KEY POINTS

- The term no reflow describes inadequate myocardial perfusion of a given segment without angiographic evidence of persistent mechanical obstruction of epicardial vessels.
- No reflow represents an independent predictor of death and myocardial infarction.
- Several strategies have been tested to treat the no-reflow phenomenon but none has been shown to be effective to revert it.

INTRODUCTION

The term no reflow refers to a state of myocardial tissue hypoperfusion in the presence of a patent epicardial coronary artery.[1] The underlying mechanism is microvascular obstruction (MVO). It can typically occur during primary percutaneous coronary intervention (PCI) in the setting of acute myocardial infarction (AMI) or, less frequently, during a PCI on a non–infarct-related artery.[2]

The coronary no-reflow phenomenon is an independent predictor of adverse clinical outcomes after AMI regardless of infarct size and is associated with heart failure, increased mortality, and malignant arrhythmias.[3,4] The incidence of the no-reflow phenomenon varies widely depending on available studies, patient complexity,[5,6] and the diagnostic methods used.

PREDISPOSING FACTORS

Several cardiovascular risk factors have been identified to portend a higher risk of no reflow, such as hypertension, smoking, dyslipidemia, diabetes, renal insufficiency, and other inflammatory processes.[7,8] Recent studies investigating the relationship between the inflammatory profile and the no-reflow phenomenon showed that elderly patients (>65 years old) have higher rates of no reflow, owing to their pronounced proinflammatory state.[9]

The concept that a higher thrombotic burden is associated with a higher risk of slow/no reflow has been confirmed by Kaya and colleagues,[10] showing that the presence of atrial fibrillation is associated with a 2-fold increase of risk to develop no reflow in patients with ST-segment elevation myocardial infarction (STEMI). However, other

[a] ICCU, San Giuseppe Moscati Hospital, ASL CE, Via Gramsci 1, Aversa 81031, Italy; [b] Department of Cardiology, Azienda Ospedaliera Bonomo, Viale Istria, Andria BT 76123, Italy; [c] Department of Cardiology, Livorno Hospital, Azienda Usl Toscana Nord-Ovest, Ospedali Riuniti di Livorno, Viale Vittorio Alfieri, 36, Livorno LI 57124, Italy; [d] Department of Cardiology, Collegium Medicum, Nicolaus Copernicus University, Bydgoszcz, SIRIO MEDICINE Network, ul. Jagiellońska 13-15, Bydgoszcz 85-067, Poland; [e] Division of Cardiology and Structural Heart Diseases, Medical University of Silesia, ul. Józefa Poniatowskiego 15, Kato 40–055, Katowice, Poland; [f] Department of Cardiology, Medical University of Warsaw, Żwirki i Wigury 61, Warszawa 02-091, Poland; [g] University of Alberta, 116 Street & 85 Avenue, Edmonton, AB T6G 2R3, Canada
* Corresponding author. 9 Skłodowskiej-Curie Street, Bydgoszcz 85-094, Poland.
E-mail address: elianonavarese@gmail.com

Cardiol Clin 38 (2020) 563–573
https://doi.org/10.1016/j.ccl.2020.07.001

patient-specific factors are more closely related to the no-reflow phenomenon, such as delayed presentation to the catheterization laboratory during STEMI.[11] Based on this, evidence has been accumulated that a shorter door-to-balloon time is associated with less myocardial injury and a lower incidence of no reflow.[12]

Polymorphisms of the gene coding for vascular endothelial growth factor A were shown to be associated with impaired microvascular tone.[13]

Barman and colleagues[14] showed an association between CHA2DS2-VASc (congestive heart failure; hypertension; age ≥75 years; diabetes mellitus; prior stroke, transient ischemic attack, or thromboembolism; vascular disease; age 65–74 years; sex category) score and a higher risk of no reflow in patients with non–ST-elevation myocardial infarction undergoing PCI.

MECHANISMS OF NO REFLOW

The no-reflow phenomenon was first described by Krug and colleagues[15] in 1966. Later, it was shown in experimental animal models that prolonged ischemia impairs perfusion and leads to damage of the arterial microvasculature, which is proportionally greater for longer time periods of ischemia.[16] Such impairment is caused by the swelling of endothelial cells of the small blood vessels leading to obstruction and consequent slow flow. As a consequence of the ischemia-reperfusion damage, the endothelial dysfunction, and the distal thromboembolism, the clearance of debris by macrophages is inhibited and this event results in poor healing of the infarcted area and adverse remodeling.[17] Infarct size is a major determinant of patients' prognosis and is associated with clinical events and cardiovascular mortality.[18] The angiographic feature of no reflow was first reported by Bates and colleagues[19] as abnormal slow antegrade flow of contrast in a culprit vessel, whereas the first clinical case of no reflow during PCI for myocardial infarction (MI) was reported by Feld and colleagues[20]. It has been widely shown that the no-reflow phenomenon is significantly correlated with poor clinical outcomes and, although advances in interventional techniques have reduced its incidence,[21] still represents an independent predictor of death and MI.[3,4]

Distal embolization has been identified as one of the most intuitive causes of no reflow. Thromboembolic material can originate from epicardial coronary thrombus and from fissured plaques during primary PCI (pPCI).[22] As an experimental confirmation of this, old studies have shown that myocardial blood flow decreases irreversibly when microspheres obstruct more than 50% of coronary capillaries.[23] Another mechanism subtending the no-reflow phenomenon has been identified with prolonged ischemia. The ischemic injury produces morphologic changes of the endothelial cells (protrusions and membrane-bound bodies), which can contribute to luminal obliteration. The consequent loss of vascular tone causes extravasation of erythrocytes, resulting in interstitial edema further compressing the microvascular circulation.[15] Reperfusion after ischemia represent a traumatic stage for coronary microcirculation, with platelets and neutrophils extensively infiltrating it and forming aggregates that obstruct capillaries and consequently block flow.[24] Reperfusion-related injury develops from this step, with activated neutrophils releasing oxygen free radicals and proinflammatory mediators that can directly cause tissue and endothelial damage. Also, damaged endothelial cells, neutrophils, and platelets contribute to sustained vasoconstriction of coronary microcirculation.[25]

Therefore, based on the underlying mechanisms, 2 types of no reflow can be identified: structural and functional no reflow.

Structural no reflow occurs when microvessels within the necrotic myocardium region under prolonged ischemia show damage and loss of capillary integrity with endothelial swelling, edema, and MVO. Structural no reflow is largely irreversible.[26]

Functional no reflow is observed when the patency of microvasculature is compromised because of spasm, microthrombotic embolization, and reperfusion injury, with accumulation of neutrophils and platelets and activation of the neurohumoral system. At variance with the structural counterpart, functional no reflow may be reversible to a varying degree.[26]

DIAGNOSTIC METHODS
Angiographic Methods

Not all no-reflow types are created equal. The causes subtending this phenomenon can be various and multifactorial, and their identification has an effect on the following therapeutic options. The classification of different grades of angiographic coronary blood flow has been established according to the Thrombolysis in Myocardial Infarction (TIMI) scale.[27] No reflow can initially be shown by the analysis of TIMI flow grade. TIMI flow grade 0 to 2, observed in 5% to 10% of patients, is predictably associated with no reflow. However, no reflow also occurs in a sizable proportion of patients with apparently successful large epicardial vessel reopening resulting in TIMI flow grade 3, caused by microvasculature and not epicardial vessel involvement. In addition to the TIMI scale, another imaging technique can be useful to confirm the angiographic diagnosis and assess myocardial microvasculature, and this is the myocardial blush grade (MBG).[28] With this method, angiographers assess the myocardial tissue opacification intensity with longer angiographic runs, performed until the venous phase of contrast passage. According to visual or computerized signal intensity automatic assessment, myocardial blush is graded using a scale with 4 intensity grades: 0, no myocardial blush; 1, minimal myocardial blush or contrast density; 2, moderate myocardial blush or contrast density, but less than that obtained during angiography of a contralateral non–infarct-related coronary artery; 3, normal myocardial blush or contrast density, similar to that obtained during angiography of a contralateral non–infarct-related coronary artery. Using the combined angiographic criteria of TIMI and MBG, no reflow can be classified as TIMI flow grade less than or equal to 2 and with MBG from 0 to 1.

Non Angiographic Methods

Several noninvasive diagnostic methods have been shown to be able to identify MVO, among them ST resolution at electrocardiogram (ECG), myocardial contrast echocardiography, cardiac magnetic resonance (CMR), and coronary flow velocity and coronary flow reserve (by means of intracoronary Doppler wires).[19] ST resolution at ECG is an easy bedside method of assessing myocardial perfusion following PCI. An ST resolution less than 70% at 60 minutes is a marker of no reflow.[29] Myocardial contrast echocardiography uses ultrasonography to visualize contrast microbubbles that flow through patent coronary microvessels. Lack of intramyocardial contrast can reveal MVO and correlates with the extent of no reflow.[30] CMR is regarded as the most sensitive and specific method to assess the extent of no reflow. The best timing, in terms of predictive value, seems to be 1 week after MI, when the resolution of the MI-related edema occurs.

No reflow can be diagnosed as (1) lack of gadolinium enhancement during the first pass; and (2) lack of gadolinium enhancement within a necrotic region, identified by late gadolinium hyperenhancement.[31]

Intracoronary Doppler guidewire is used to measure coronary flow velocity and coronary flow reserve. These parameters are standard methods for assessing microvascular function. During no reflow, this technique usually shows systolic flow reversal, reduced antegrade flow, and forward diastolic flow with rapid deceleration slope.[32]

STAGES OF NO-REFLOW AND THERAPEUTIC MEASURES
Prevention Before Reperfusion

Different therapeutic strategies can be implemented in a temporal phase occurring before and during no-reflow onset (**Fig. 1**). They are based on the treatment of predisposing factors of no reflow, such as increased lipid levels and glucose plasma concentrations, and smoking cessation. After chest pain onset, in patients with STEMI the goal is to reduce the time to ischemia, shortening the arrival to the catheterization laboratory to guarantee timely reperfusion with pPCI.

Within this temporal phase, the adoption of noninvasive therapies as remote ischemic preconditioning (IPC) may offer some degree of cardioprotection. Brief ischemia in an organ that is distant or remote from the heart, such as a limb, also reduces MI in experimental models. Cycles of intermittent limb ischemia provide an acceptable method for inducing cardioprotection, and early experimental studies have confirmed the effectiveness of remote IPC in cardiac surgery and coronary angioplasty, as assessed by reduced markers of cardiac injury.[33,34]

In the Catheterization Laboratory

Identified procedural predictors of angiographic no reflow are high thrombus burden,[35] predilatation,[36] long coronary lesions (>15 mm),[37] and reperfusion time greater than 6 hours.[38,39] During the primary PCI, distal microvascular plugs in the microcirculation, local inflammation, and hemorrhage can occur, leading to the angiographic appearance of no reflow. To counteract this significant flow impairment, both interventional and pharmacologic therapies have been tested.

NON PHARMACOLOGIC THERAPIES

Among procedural strategies for no-reflow prevention, direct stenting, nominal pressure stent deployment, stent postdilation avoidance, and manual thrombectomy before the intervention are included. Manual thrombectomy has been shown to be correlated to lower no-reflow incidence in several studies, although a positive significant impact on clinical outcomes is still debated.[40–42] Some recent meta-analyses and trials questioned its beneficial effect on mortality, raising safety concerns in terms of stroke.[43,44] For this reason, manual thrombectomy is not recommended as a routine approach during STEMI and should

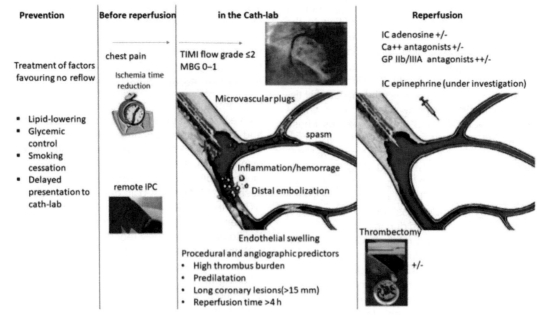

Fig. 1. Therapeutic measures applied at different stages to prevent or treat the no-reflow phenomenon. Cath-lab, catheterization laboratory; GP, glycoprotein; IC, intracoronary; IPC, ischemic preconditioning.

probably be limited to the presence of angiographically large thrombotic burden.[45] Also, different devices for embolic protection have been tested in the past but the effectiveness of their routine use during primary PCI for STEMI in terms of microvascular flow improvement has not been shown.[46,47] Of note, in a recent randomized trial, the use of distal embolic protection applied with a filter device decreased the incidence of the no-reflow phenomenon after revascularization compared with conventional PCI in patients with acute coronary syndrome with attenuated plaque identified by intravascular ultrasonography[48] (**Table 1**).

PHARMACOLOGIC THERAPIES

Pharmacologic management has probably been the most used therapeutic option for functional slow-flow/no-reflow phenomenon and still represents the most effective strategy in the catheterization laboratory to counteract no reflow in the acute setting (**Table 2**). Antiplatelet therapy is a cornerstone for AMI management and is essential as baseline therapy in order to prevent no reflow.[49]

Common oral antiplatelet drugs such as aspirin, clopidogrel, prasugrel, and ticagrelor are of paramount importance in order to counteract the early phase of thrombus formation.[50–52] However, they may not be sufficient as preventive therapies, and some evidence exists in favor of glycoprotein (GP) IIb/IIIa inhibitors as bailout therapy in the event of angiographic evidence of a large

thrombus, slow flow, or no reflow, and a mortality reduction is observed with the intracoronary compared with the intravenous administration.[53–55] No evidence is available with regard to the new intravenous P2Y12 receptor inhibitor cangrelor on this topic.

Adenosine and sodium nitroprusside (SNP) are probably the most evaluated adjunctive therapies designed to attenuate MVO and infarct size.

Adenosine produces smooth muscle relaxation in the coronary circulation, although evidence also suggests antiplatelet properties[56] as well as reduction of oxygen free radical formation. Initial studies focused on the use of adenosine following intervention for STEMI. The AMISTAD (Acute Myocardial Infarction Study of Adenosine) and AMISTAD-II trials (**Table 3**)[57,58] showed a significant reduction in infarct size, with high-dose adenosine administration not translating into better clinical outcomes. Recent meta-analyses reported discordant findings,[59,60] whereas the most recent randomized trial on the topic, the REFLO-STEMI (Reperfusion Facilitated by Local Adjunctive Therapy in STEMI) trial, comparing intracoronary administration of adenosine or SNP following thrombus aspiration, found that high-dose intracoronary adenosine and SNP during pPCI did not reduce infarct size or MVO measured by CMR imaging.[61] When sodium nitroprusside is injected distally in the coronary artery, it has negligible systemic effect on the blood pressure but

Table 1
Clinical and angiographic outcomes of interventional studies for prevention of coronary no-reflow phenomenon following primary percutaneous coronary intervention

Intervention		Study	Study Type	Patients (n)	Results
Nonphar-macologic therapies	Thrombus aspiration/ thrombectomy	Svilaas et al,[40] 2008	Randomized trial	1071	Lower myocardial blush grade of 0 or 1 in the thrombus-aspiration group
		De Vita et al,[41] 2009	Meta-analysis	2686	Lower all-cause mortality, reduced MACE, death, and MI rate
					Improved survival in patients treated with GP IIb/IIIa inhibitors
		Mongeon et al,[42] 2010	Meta-analysis	4299	Less no-reflow phenomenon, higher ST-segment resolution in the thrombus-aspiration group
					No 30-d benefit on mortality, reinfarction, and stroke
		Jolly et al,[43] 2015	Randomized trial	10,732	No 180-d benefit on CV death, recurrent MI, cardiogenic shock, or NYHA class IV
					Increased rate of stroke within 30 d
		Elgendy et al,[44] 2015	Meta-analysis	20,960	No benefit on clinical end points. Possible increase of risk of stroke
		De Luca et al,[45] 2013	Meta-analysis	18,306	Clinical outcomes not improved. Patients with thrombus grade >3: trend toward reduced CV death and increased stroke or transient ischemic attack
	Distal protection	Stone et al,[47] 2005	Randomized trial	501	Similar ST-segment resolution, infarct size, and clinical outcomes between groups (balloon occlusion and aspiration distal microcirculatory protection system vs angioplasty without distal protection)
		Kelbaek et al,[46] 2008	Randomized trial	626	Similar microvascular perfusion, infarct size, MACCE between groups (pPCI with distal protection vs conventional pPCI)
		Hibi et al,[48] 2018	Randomized trial	200	Lower incidence of no-reflow phenomenon, fewer serious adverse cardiac events in patients with ACS and attenuated plaque ≥5 mm in length at IVUS in the distal protection group vs conventional PCI

Abbreviations: ACS, acute coronary syndrome; CV, cardiovascular; GP IIb/IIIa, glycoprotein IIb/IIIa inhibitors; IVUS, intravascular ultrasonography; MACCE, major adverse cerebral and cardiovascular events; MACE, major adverse cardiovascular events; NYHA, New York Heart Association.
Data from Refs.[40–48]

Table 2
Pharmacologic agents currently used for no-reflow phenomenon treatment and principal characteristics

Drug	Dose	Mechanism of Action	Effects on Coronary Circulation	Side Effects
Antiplatelet Therapy				
Anti-GP IIb/IIIa		Inhibition of GP IIb-IIIa receptors	• Inhibition of platelet activation • Reduction of downstream embolization/local thrombus • No release of vasoactive-chemotactic mediators	Bleeding
Abciximab	IV bolus: 0.25 mg/kg; IV infusion: 0.125 µg/kg/min			
Eptifibatide	IV bolus: 180 µg/kg; IV infusion: 2 µg/kg/min			
Tirofiban	IV bolus: 25 µg/kg; IV infusion: 0.15 µg/kg/min			
Vasodilators				
Adenosine	IV: 70 µg/kg/min for 3 h IC: 48–200-µg bolus	Adenosine receptors activation	• Vasodilatation • PLTs: neutrophils inhibition • Reduction Ca^{2+} overload: ROS	Bradycardia, transient AV block, chest pain, dyspnea, headache, flushing, bronchospasm
Verapamil	IC: 100–250-µg bolus or 100-µg/min up to 1000 µg	Calcium-channel blocker	• Vasodilatation endothelium mediated • Reduction of myocardial O_2 demand	Hypotension, heart block
Diltiazem	IC: 400 µg			
Nicardipine	IC: 50–200-µg bolus (up to 500 µg)			
Nitroprusside	IC: 50–200-µg bolus	Nitric oxide donor Activation of guanylate cyclase	• Vasodilatation • Antiplatelet effects	Hypotension, cyanide toxicity
Nicorandil	IV: 8-mg/h infusion IC: 2-mg bolus	KATP channel opener Nicotinamide nitrate	• Vasodilatation • Reduction of Ca^{2+} overload • Neutrophil inhibition	Headaches, nausea, vomiting, flushing
Hormones				
Epinephrine	IC: 50–200 µg	β2-receptor activation	• Reduction of Ca^{2+} overload • Coronary vasodilatation	Arrhythmias
Mitochondrial Permeability Transition Pore Blocker				
Cyclosporine-a	IC: 2.5–10 mg/kg	Inhibition of opening of mitochondrial permeability transition pores	• Protective effect on mitochondrial function • Reduction of ROS	Kidney damage, hypertension, infection

Novel Therapies

| Liraglutide | Glucagonlike peptide-1 analogue | • Before reperfusion 1.8 mg
• 0.6 mg/2 days
• 1.2 mg/2 days
• 1.8 mg/3 days | • Inflammation reduction
• Vasodilatation, endothelial dependent
• Reduced monocyte adhesion
• Improved endothelial viability | Nausea, loss of appetite, runny nose, rash |

Abbreviations: AV, atrioventricular; IC, intracoronary; IV, intravenous; PLTs, platelets; ROS, reactive oxygen species.

Table 3
Clinical and angiographic outcomes of pharmacologic studies for prevention and/or treatment of coronary no-reflow phenomenon following primary percutaneous coronary intervention

	Drug	Study	Study Type	Patients (n)	Results
Pharmacologic therapies	GP IIb/IIIa inhibitors	Navarese et al,[53] 2012	Meta-analysis	1246	Intracoronary administration of abciximab is associated with significant benefits in mortality at short-term follow-up compared to IV abciximab administration, in STEMI patients undergoing PPCI
		Van't Hof et al,[54] 2008	Randomized trial	984	Routine prehospital initiation of high-bolus-dose tirofiban improved ST-segment resolution and clinical outcome after PCI
	Vasodilators (adenosine, nitroprusside)	Mahaffey et al,[57] 1999	Randomized trial	236	Adenosine resulted in a significant reduction in infarct size
		Ross et al,[58] 2005	Randomized trial	2118	Adenosine did not improve clinical outcomes in patients with STEMI undergoing reperfusion; infarct size was reduced
		Navarese et al,[59] 2012	Meta-analysis	3821	Adenosine showed beneficial effect on postprocedural coronary flow not associated with consistent advantages on clinical outcomes
		Polimeni et al,[60] 2016	Meta-analysis	1487	Intracoronary adenosine associated with lower incidence MACE
		Nazir et al,[61] 2016	Randomized trial	247	High-dose intracoronary adenosine and SNP during pPCI did not reduce infarct size or MVO measured by CMR. Adenosine may adversely affect midterm clinical outcome
		Zaho et al,[62] 2014	Meta-analysis	781	Intracoronary nitroprusside reduces the incidence of no-reflow during pPCI as well as the incidence of MACE
	Nicorandil	Iwakura et al,[63] 2009	Meta-analysis	1337	Nicorandil reduced the incidence of TIMI flow grade ≥2
	Cyclosporine	Cung et al,[64] 2015	Randomized trial	970	IV cyclosporine did not show better clinical outcomes and did not prevent adverse left ventricular remodeling at 1 y
	Liraglutide	Chen et al,[66] 2016	Randomized trial	284	Lower no-reflow prevalence

Data from Refs.[53,54,57–64,66]

induces marked improvement in coronary flow and myocardial tissue blush. Recent meta-analyses confirmed a clear benefit of nitroprusside in the management of no reflow during PCI.[62] Calcium-channel blockers, nicorandil, cyclosporine-A, and dabigatran have also been investigated as pharmacologic therapy in the context of no reflow, but no definitive conclusions exist regarding their efficacy.[63–65] Recently, the results of a small randomized trial have been reported, showing a potential for the glucagonlike peptide (GLP)-1 analogue liraglutide to reduce no reflow.[66] Adrenaline (epinephrine) also represents an interesting drug in the context of the no-reflow phenomenon, given its potent β2-receptor agonist properties that mediate coronary vasodilatation, increasing coronary blood flow. Several observational data show the significantly positive impact on coronary circulation mediated by adrenaline.[67] For these reasons, intracoronary adrenaline might have the potential to revert no-reflow instances.

SUMMARY

The occurrence of the no-reflow phenomenon still represents an important clinical issue during pPCI and can negate the benefits of restoring culprit-vessel patency. Novel promising therapeutic options are on the horizon, such as intracoronary adrenaline, which will be tested in future studies.

DISCLOSURE

The authors have no commercial or financial conflicts of interest; no funding has been received for this article.

REFERENCES

1. Rezkalla SH, Kloner RA. Coronary no-reflow phenomenon: from the experimental laboratory to the cardiac catheterization laboratory. Catheter Cardiovasc Interv 2008;72(7):950–7.
2. Rezkalla SH, Stankowski RV, Hanna J, et al. Management of no-reflow phenomenon in the catheterization laboratory. JACC Cardiovasc Interv 2017; 10(3):215–23.
3. Ndrepepa G, Tiroch K, Fusaro M, et al. 5-year prognostic value of no-reflow phenomenon after percutaneous coronary intervention in patients with acute myocardial infarction. J Am Coll Cardiol 2010;55: 2383–9.
4. Wu KC, Zerhouni EA, Judd RM, et al. Prognostic significance of microvascular obstruction by magnetic resonance imaging in patients with acute myocardial infarction. Circulation 1998;97:765–72.
5. Morishima I, Sone T, Okumura K, et al. Angiographic no-reflow phenomenon as a predictor of adverse long-term outcome in patients treated with percutaneous transluminal coronary angioplasty for first acute myocardial infarction. J Am Coll Cardiol 2000;36:1202–9.
6. Durante A, Camici PG. Novel insights into an "old" phenomenon: the no-reflow. Int J Cardiol 2015;187: 273–80.
7. Iwakura K, Ito H, Ikushima M, et al. Association between hyperglycemia and the no-reflow phenomenon in patients with acute myocardial infarction. J Am Coll Cardiol 2003;41:1–7.
8. Navarese EP, Kowalewski M, Andreotti F, et al. Meta-analysis of time-related benefits of statin therapy in patients with acute coronary syndrome undergoing percutaneous coronary intervention. Am J Cardiol 2014;113(10):1753–64.
9. Del Turco S, Basta G, De Caterina AR, et al. Different inflammatory profile in young and elderly STEMI patients undergoing primary percutaneous coronary intervention (PPCI): its influence on no-reflow and mortality. Int J Cardiol 2019;290:34–9.
10. Kaya A, Keskin M, Tatlisu MA, et al. Atrial fibrillation: a novel risk factor for no-reflow following primary percutaneous coronary intervention. Angiology 2020;71(2):175–82.
11. Rezkalla SH, Dharmashankar KC, Abdalrahman IB, et al. No-reflow phenomenon following percutaneous coronary intervention for acute myocardial infarction: incidence, outcome, and effect of pharmacologic therapy. J Interv Cardiol 2010;23: 429–36.
12. Magro M, Springeling T, Jan van Geuns R, et al. Myocardial 'no-reflow' prevention. Curr Vasc Pharmacol 2013;11:263–77.
13. Yoshino S, Ciluffo R, Best PJ, et al. A single nucleotide polymorphism associated with abnormal coronary micro-vascular function. Coron Artery Dis 2014;25:281–9.
14. Barman HA, Kahyaoglu S, Durmaz E, et al. The CHADS-VASc score is a predictor of no-reflow in patients with non-ST-segment elevation myocardial infarction. Coron Artery Dis 2020;31(1):7–12.
15. Krug A, de Rochemont WM, Korb G. Blood supply of the myocardium after temporary coronary occlusion. Circ Res 1996;19:57–62.
16. Kloner RA, Ganote CE, Jennings RB. The "no-reflow" phenomenon after temporary coronary occlusion in the dog. J Clin Invest 1974;54:1496–506.
17. Bolognese L, Carrabba N, Parodi G, et al. Impact of microvascular dysfunction on left ventricular remodeling and long-term clinical outcome after primary coronary angioplasty for acute myocardial infarction. Circulation 2004;109:1121–6.
18. Stone GW, Selker HP, Thiele H, et al. Relationship between infarct size and outcomes following primary PCI: patient-level analysis from 10 randomized trials. J Am Coll Cardiol 2016;67:1674–83.

19. Bates ER, Krell MJ, Dean EN, et al. Demonstration of 'no-reflow' phenomenon by digital coronary arteriography. Am J Cardiol 1986;57:177–8.

20. Feld H, Lichstien E, Schachter J, et al. Early and late angiographic findings of the 'no-reflow' phenomenon following direct angioplasty as the primary treatment for acute myocardial infarction. Am Heart J 1992;123:782–4.

21. Salinas P, Jimenez-Valero S, Moreno R, et al. Update in pharmacological management of coronary no-reflow phenomenon. Cardiovasc Hematol Agents Med Chem 2012;10(3):256–64.

22. Skyschally A, Leineweber K, Gres P, et al. Coronary microembolization. Basic Res Cardiol 2006;101:373–82.

23. Hori M, Inoue M, Kitakaze M, et al. Role of adenosine in hyperemic response of coronary blood flow in microembolization. Am J Physiol 1986;250:H509–18.

24. Tantry US, Navarese EP, Myat A, et al. Combination oral antithrombotic therapy for the treatment of myocardial infarction: recent developments. Expert Opin Pharmacother 2018;19:653–65.

25. Ito BR, Schmid-Schönbein G, Engler RL. Effects of leukocyte activation on myocardial vascular resistance. Blood Cells 1990;16:145–63.

26. Galiuto L. Optimal therapeutic strategies in the setting of post-infarct no-reflow: the need for a pathological classification. Heart 2004;90:123–5.

27. The TIMI Study Group. The Thrombolysis in myocardial infarction [TIMI] trial. Phase I findings. N Engl J Med 1985;312:932–6.

28. Van't Hof AW, Liem A, Suryapranata H, et al, Zwolle Myocardial Infarction Study Group. Angiographic assessment of myocardial reperfusion in patients treated with primary angioplasty for acute myocardial infarction: myocardial blush grade. Circulation 1998;97:2302–6.

29. Schroder R. Prognostic impact of early ST-segment resolution in acute ST-elevation myocardial infarction. Circulation 2004;110:e506–10.

30. Iliceto S, Marangelli V, Marchese A, et al. Myocardial contrast echocardiography in acute myocardial infarction. Pathophysiological background and clinical applications. Eur Heart J 1996;17:344–53.

31. Albert TS, Kim RJ, Judd RM. Assessment of no-reflow regions using cardiac MRI. Basic Res Cardiol 2006;101:383–90.

32. Yamamuro A, Akasaka T, Tamita K, et al. Coronary flow velocity pattern immediately after percutaneous coronary intervention as a predictor of complications and in-hospital survival after acute myocardial infarction. Circulation 2002;106:3051–6.

33. Kharbanda RK, Mortensen UM, White PA, et al. Transient limb ischemia induces remote ischemic preconditioning in vivo. Circulation 2002;106:2881–3.

34. Kharbanda RK, Nielsen TT, Redington AN. Translation of remote ischaemic preconditioning into clinical practice. Lancet 2009;374:1557–65.

35. Yip HK, Chen MC, Chang HW, et al. Angiographic morphologic features of infarct-related arteries and timely reperfusion in acute myocardial infarction: predictors of slow-flow and no-reflow phenomenon. Chest 2002;122:1322–32.

36. Piscione F, Piccolo R, Cassese S, et al. Is direct stenting superior to stenting with predilation in patients treated with percutaneous coronary intervention? Results from a meta-analysis of 24 randomised controlled trials. Heart 2010;96(8):588–94.

37. Tasar O, Karabay AK, Oduncu V, et al. Predictors and outcomes of no-reflow phenomenon in patients with acute ST-segment elevation myocardial infarction undergoing primary percutaneous coronary intervention. Coron Artery Dis 2019;30(4):270–6.

38. Mazhar J, Mashicharan M, Farshid A. Predictors and outcome of no-reflow post primary percutaneous coronary intervention for ST elevation myocardial infarction. Int J Cardiol Heart Vasc 2015;10:8–12.

39. Nallamothu BK, Bradley EH, Krumholz HM. Time to treatment in primary percutaneous coronary intervention. N Engl J Med 2007;357:1631–8.

40. Svilaas T, Vlaar PJ, van der Horst IC, et al. Thrombus aspiration during primary percutaneous coronary intervention. N Engl J Med 2008;358:557–67.

41. De Vita M, Burzotta F, Biondi-Zoccai GG, et al. Individual patient-date meta-analysis comparing clinical outcome in patients with ST-elevation myocardial infarction treated with percutaneous coronary intervention with or without prior thrombectomy. ATTEMPT study: a pooled Analysis of Trials on ThrombEctomy in Acute Myocardial infarction based on individual PatienT data. Vasc Health Risk Manag 2009;5:243–7.

42. Mongeon FP, Bélisle P, Joseph L, et al. Adjunctive thrombectomy for acute myocardial infarction: a Bayesian meta- analysis. Circ Cardiovasc Interv 2010;3:6–16.

43. Jolly SS, Cairns JA, Yusuf S, et al. Stroke in the TOTAL trial: a randomized trial of routine thrombectomy vs. percutaneous coronary intervention alone in ST elevation myocardial infarction. Eur Heart J 2015;36:2364–72.

44. Navarese EP, Tarantini T, Musumeci G, et al. Manual vs mechanical thrombectomy during PCI for STEMI: a comprehensive direct and adjusted indirect meta-analysis of randomized trials. Am J Cardiovasc Dis 2013;3(3):146–57.

45. De Luca G, Navarese EP, Suryapranata H. A meta-analytic overview of thrombectomy during primary angioplasty. Int J Cardiol 2013;166(3):606–12.

46. Kelbaek H, Terkelsen CJ, Helqvist S, et al. Randomized comparison of distal protection versus conventional treatment in primary percutaneous coronary intervention: the drug elution and distal protection

in ST-elevation myocardial infarction (DEDICATION) trial. J Am Coll Cardiol 2008;51:899–905.

47. Stone GW, Webb J, Cox DA, et al. Distal microcirculatory protection during percutaneous coronary intervention in acute ST-segment elevation myocardial infarction: a randomized controlled trial. JAMA 2005;293:1063–72.

48. Hibi K, Kozuma K, Sonoda S, et al, VAMPIRE 3 Investigators. A randomized study of distal filter protection versus conventional treatment during percutaneous coronary intervention in patients with attenuated plaque identified by intravascular ultrasound. JACC Cardiovasc Interv 2018;11(16): 1545–55.

49. Gurbel PA, Jeong YH, Navarese EP, et al. Platelet-mediated thrombosis: from bench to bedside. Circ Res 2016;118(9):1380–91.

50. Adamski P, Adamska U, Ostrowska M, et al. Evaluating current and emerging antithrombotic therapy currently available for the treatment of acute coronary syndrome in geriatric populations. Expert Opin Pharmacother 2018;19(13):1415–25.

51. Navarese EP, Buffon A, Kozinski M, et al. A critical overview on ticagrelor in acute coronary syndromes. QJM 2013;106(2):105–15.

52. Tantry US, Navarese EP, Myat A, et al. Selection of P2Y12 inhibitor in percutaneous coronary intervention and/or acute coronary syndrome. Prog Cardiovasc Dis 2018;60(4–5):460–70.

53. Navarese EP, Kozinski M, Obonska K, et al. Clinical efficacy and safety of intracoronary vs. intravenous abciximab administration in STEMI patients undergoing primary percutaneous coronary intervention: a meta-analysis of randomized trials. Platelets 2012;23(4):274–81.

54. Van't Hof AW, Ten Berg J, Heestermans T, et al, Ongoing Tirofiban in Myocardial infarction Evaluation (On-TIME) 2 Study Group. Prehospital initiation of tirofiban in patients with ST-elevation myocardial infarction undergoing primary angioplasty (On-TIME 2): a multicentre, double-blind, randomised controlled trial. Lancet 2008;372(9638):537–46.

55. De Luca G, Navarese E, Marino P. Risk profile and benefits from Gp IIb-IIIa inhibitors among patients with ST-segment elevation myocardial infarction treated with primary angioplasty: a meta-regression analysis of randomized trials. Eur Heart J 2009;30:2705–13.

56. Johnson-Cox HA, Yang D, Ravid K. Physiological implications of adenosine receptor- mediated platelet aggregation. J Cell Physiol 2011;226:46–51.

57. Mahaffey KW, Puma JA, Barbagelata NA, et al. Adenosine as an adjunct to thrombolytic therapy for acute myocardial infarction: results of a multicenter, randomized, placebo-controlled trial: the Acute Myocardial Infarction STudy of Adenosine (AMISTAD) trial. J Am Coll Cardiol 1999;34:1711–20.

58. Ross AM, Gibbons RJ, Stone GW, et al. AMISTAD-II Investigators. A randomized, double-blinded, placebo- controlled multicenter trial of adenosine as an adjunct to reperfusion in the treatment of acute myocardial infarction (AMISTAD-II). J Am Coll Cardiol 2005;45:1775–80.

59. Navarese EP, Buffon A, Andreotti F, et al. Adenosine improves post-procedural coronary flow but not clinical outcomes in patients with acute coronary syndrome: a meta-analysis of randomized trials. Atherosclerosis 2012;222:1–7.

60. Polimeni A, De Rosa S, Sabatino J, et al. Impact of intracoronary adenosine administration during primary PCI: a meta-analysis. Int J Cardiol 2016;203: 1032–41.

61. Nazir SA, Khan JN, Mahmoud IZ, et al. The REFLO-STEMI (REperfusion Facilitated by LOcal adjunctive therapy in ST-Elevation Myocardial Infarction) trial: a randomised controlled trial comparing intracoronary administration of adenosine or sodium nitroprusside with control for attenuation of microvascular obstruction during primary percutaneous coronary intervention. Southampton (United Kingdom): NIHR Journals Library; 2016.

62. Zhao S, Qi G, Tian W, et al. Effect of intracoronary nitroprusside in preventing no-reflow phenomenon during primary percutaneous coronary intervention: a meta-analysis. J Interv Cardiol 2014;27:356–64.

63. Iwakura J, Ito H, Okamura A, et al. Nicorandil treatment in patients with acute myocardial infarction: a meta-analysis. Circ J 2009;73:925–31.

64. Cung TT, Morel O, Cayla G, et al. Cyclosporine before PCI in patients with acute myocardial infarction. N Engl J Med 2015;373:1021–31.

65. Hale SL, Kloner RA. Dabigatran treatment: effects on infarct size and the no-reflow phenomenon in a model of acute myocardial ischemia/reperfusion. J Thromb Thrombolysis 2015;39:50–4.

66. Chen WR, Tian F, Chen YD, et al. Effects of liraglutide on no-reflow in patients with acute ST-segment elevation myocardial infarction. Int J Cardiol 2016; 208:109–14.

67. Navarese EP, Frediani L, Kandzari DE, et al. Efficacy and safety of intracoronary epinephrine versus conventional treatments alone in STEMI patients with refractory coronary no-reflow during primary PCI: The RESTORE observational study. Catheter Cardiovasc Interv 2020. [Epub ahead of print].

Coronary Physiology Assessment for the Diagnosis and Treatment of Coronary Artery Disease

Elisabetta Moscarella, MD[a,b],*, Felice Gragnano, MD[a,b],
Arturo Cesaro, MD[a,b], Alfonso Ielasi, MD[c], Vincenzo Diana, MD[a,b],
Matteo Conte, MD[a,b], Alessandra Schiavo, MD[a,b], Silvio Coletta, MD[a,b],
Dario Di Maio, MD[a,b], Fabio Fimiani, MD[a,b], Paolo Calabrò, MD, PhD[a,b]

KEYWORDS

- Percutaneous coronary intervention • Physiologic assessment • FFR • IFR • QFR

KEY POINTS

- Percutaneous coronary intervention is a well-established treatment option in patients with coronary artery disease. Survival benefit has been demonstrated, however, only by treating coronary lesions responsible for myocardial ischemia.
- Fractional flow reserve (FFR) is the gold standard for the analysis of lesion severity. Its use is limited, however, by reimbursement (not available in some countries, such as Italy) and the need for adenosine, which adds time, complexity, and potential side effects to the procedure.
- Nonhyperemic instantaneous wave-free ratio (iFR)-guided revascularization showed safety and effectiveness with respect to adverse events at 12-month. Newer tools, such as resting full-cycle ratio, diastolic hyperemia-free ratio (DFR), and the diastolic pressure ratio (dPR), showed good accuracy compared with FFR and iFR.
- Less invasive quantitative flow ratio (QFR) enables FFR computation from 3-dimensional quantitative coronary angiography and thrombolysis in myocardial infarction frame counting. Data showed a good performance of QFR with an excellent agreement and correlation with FFR.
- Nowadays, simple physiologic assessment of coronary stenosis is essential for interventional cardiologists. The use of any of these tools needs to be implemented to improve patient care.

INTRODUCTION

Coronary artery disease (CAD) and its consequences remain the leading causes of premature death and lifelong disability in most countries.[1] The main issue in treating CAD by percutaneous coronary intervention (PCI) is to distinguish lesions that are responsible for ischemia from those that are not. Although stenting functionally significant coronary lesions provides survival benefit and relief of symptoms, no benefit has been shown in treating nonfunctionally significant lesions.[2,3] So, demonstration of myocardial ischemia is the key aspect to decide whether or not PCI has to be performed.

Angiographic assessment of disease severity is weakened numerous limitations, because both physician visual assessment and quantitative

[a] Division of Clinical Cardiology, A.O.R.N. "Sant'Anna e San Sebastiano", Via F. Palasciano, Caserta 81100, Italy;
[b] Department of Translational Medical Sciences, University of Campania "Luigi Vanvitelli", Naples 80131, Italy;
[c] Clinical and Interventional Cardiology Unit, Istituto Clinico S. Ambrogio, Via Faravelli 16, Milan 20149, Italy
* Corresponding author. Division of Clinical Cardiology, A.O.R.N. "Sant'Anna e San Sebastiano", Via F. Palasciano, Caserta 81100, Italy.
E-mail address: elisabetta.moscarella@gmail.com

Cardiol Clin 38 (2020) 575–588
https://doi.org/10.1016/j.ccl.2020.07.003

coronary analysis (QCA) have shown poor correlation with functional stenosis severity. For these reasons, invasive functional assessment must be available and used before revascularization in patients with a high likelihood of CAD undergoing early angiography or when noninvasive functional imaging tests either are not available or are inconclusive.[4]

Intracoronary transgradient pressure measurement through fractional flow reserve (FFR) has become the gold standard for the assessment of lesion severity.[5] FFR measurement, however, requires adenosine administration to induce hyperemia, which limits its use in clinical practice. Thus, interest has been focused on indices derived from resting gradient alone, not requiring hyperemia, such as distal coronary pressure–to–aortic pressure (Pd/Pa), the Pd/Pa measured during contrast-induced hyperemia (cFFR) or instantaneous wave-free ratio (iFR), and resting full-cycle ratio (RFR). Both hyperemic and nonhyperemic indices, however, require invasive pressure guide wire utilization. More recently, the less invasive quantitative flow ratio (QFR) has emerged as a new tool to assess the functional significance of coronary lesions, showing excellent correlation with FFR.

The aim of this review is to provide a comprehensive overview of existing evidence regarding the physiologic assessment of coronary lesions and highlight newly available options in the field.

IMPORTANCE OF ISCHEMIA AND RATIONALE FOR PERCUTANEOUS CORONARY INTERVENTION

Coronary stenosis are defined as functionally significant if they are resposible for inducible myocardial ischemia. Several studies demonstrated that the presence of ischemia correlates with adverse clinical outcomes[6] and that the greater the extent of jeopardized myocardium, the higher the risk of death or myocardial infarction (MI).

Correct identification of functionally significant coronary lesions is of paramount is mandatory to properly pose indication for revascularization. In patients with non–functionally significant coronary stenosis, no benefits have been demonstrated compared with optimal medical therapy, even at 15-year follow-up.[2,3]

It has been shown that revascularization with PCI of ischemic lesions allows relief of symptoms more effectively than medical therapy alone.[7] The 5-year follow-up of the Percutaneous Coronary Intervention of Functionally Nonsignificant Stenosis (DEFER) trial[8] showed that stenting ischemia-producing lesions (FFR <0.75) improves

symptoms. At baseline, 90% of patients had angina, whereas at 5-year follow-up after stenting, 72% of patients were free from symptoms. Similarly, the Fractional Flow Reserve Versus Angiography for Guiding Percutaneous Coronary Intervention (FAME)[9] study showed that 80% of patients were free from angina 2 years after stenting.

Recently the International Study of Comparative Health Effectiveness With Medical and Invasive Approaches (ISCHEMIA) trial[10,11] questioned the role of PCI in reducing the rate of cardiac death and MI. The trial randomized more than 5000 patients with demonstrated obstructive CAD (at coronary computed tomography) and moderate to severe ischemia (>10% in physiologic tests; nuclear imaging was used most frequently) to percutaneous or surgical revascularization versus optimal medical therapy. No difference in the primary composite endpoint of cardiovascular death, MI, hospitalization for unstable angina, heart failure, or resuscitated cardiac arrest was noticed between the 2 strategies. The trial initially was designed, however, to include objective endpoints, such as cardiovascular death and MI, but then was changed to a composite endpoint to accrue more events. Cardiovascular death or MI did not differ over the 4 years, but the curves initially higher in the invasive group crossed at approximately 2 years and were lower in the invasive group at 2 years. Total MI rate did not differ between groups, but the invasive group had significantly higher rate of periprocedural MI and lower rate of spontaneous MI. It has been shown that spontaneous MIs not related to the PCI are independent predictors of mortality whereas periprocedural MIs are not related to the prognosis.[12] Moreover, the trial findings were sensitive to the definition of MI adopted. The quality-of-life outcomes analysis also reported significant improvement in angina control and quality of life with the invasive strategy in patients symptomatic at baseline.

FRACTIONAL FLOW RESERVE

FFR is defined as the ratio between the maximal blood flow in a coronary artery with a stenotic lesion and the maximal blood flow in the same artery if the stenosis would not be present. The ratio of these 2 flows is expressed as ratio between 2 pressures. FFR is calculated as the ratio between the Pd and the Pa at maximum blood flow. The derived Pd/Pa represents the relative fraction of total flow across the stenosis. FFR can be measured by coronary guidewires equipped with a pressure sensor located near the tip. Hyperemia is required for FFR calculation and it can be obtained minimizing microvascular resistance through adenosine administration by either continuous intravenous infusion (140 μg/kg/min) or intracoronary bolus (right coronary artery 50–100 μg, left coronary artery 100–200 μg). Although associated with potential drawbacks, intravenous administration enables achieving a more consistent hyperemic effect, which allows a pressure pull back during steady-state hyperemia for the hemodynamic analysis of all abnormalities along the length of the coronary artery.[13] In normal coronary arteries, the expected FFR value is 1.0, meaning the absence of obstacles to the coronary flow. In diseased coronary arteries, an FFR value below the threshold of 0.80 indicates hemodynamically significant stenoses, causing myocardial ischemia, with an accuracy of 90%.[14,15] To date, FFR is the gold standard for the detection of myocardial ischemia because it is much more accurate in distinguishing functionally significant stenoses than noninvasive provocative tests, such as exercise electrocardiogram, myocardial perfusion scintigraphy, and stress echocardiography.[14] Despite the class IA recommendation by current guidelines,[5] however, real-life data showed that the use of physiology-based guidance to assist coronary revascularization decisions is performed in lower than 10% of the procedures.[16]

EVIDENCE FOR FRACTIONAL FLOW RESERVE–GUIDED PERCUTANEOUS CORONARY INTERVENTION STRATEGY IN STABLE CORONARY ARTERY DISEASE PATIENTS

Currently, FFR is a diagnostic tool routinely available and used in most catheterization laboratories for clinical decision making. Several studies have validated that FFR-guided PCI is safe and reduces the rate of major adverse cardiovascular events, including the need for urgent revascularization. The DEFER[8] study randomized nonsignificant stenoses (FFR >0.75) to be treated either medically or by stenting. The 15-year follow-up showed that the rate of MI was significantly lower in the deferred group (2.2%) compared with patients who underwent revascularization (10%).[3] The FAME[9,17] study showed that in patients with multivessel disease (MVD) a strategy of FFR-guided PCI resulted in a significant decrease of major adverse cardiac events for up to 2 years after the index procedure. The FAME 2[18] study was the first large randomized trial in which patients in whom at least 1 stenosis was functionally significant (FFR ≤0.80) were randomly assigned to FFR-guided PCI plus the best available medical therapy (PCI group) or the best available medical therapy alone (medical

therapy group), whereas patients with nonfunctionally significant stenosis (FFR >0.80) were entered into a registry and treated with medical treatment only. A total of 888 patients were randomized between PCI and medical therapy. The trial was stopped prematurely due to an increased rate of major adverse cardiovascular events in the medical-therapy group compared with the PCI group. Also, the 5-year results confirmed that FFR-guided PCI plus the best available medical therapy improved outcomes, with a significantly lower rate of the primary composite endpoint of death, MI, or urgent revascularization compared with the best available medical therapy alone.[19] The ongoing FAME 3[20] trial will investigate whether in patients with MVD an FFR-guided PCI approach using contemporary drug-eluting stents is noninferior compared with surgical revascularization. Finally, a large individual patient data meta-analysis[2] provided strong evidence that an FFR-guided strategy improves both clinical outcomes (with a significant reduction in death and MI) and quality of life. Conversely to this, large amount of data favoring and FFR based PCI strategy, the Functional Testing Underlying Coronary Revascularisation study was prematurely halted due to a doubling in the risk of death within the first year, with no beneficial impact seen on other outcomes, in patients with MVD undergoing FFR-guided PCI.

FRACTIONAL FLOW RESERVE IN ACUTE CORONARY SYNDROME PATIENTS

Physiologic evaluation by FFR of infarct-related artery (IRA) is neither practical nor valid due to heightened microvascular resistance after MI that falsely increases the FFR measurement of the culprit vessel. In acute coronary syndrome (ACS) patients with MVD, however, FFR evaluation of nonculprit lesions has theoretic appeal and several data showed the feasibility of FFR use in this setting (**Table 1**).

In the Fractional Flow Reserve vs Angiography in Guiding Management To Optimize Outcomes in Non-ST-Segment Elevation Myocardial Infarction study,[21] 350 patients with non–ST-elevation MI (STEMI) and MVD, were randomly assigned to an FFR-guided PCI or angiography-guided standard care. Revascularization rate was significantly lower in the FFR-guided group compared with angiography guidance alone, with otherwise no detectable difference in health outcomes and quality of life between the 2 populations, underlying the feasibility and safety of this strategy in these patients.

Also, in patients presenting with STEMI and MVD, incomplete revascularization showed to be

Table 1
Main studies of validation and outcomes of physiologic diagnostic tools

Study	Tool	Patients, n	Study Design	Population	Primary Endpoint	Follow-up	Outcomes
DEFER[8,3]	FFR	325	Prospective, randomized comparing medical therapy vs PCI for non-ischemic lesions (FFR>0.75)	Stable CAD	Adverse cardiac events	15 y	No differences in rate of death MI significantly lower in defer group
FAME[9,16]	FFR	1005	Prospective, randomized comparing FFR-guided (FFR<0.80) vs angio-guided PCI	Multivessel disease	Composite of death, MI and repeat revascularization	5 y	Lower rate of the composite endpoint in the FFR-guided vs angiography-guided group
FAME 2[17,18]	FFR	888	Prospective, randomized comparing OMT vs PCI + OMT in significant lesions (FFR<0.80)	Stable CAD	Composite of death from any cause, nonfatal MI and urgent revascularization	5 y	Significantly lower rate of priary endpoint in PCI group vs OMT group
FAMOUS NSTEMI[20]	FFR	350	Prospective, randomized comparing FFR-guided (FFR<0.80) vs angiography guided PCI	NSTEMI and Multivessel disease	The between-group difference in the proportion of patients allocated to medical management	12 mo	Higher rate of medically managed patients in the FFR- vs angiography group.
DANAMI 3 PRIMULTI[23]	FFR	627	Prospective, randomized comparing complete FFR-guided (FFR<0.80) PCI vs IRA-only PCI	STEMI and Multivessel disease	Composite of all-cause mortality, non-fatal reinfarction, and ischaemia-driven revascularisation of lesions in non-IRA	27 mo	Significantly fewer repeat revascularisations in the FFR-guided PCI group No differences in all-cause mortality and non-fatal reinfarction

Study	Index	N	Study design	Population	Endpoint	Follow-up	Findings
COMPARE-ACUTE[24,25]	FFR	885	Prospective, randomized comparing complete FFR-guided (FFR<0.80) PCI vs IRA-only PCI	STEMI and Multivessel disease	Composite of all-cause death, MI, any revascularization and cerebrovascular event	3 y	FFR-guided complete revascularization is more beneficial in terms of outcome and health-care costs compared to IRA-only revascularization
RESOLVE[27]	Pd/Pa, iFR and FFR	1768	Non-randomized, retrospective	Coronary artery disease undergoing physiologic assessment	Level of diagnostic accuracy of iFR and Pd/Pa compared with FFR	-	iFR and Pd/Pa compared with FFR demonstrated an overall accuracy of ~80%
RINASCI[28]	cFFR vs FFR	104	Observational, prospective evaluating diagnostic accuracy of cFFR (<0.83) vs FFR	Intermediate coronary stenoses	Accuracy of cFFR in comparison to FFR	-	Strong correlation between cFFR and FFR values
DEFINE-FLAIR[29]	iFR vs FFR	2492	Prospective, randomized study comparing iFR (iFR<0.89) vs FFR-guided PCI	CAD with at least one intermediate stenosis in a native artery	Composite of death, nonfatal MI or unplanned revascularization	12 mo	iFR guided PCI was noninferior to FFR-guided PCI with respect to primary endpoint rate
iFR-SWEDEHEART[30]	iFR vs FFR	2037	Prospective, randomized evaluating non inferiority of iFR (iFR<0.89) vs FFR in detecting functionally significant lesions	Stable angina or acute coronary syndromes	Composite of death from any cause, nonfatal MI or unplanned revascularization	12 mo	iFR-guided revascularization strategy was non-inferior to FFR-guided PCI with respect to primary endpoint rate
VALIDATE RFR[31]	RFR vs iFR	651	Retrospective, designed to derive and validate the RFR	Intermediate coronary stenoses	Agreement between RFR and iFR	-	RFR was highly correlated to iFR

(continued on next page)

Table 1
(continued)

Study	Tool	Patients, n	Study Design	Population	Primary Endpoint	Follow-up	Outcomes
Lee et al,[32] 2019	RFR or dPR	435 (1024 vessels)	Study population derived from the 3 V FFR-FRIENDS study (3-Vessel Fractional Flow Reserve for the Assessment of Total Stenosis Burden and Its Clinical Impact in Patients With Coronary Artery Disease; NCT01621438) and the 13N-ammonia PET registry.	Intermediate coronary stenoses	Agreement of RFR or dPR with IFR and FFR and the risk of composite endopinf of cardiac death, vessel-related MI, and vessel-related ischemia-driven revascularization	2 y	Both RFR and dPR showed a significant correlation with iFR which was higher than that FFR. All tools showed significant association with the risk of 2-y vessel-oriented composite outcomes
FAVOR[38]	QFR and FFR	73 (84 vessels)	Prospective, observational	Intermediate coronary stenoses	Correlation and agreement between QFR and FFR	-	fQFR, cQFR and aQFR showed a good correlation with FFR
WIFI II[39]	QFR and FFR	362	Prospective, observational	Unselected consecutive patients	Feasibility and diagnostic performance of QFR	-	QFR assessment showed good agreement and diagnostic accuracy compared with FFR
FAVOR II China[40]	QFR and FFR	308	Prospective, multicenter	Intermediate coronary stenoses	Improvement of the diagnostic accuracy of coronary angiography by QFR	-	Sensitivity and specificity in identifying hemodynamically significant stenosis were significantly higher for QFR than for QCA

an independent risk factor for non–target vessel–related adverse events[22] and FFR showed to be useful a tool for the identification of nonculprit lesions needing revascularization.[23] The Complete Revascularisation vs Treatment of the Culprit Lesion Only in Patients with ST-Segment Elevation Myocardial Infarction and Multivessel Disease trial[24] (n = 627) showed a reduction in composite endpoint with FFR-guided complete revascularization performed as a staged procedure during the hospitalization versus IRA-PCI only, and similarly the Fractional Flow Reserve–Guided Multivessel Angioplasty in Myocardial Infarction trial[25,26] (n = 885; 12-month follow-up) showed that FFR-guided complete revascularization during the index procedure significantly reduced the primary endpoint rate compared with IRA-only PCI. The ongoing Functional vs Culprit-only Revascularization in Elderly Patients with Myocardial Infarction and Multivessel Disease randomized trial (NCT03772743) will investigate if, in elderly patients (>75 years) with MI and MVD, a functional-guided PCI (FFR, iFR, cFFR, and QFR all are allowed and left to operator discretion) is superior to a culprit-only strategy in the reduction of 1-year adverse cardiovascular events.

NONHYPEREMIC INDICES FOR CORONARY STENOSIS ASSESSMENT

Although a critical mass of evidence supports the use of FFR for guiding revascularization strategy in patients with CAD, this tool remains flawed by substantial underutilization in clinical practice.[27] Among the barriers preventing more extensive use of FFR, the requirement of adenosine administration to achieve maximal hyperemia often is flagged, because it adds time and complexity to the procedure and exposes patients to adverse side effects.[27] Moreover, the usefulness of FFR is limited in the presence of true bifurcations and/or tandem lesions, which are challenging to interrogate properly.[27] To overtake these limits, in recent years numerous studies investigated the use of nonhyperemic indices alternative to FFR, such as the simple resting Pd/Pa measurement, cFFR,[28] iFR (the most widely validated after FFR[27,29,30]), RFR,[31,32] diastolic hyperemia-free ratio (DFR), and the diastolic pressure ratio (dPR) (**Table 2**).[32]

The iFR grounds on the concept that at a specific time in diastole—the so-called wave-free period—intracoronary pressure and flow decline together in a linear fashion, whereas microvascular resistance remains more stable and significantly lower than the rest of cardiac cycle.[27] Therefore, over this period, the pressure gradient across coronary stenosis can be measured obviating generating

hyperemia through adenosine infusion. Another advantage of iFR is the ability to individually assess lesions severity in the context of diffuse vessel disease, thus minimizing FFR limitations in the setting of serial coronary stenoses. Specifically, by using the coregistration of the iFR pullback trace and the coronary angiogram (ie, plotting measured values directly over angiographic views), iFR is able to detect lesion-specific pressure drop along the whole length of the vessel and differentiate focal from diffuse coronary disease.[27] This allows the cardiologist to (1) properly identify which lesion/s should be treated (if any), (2) accurately predict to what extent coronary physiology will improve after PCI per each lesion, and (3) confidently decide the number, length, and position of stents to be used to pursue a successful procedure.[27] When its performance has been tested by meta-analyzed data,[33] iFR showed a significant correlation (0.79 [0.78–0.82]) with the gold-standard of FFR and good diagnostic accuracy for the identification of FFR-positive stenoses (area under the curve = 0.88 [0.86–0.90]), confirming its role of reliable adenosine-free alternative in practice.[33] Recently, 2 large randomized, controlled trials, the blinded Functional Lesion Assessment of Intermediate Stenosis to Guide Revascularisation[29] and the open-label Instantaneous Wave-free Ratio versus Fractional Flow Reserve in Patients with Stable Angina Pectoris or Acute Coronary Syndrome,[30] established that iFR-guided revascularization (cutoff point of 0.89) is as safe and effective as FFR-guided revascularization (cutoff point of 0.80) with respect to adverse cardiac events at 12 months.[29,30] Besides patients with stable CAD, both studies tested iFR for nonculprit lesions evaluation in patients with ACS, proving the noninferiority of iFR to FFR in this setting.[29,30] Although evidence overall speaks in favor of substantial equivalence of the 2 techniques,[29,30,33] the enduring controversy on how to manage patients with iFR values that are borderline or discordant with FFR[34] (especially for left main and proximal left anterior descending artery lesions)[35] warrants further investigations for a full understanding of their synergistic use (**Figs. 1** and **2**).

The rise of iFR encouraged the development of additional hyperemia-free indices, intending to overcome potential iFR limitations, such as the sensitive automated landmarking of pressure waveform components and the assumption that maximal flow and minimal resistance occur during a specific (fixed) period of diastole.[27] In this background, the RFR has been proposed as a novel hyperemia-free tool able to measure coronary pressure at the point of absolute lowest resting Pd/Pa in the cardiac cycle.[31] In other words, the

Table 2
Main features, strengths, and limitations of actually available tools for coronary lesions severity assessment

Tool	Definition	Ischemia Cut-off	Need of Pressure Wire	Need of Hyperemia	Strengths	Limits
FFR	Average Pd/Pa during adenosine induced hyperemia	≤ 0.80	Yes	Yes	Gold standard for lesion severity assessment Supported by outcome studies	Invasive Need of guidewire use and adenosine administration
Pd/Pa	Average Pd/Pa during the entire cardiac cycle	≤ 0.91	Yes	No	Adenosine not required	Invasive Need of guidewire No outcomes studies available
cFFR	Average Pd/Pa during contrast-induced hyperemia	≤ 0.83	Yes	Contrast-induced hyperemia	Adenosine not required	Invasive Need of guidewire No outcomes studies available
iFR	Average Pd/Pa during the WFP	≤ 0.89	Yes	No	Adenosine not required Supported by outcomes studies	Invasive Need of guidewire
RFR	Lowest mean Pd/Pa during the entire cardiac cycle	≤ 0.89	Yes	No	Adenosine not required	Invasive Need of guidewire No outcomes studies available
DFR	Average Pd/Pa during diastolic period when Pa < mean Pa	≤ 0.89	Yes	No	Adenosine not required	Invasive Need of guidewire No outcomes studies available
DPR	Average Pd/Pa during the entire diastolic period	≤ 0.89	Yes	No	Adenosine not required	Invasive Need of guidewire No outcomes studies available
dPR	Pd/Pa during the flat period (identified using dP/dt) of WFP	≤ 0.89	Yes	No	Adenosine not required	Invasive Need of guidewire No outcomes studies available
QFR	Fluid dynamic equations, emulating hyperaemic flow velocity	≤ 0.80	No	Adenosine needed only for aQFR	Less invasive Not requiring pressure wire No need for adenosine (aQFR only). Faster than FFR and iFR.	Outcome studies not available yet

Abbreviations: aQFR, adenosine quantitative flow ratio; cFFR, contrast FFR; DFR, diastolic hyperemia-free ratio; dP/dt, change in pressure/change in tim; DPR, diastolic pressure ratio; FFR, fractional flow reserve; iFR, instantaneous wave-free ratio; Pd/Pa, pressure $_{distal}$/pressure $_{aorta}$; QFR, quantitative flow ratio; RFR, resting full-cycle ratio.

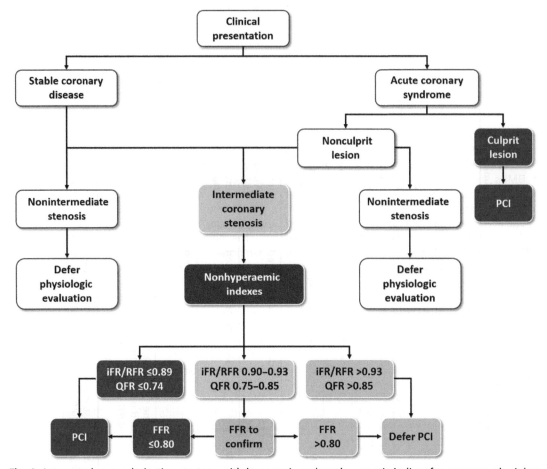

Fig. 1. Integrated revascularization strategy with hyperemic and nonhyperemic indices for coronary physiology evaluation.

RFR measures the maximal relative pressure difference during the entire cardiac cycle (and not limited to diastole), aiming at simplifying iFR assumptions and limiting potential biases.[31] The diagnostic performance of RFR (at a cutoff point of 0.89) has been tested and validated in large population studies,[31,32] suggesting its potential use as an alternative to iFR or FFR to guide revascularization in patients with CAD.[31,32] Considering the current lack of randomized clinical trials, however, as well as its potential inaccuracies in specific (and more complex) settings,[36] while awaiting solid evidence, RFR-guided strategy cannot be yet considered as interchangeable to FFR on iFR in clinical practice.

THREE-DIMENSIONAL QUANTITATIVE CORONARY ANGIOGRAPHY AND BLOOD FLOW SIMULATION DERIVED INDEX: QUANTITATIVE FLOW RATIO

Although hyperemic and nonhyperemic indices for coronary stenosis assessment have proved their undisputable benefit, their penetration in clinical practice remains low. In recent years, modern software for 3-dimensional (3-D) vessel reconstruction and flow model calculation has been developed for functional assessment of coronary stenosis. QFR is an innovative angiographic-based technique allowing computation of FFR from 3-D–QCA and thrombolysis in MI frame counting based on computational fluid dynamics technology.[37]

For 3-D reconstruction, 2 diagnostic angiographic projections (at least 25° apart) must be obtained; frame rate count is analyzed in both angiographic views to obtain patient-specific hyperemic flow velocity evaluation during contrast injection and/or adenosine administration. QFR uses 3 different flow simulation models: (1) fixed-flow QFR (fQFR), with a fixed empiric hyperemic flow velocity of 0.35 m/s; (2) contrast-flow QFR (cQFR), with a modeled virtual hyperemic flow velocity derived from contrast flow without adenosine use; and (3) adenosine-flow QFR (aQFR),

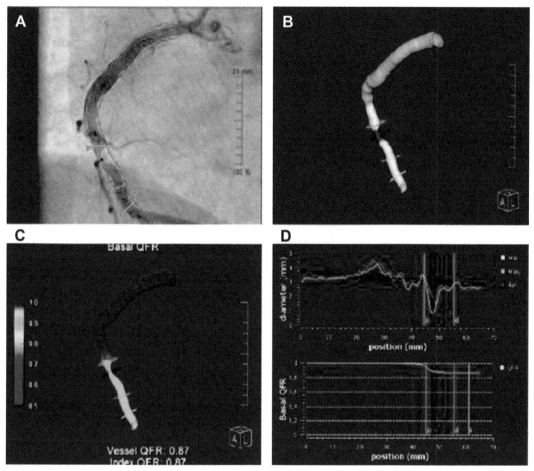

Fig. 2. Discordance between angiographic and functional severity of a lesion in the right coronary artery. (*A*) Oblique left projection of the right coronary artery. (*B*) 3-D QCA derived with diameter stenosis of 73.6%. (*C*) QFR = 0.87. (*D*) Luminal diameter and QFR pull-back.

with adenosine administration to induce maximum hyperemia. The cutoff point has been set at 0.80 and these 3 models were compared with the measured FFR. In the Functional Assessment by Various Flow Reconstructions (FAVOR) pilot trial, fQFR, cQFR, and aQFR showed good correlation with FFR (r = 0.69, *P*<.001; r = 0.77, *P*<.001; and r = 0.72, *P*<.001; respectively).[38] Similar results were obtained in the Wire-Free Functional Imaging II, where QFR showed a good correlation with FFR (r = 0.70, *P*<.0001).[39]

Diagnostic accuracy of QFR was evaluated in both the FAVOR II China and FAVOR II Europe and Japan studies.[40,41] In the first, QFR analysis showed diagnostic accuracy of 92.7% and 93.3% when it was performed online and offline, respectively, using FFR as reference. In the European-Japanese study, online QFR proved e more effective than 2-dimensional QCA in

detecting severe coronary stenosis, with sensitivity and specificity of 87% and positive and negative predictive values of 78% and 94%, respectively, with FFR as reference. Several recent meta-analyses[42–44] confirmed good performance of QFR with an excellent agreement and correlation with FFR.

QFR computation can be applied in several clinical scenarios. In patients with prior MI, QFR accuracy in assessing functional lesion severity might be reduced[45] (not considering the vital myocardium). In STEMI, however, it can be a useful tool to assess nonculprit lesions in patients with MVD[46] as well as residual microvascular dysfunction.[47] Furthermore, QFR appears to be a reliable tool in assessing the functional relevance of coronary stenosis in patients with concomitant severe aortic stenosis scheduled for transcatheter aortic-valve implantation.[48]

Focusing on outcomes, the Angio-based Fractional Flow Reserve to Predict Adverse Events After Stent Implantation[49] study showed that lower QFR values after complete revascularization could predict subsequent adverse events. In daily practice, QFR also can be useful in risk stratification of patients without coronary stenosis, because low QFR values correspond to an increased risk of developing future cardiovascular events.[50] The ongoing FAVOR III study (NCT03656848) is adequately powered to investigate if a strategy QFR-guided PCI provides superior clinical outcome and cost-effectiveness compared with standard coronary angiography–guided PCI in CAD patients.

The reliability of QFR and its benefits in terms of cost-effectiveness and less invasiveness make this technique attractive for interventional cardiologists in assessing intermediate coronary stenosis, and its routine use in the catheterization laboratory is expected to increase in the near future.

SUMMARY

Thanks to the advantages in pharmacologic treatment and procedural techniques that significantly reduced complications rates,[51,52] PCI is one of the most wildly performed interventional procedures worldwide. Stenting nonischemic lesions is not cost effective, however, and worsens the outcomes. Detecting functionally significant stenosis is a key aspect to decide which lesion (if any) need to be treated. FFR is considered the gold standard but is still underutilized in practice. Nowadays, technological advances have led to the development of new invasive physiology techniques, such as the nonhyperemic indices as well as the less invasive QFR, which showed good reproducibility and correlation with FFR. In modern catheterization, laboratory physiologic assessment with any of these tools (according to operator expertise) should be routinely available and used to improve the appropriateness of revascularization and define the optimal intervention strategy to increase safety, efficiency, and successful outcomes after PCI.

CONFLICTS OF INTEREST

None.

REFERENCES

1. Kaptoge S, Pennells L, De Bacquer D, et al. World Health Organization cardiovascular disease risk charts: revised models to estimate risk in 21 global regions. Lancet Glob Health 2019;7(10):e1332–45.
2. Zimmermann FM, Omerovic E, Fournier S, et al. Fractional flow reserve-guided percutaneous coronary intervention vs. medical therapy for patients with stable coronary lesions: meta-analysis of individual patient data. Eur Heart J 2019;40(2): 180–6.
3. Zimmermann FM, Ferrara A, Johnson NP, et al. Deferral vs. performance of percutaneous coronary intervention of functionally non-significant coronary stenosis: 15-year follow-up of the DEFER trial. Eur Heart J 2015;36(45):3182–8.
4. Knuuti J, Wijns W, Achenbach S, et al. 2019 ESC guidelines for the diagnosis and management of chronic coronary syndromes. Eur Heart J 2020; 41(3):407–77.
5. Neumann F-J, Sousa-Uva M, Ahlsson A, et al. 2018 ESC/EACTS Guidelines on myocardial revascularization. Eur Heart J 2018. https://doi.org/10.1093/eurheartj/ehy394.
6. Shaw LJ, Berman DS, Maron DJ, et al. Optimal medical therapy with or without percutaneous coronary intervention to reduce ischemic burden: results from the Clinical Outcomes Utilizing Revascularization and Aggressive Drug Evaluation (COURAGE) trial nuclear substudy. Circulation 2008;117(10): 1283–91.
7. Johnson NP, Tóth GG, Lai D, et al. Prognostic value of fractional flow reserve: linking physiologic severity to clinical outcomes. J Am Coll Cardiol 2014;64(16): 1641–54.
8. Bech GJW, De Bruyne B, Pijls NHJ, et al. Fractional flow reserve to determine the appropriateness of angioplasty in moderate coronary stenosis. Circulation 2001;103(24):2928–34.
9. Tonino PAL, De Bruyne B, Pijls NHJ, et al. Fractional flow reserve versus angiography for guiding percutaneous coronary intervention. N Engl J Med 2009; 360(3):213–24.
10. Maron DJ, Hochman JS, Reynolds HR, et al. Initial invasive or conservative strategy for stable coronary disease. N Engl J Med 2020. https://doi.org/10.1056/NEJMoa1915922.
11. Spertus JA, Jones PG, Maron DJ, et al. Health-status outcomes with invasive or conservative care in coronary disease. N Engl J Med 2020. https://doi.org/10.1056/NEJMoa1916370.
12. Prasad A, Gersh BJ, Bertrand ME, et al. Prognostic significance of periprocedural versus spontaneously occurring myocardial infarction after percutaneous coronary intervention in patients with acute coronary syndromes. An analysis from the ACUITY (acute catheterization and urgent intervention triage strategy) trial. J Am Coll Cardiol 2009; 54(5):477–86.
13. De Bruyne B, Pijls NHJ, Barbato E, et al. Intracoronary and intravenous adenosine 5′-triphosphate, adenosine, papaverine, and contrast medium to assess fractional flow reserve in humans. Circulation 2003;107(14):1877–83.

14. Pijls NHJ, De Bruyne B, Peels K, et al. Measurement of fractional flow reserve to assess the functional severity of coronary-artery stenoses. N Engl J Med 1996;334(26):1703–8.

15. Pijls NHJ, Van Gelder B, Van Der Voort P, et al. Fractional flow reserve: a useful index to evaluate the influence of an epicardial coronary stenosis on myocardial blood flow. Circulation 1995;92(11): 3183–93.

16. Tebaldi M, Biscaglia S, Fineschi M, et al. Evolving routine standards in invasive hemodynamic assessment of coronary stenosis: the nationwide Italian SICI-GISE cross-sectional ERIS study. JACC Cardiovasc Interv 2018;11(15):1482–91.

17. Van Nunen LX, Zimmermann FM, Tonino PAL, et al. Fractional flow reserve versus angiography for guidance of PCI in patients with multivessel coronary artery disease (FAME): 5-year follow-up of a randomised controlled trial. Lancet 2015; 386(10006):1853–60.

18. De Bruyne B, Fearon WF, Pijls NHJ, et al. Fractional flow reserve-guided PCI for stable coronary artery disease. N Engl J Med 2014;371(13):1208–17.

19. Xaplanteris P, Fournier S, Pijls NHJ, et al. Five-year outcomes with PCI guided by fractional flow reserve. N Engl J Med 2018;379(3):250–9.

20. Zimmermann FM, De Bruyne B, Pijls NHJ, et al. Rationale and design of the Fractional Flow Reserve versus Angiography for Multivessel Evaluation (FAME) 3 Trial: a comparison of fractional flow reserve-guided percutaneous coronary intervention and coronary artery bypass graft surgery in patients with multivessel coronary artery disease. Am Heart J 2015;170(4):619–26.e2.

21. Layland J, Oldroyd KG, Curzen N, et al. Fractional flow reserve vs. angiography in guiding management to optimize outcomes in non-ST-segment elevation myocardial infarction: the British Heart Foundation FAMOUS-NSTEMI randomized trial. Eur Heart J 2015;36(2):100–11.

22. Spitaleri G, Moscarella E, Brugaletta S, et al. Correlates of non-target vessel-related adverse events in patients with ST-segment elevation myocardial infarction: Insights from five-year follow-up of the EX-AMINATION trial. Eurointervention 2018;13(16): 1939–45.

23. Moscarella E, Brugaletta S, Sabaté M. Latest STEMI treatment: a focus on current and upcoming devices. Expert Rev Med Devices 2018;15(11):807–17.

24. Engstrøm T, Kelbæk H, Helqvist S, et al. Complete revascularisation versus treatment of the culprit lesion only in patients with ST-segment elevation myocardial infarction and multivessel disease (DA-NAMI-3—PRIMULTI): an open-label, randomised controlled trial. Lancet 2015;386(9994):665–71. Available at: http://www.ncbi.nlm.nih.gov/pubmed/26347918. Accessed February 1, 2018.

25. Smits PC, Abdel-Wahab M, Neumann F-J, et al. Fractional flow reserve–guided multivessel angioplasty in myocardial infarction. N Engl J Med 2017; 376(13):1234–44.

26. Smits PC, Laforgia PL, Abdel-Wahab M, et al. Fractional flow reserve-guided multivessel angioplasty in myocardial infarction: 3-year follow-up with cost benefit analysis of the compare-acute trial. EuroIntervention 2020. https://doi.org/10.4244/EIJ-D-20-00012.

27. Götberg M, Cook CM, Sen S, et al. The evolving future of instantaneous wave-free ratio and fractional flow reserve. J Am Coll Cardiol 2017;70(11): 1379–402.

28. Leone AM, Scalone G, De Maria GL, et al. Efficacy of contrast medium induced Pd/Pa ratio in predicting functional significance of intermediate coronary artery stenosis assessed by fractional flow reserve: Insights from the RINASCI study. EuroIntervention 2015;11(4):421–7.

29. Davies JE, Sen S, Dehbi HM, et al. Use of the instantaneous wave-free ratio or fractional flow reserve in PCI. N Engl J Med 2017;376(19):1824–34.

30. Götberg M, Christiansen EH, Gudmundsdottir IJ, et al. Instantaneous wave-free ratio versus fractional flow reserve to guide PCI. N Engl J Med 2017; 376(19):1813–23.

31. Svanerud J, Ahn JM, Jeremias A, et al. Validation of a novel non-hyperaemic index of coronary artery stenosis severity: the Resting Full-cycle Ratio (VALIDATE RFR) study. EuroIntervention 2018;14(7): 806–14.

32. Lee JM, Choi KH, Park J, et al. Physiological and clinical assessment of resting physiological Indexes: resting full-cycle ratio, diastolic pressure ratio, and instantaneous wave-free ratio. Circulation 2019; 139(7):889–900.

33. De Rosa S, Polimeni A, Petraco R, et al. Diagnostic performance of the instantaneous wave-free ratio: comparison with fractional flow reserve. Circ Cardiovasc Interv 2018;11(1):e004613.

34. Lee SH, Choi KH, Lee JM, et al. Physiologic characteristics and clinical outcomes of patients with discordance between FFR and iFR. JACC Cardiovasc Interv 2019;12(20):2018–31.

35. Kobayashi Y, Johnson NP, Berry C, et al. The influence of lesion location on the diagnostic accuracy of adenosine-free coronary pressure wire measurements. JACC Cardiovasc Interv 2016;9(23): 2390–9.

36. Liou K, Ooi S-Y. Resting full-cycle ratio (RFR) in the assessment of left main coronary disease: caution required. Heart Lung Circ 2020. https://doi.org/10.1016/j.hlc.2019.12.014.

37. Cesaro A, Gragnano F, Di Girolamo D, et al. Functional assessment of coronary stenosis: an overview of available techniques. Is quantitative flow ratio a

step to the future? Expert Rev Cardiovasc Ther 2018;16(12):951–62.

38. Tu S, Westra J, Yang J, et al. Diagnostic accuracy of fast computational approaches to derive fractional flow reserve from diagnostic coronary angiography: the International Multicenter FAVOR Pilot Study. JACC Cardiovasc Interv 2016;9(19):2024–35.

39. Westra J, Tu S, Winther S, et al. Evaluation of coronary artery stenosis by quantitative flow ratio during invasive coronary angiography the WIFI II study (Wire-Free functional imaging II). Circ Cardiovasc Imaging 2018;11(3):e007107.

40. Xu B, Tu S, Qiao S, et al. Diagnostic accuracy of angiography-based quantitative flow ratio measurements for online assessment of coronary stenosis. J Am Coll Cardiol 2017;70(25):3077–87.

41. Westra J, Andersen BK, Campo G, et al. Diagnostic performance of in-procedure angiography-derived quantitative flow reserve compared to pressure-derived fractional flow reserve: the FAVOR II Europe-Japan study. J Am Heart Assoc 2018;7(14): e009603.

42. Westra J, Tu S, Campo G, et al. Diagnostic performance of quantitative flow ratio in prospectively enrolled patients: an individual patient-data meta-analysis. Catheter Cardiovasc Interv 2019;94(5): 693–701.

43. Cortés C, Carrasco-Moraleja M, Aparisi A, et al. Quantitative flow ratio-Meta-analysis and systematic review. Catheter Cardiovasc Interv 2020;1–8. https:// doi.org/10.1002/ccd.28857.

44. Xing Z, Pei J, Huang J, et al. Diagnostic performance of qfr for the evaluation of intermediate coronary artery stenosis confirmed by fractional flow reserve. Braz J Cardiovasc Surg 2019;34(2):165–72.

45. Emori H, Kubo T, Kameyama T, et al. Diagnostic accuracy of quantitative flow ratio for assessing myocardial ischemia in prior myocardial infarction. Circ J 2018;82(3):807–14.

46. Spitaleri G, Tebaldi M, Biscaglia S, et al. Quantitative flow ratio Identifies nonculprit coronary lesions requiring revascularization in patients with ST-segment-elevation myocardial infarction and multi-vessel disease. Circ Cardiovasc Interv 2018;11(2): e006023.

47. Sheng X, Qiao Z, Ge H, et al. Novel application of quantitative flow ratio for predicting microvascular dysfunction after ST-segment-elevation myocardial infarction. Catheter Cardiovasc Interv 2020;95(S1): 624–32.

48. Mejia-Renteria H, Nombela-Franco L, Paradis J-M, et al. Title: functional assessment of coronary stenosis with angiography-based quantitative flow ratio compared with fractional flow reserve in patients with severe aortic stenosis. EuroIntervention 2020. https://doi.org/10.4244/EIJ-D-19-01001.

49. Biscaglia S, Tebaldi M, Brugaletta S, et al. Prognostic value of QFR measured Immediately after successful stent implantation: the International Multicenter Prospective HAWKEYE Study. JACC Cardiovasc Interv 2019;12(20):2079–88.

50. Buono A, Mühlenhaus A, Schäfer T, et al. QFR predicts the Incidence of long-term adverse events in patients with suspected CAD: feasibility and reproducibility of the method. J Clin Med 2020;9(1):220.

51. Cesaro A, Moscarella E, Gragnano F, et al. Transradial access versus transfemoral access: a comparison of outcomes and efficacy in reducing hemorrhagic events. Expert Rev Cardiovasc Ther 2019;17(6):435–47.

52. Andò G, Gragnano F, Calabrò P, et al. Radial vs femoral access for the prevention of acute kidney injury (AKI) after coronary angiography or intervention: a systematic review and meta-analysis. Catheter Cardiovasc Interv 2018;92(7):E518–26.

Bioresorbable Coronary Scaffold Technologies
What's New?

Giulia Masiero, MD[a],*, Giulio Rodinò, MD[a], Juji Matsuda, MD[a,b],
Giuseppe Tarantini, MD, PhD[a]

KEYWORDS

- Bioresorbable scaffold • Vascular restoration therapy • Stent thrombosis • Dismantling

KEY POINTS

- Bioresorbable scaffolds (BRS) were designed to provide temporary mechanical support and early drug delivery followed by complete resorption.
- BRS may be identified as either polymeric (composed of polylactic acid or related compounds) or metallic (composed of magnesium alloy) according to the composition of the backbone.
- Different mechanical properties and biodegradation profile of both BRS type might affect different efficacy and safety outcomes.
- Further improvement in scaffold design and deployment technique might mitigate the proven early risk of failure enhancing the late benefit of complete resorption.

INTRODUCTION

The use of new-generation drug-eluting stents (DES) is recommended in almost every clinical and angiographic scenario in patients with coronary artery disease.[1] However, the permanent delivery of a metallic device is affected by several drawbacks, such as the persistent risks of neoatherosclerosis and very late stent thrombosis, the limitation of late lumen enlargement, the lack of reactive vasomotion in the stented vessel, the jailing of branches, and the exclusion from the possibility of future graft anastomosis especially in the midportion of the left anterior descending coronary artery.[2] Bioresorbable scaffolds (BRS) were designed to provide temporary mechanical support and to prevent neointimal proliferation by eluting immunosuppressive drugs. Moreover, the following complete bioresorption was supposed to be associated with restoration of vasomotion and endothelial function (vascular restoration therapy), luminal enlargement and plaque burden reduction, suitability for future possible treatment options (either percutaneous or surgical) and, most important, a decreased risk of lesion-related events when compared with permanent metallic DES.[3] According to the composition of the backbone, BRS may be identified as either polymeric BRS (pBRS, composed of polylactic acid or related compounds) or metallic (composed of a magnesium alloy).[4] Apart from the backbone, they typically consist of a biodegradable polymer matrix and an antiproliferative drug. This review aims to discuss the lights and shadows of the current available bioresorbable devices that have been evaluated in the management of patients with coronary artery disease. To date, 5 current generations of pBRS (Absorb BVS, DESolve,

[a] Department of Cardiac, Thoracic, Vascular Sciences and Public Health, University of Padua, Via Giustiniani 2, Padua 35128, Italy; [b] Department of Cardiovascular Medicine, Graduate School of Medical and Dental Science, Tokyo Medical and Dental University, 1-5-45 Yushima, Bunkyo-ku, Tokyo 113 - 8510, Japan
* Corresponding author.
E-mail address: giulia.masiero@aopd.veneto.it

Cardiol Clin 38 (2020) 589–599
https://doi.org/10.1016/j.ccl.2020.07.004
0733-8651/20/© 2020 Elsevier Inc. All rights reserved.

ART Pure, Fantom, and MeRes 100) and 1 absorbable metal scaffold (Magmaris) have received the "Conformité Européene" (CE) mark approval (**Table 1**).

Overview of Poly-ʟ-Lactide Scaffold

The Absorb bioresorbable vascular scaffold (BVS; Abbott Vascular, Santa Clara, CA) was one of the first to enter this realm and the most thoroughly studied and widely used BRS. The device consists of a 150 μm polymer backbone of poly-ʟ-lactide (PLLA) coated with poly-D,ʟ-lactide (PDLLA), which contains and controls the release of everolimus with a similar pharmacokinetics to the newer generation metallic everolimus-eluting stents (EES).[5] Degradation occurs by stepwise hydrolysis in a progressive process with minimal inflammatory reaction. In the final stage, either PLLA or PDLLA particles degrade entirely to lactic acid, or small remnants that are phagocytized by macrophages.[2] Owing to the mechanical properties of their polymeric backbone, the struts have an increased thickness to reach an acceptable tensile strength and to decrease stiffness and the chance of deformation.[5] To date, Absorb BVS has been compared with newer generation EES in more than 10,000 patients from several randomized controlled trials (RCTs), covering a wide range of clinical and angiographic subsets.[3] The initial studies first showed late lumen enlargement as well as restoration of vasomotion and endothelial function at 2 years after the Absorb implantation.[2] In this initial, highly selected cohort of patients, excellent clinical performance with no events of very late stent thrombosis was confirmed.[6] Also, several registries have confirmed the feasibility of the Absorb implantation for the so-called off-label indications, as in acute coronary syndromes, bifurcations, saphenous vein grafts, chronic total occlusions, or long lesions.[7,8] However, additional data revealed that most promises associated with the advantage of resorption had been overestimated (**Table 2**). In a meta-analysis of 6 trials, the rates of target vessel failure (TVF), target lesion revascularization (TLR), myocardial infarction (MI), and death at 1 year were comparable for patients treated with the Absorb BVS and the Xience EES.[9] However, the risk of 1-year definite or probable scaffold thrombosis (ScT) was doubled for the Absorb BVS patients (odds ratio [OR], 3.11; 95% confidence interval [CI], 1.24–7.82; P = .02). Although the risk of TLR was much improved by applying a rigorous BVS-specific implantation protocol with routine before and after dilatation and avoiding small vessels in the following ABSORB IV and the COMPARE-ABSORB trial, the concerns

about device thrombosis continued.[10,11] Moreover, the meta-analysis by Ali and colleagues[12] of 7 RCTs showed a higher risk of 2-year TVF in patients treated with the Absorb BVS (9.4% vs 7.4%; P = .0059). This difference was driven by increased rates of target vessel MI and ischemia-driven TLR. Also, the 2-year incidence of ScT was higher for the Absorb BVS than for the Xience stent (2.3% vs 0.7%; P<.001). Interestingly, a landmark analysis between 1 and 2 years confirmed higher rates of TVF (3.3% vs 1.9%; P = .0376) and device thrombosis (0.5% vs 0.0%; P<.001) in patients treated with the pBRS. These findings were strengthened by 2 recent analyses, one being a patient-data pooled analysis of 4 ABSORB trials, the other a meta-analysis of 7 RCTs comprehensive of higher risk subset of patients.[13,14] The results of these studies confirmed a significantly higher 3-year TVF, target vessel MI, and ischemia-driven TLR rates in the Absorb BVS group, with comparable cardiac mortality. Moreover, the risk of device thrombosis at 3 years was higher for BRS, at between 1 and 3 years. The key question of whether ABSORB BVS is able to reduce adverse events beyond complete device degradation was answered by the long-term clinical follow-up results of the ABSORB III trial with relatively simple coronary lesion.[15] At 5 years, the Absorb BVS showed equal performance in terms of TLF (17.5% vs 15.2%; P = .15) and there was no difference in ischemia-driven TLR (9.5% vs 8.0%; P = .27). However, the BRS-treated patients continued to show worse TV-MI (10.4% vs 7.5%; P = .04) and doubled ScT rates (2.5% vs 1.1%; P = .03). Importantly, there were time dependent effects in device-related events: Absorb BVS induced harm during the early time period (0–3 years) and showed similar outcomes in the subsequent 2 years with a downward trend in the annualized event rates. However, it must be considered that almost one-half of these patients continued dual antiplatelet therapy (DAPT) until 5 years. Disappointingly, other promises beyond the failed improvement of device-related events could not be confirmed. At longer follow-up, the results of several studies in patients with stable coronary disease, no sign of positive vessel remodeling, late luminal enlargement, or restoration of vasomotion was found between Absorb BVS and EES.[3,16] Further evidence is needed to fully understand and confirm these results. The Absorb technology is currently under refinement, and the next Falcon BVS generation is under preclinical testing. The new scaffold is expected to have thinner struts (<100 μm) and improved deliverability and acute performance.

Table 1
Technical characteristics of principal BRS currently available for clinical studies

Scaffold	Absorb GT1	DESolve Cx	Fantom	ART Pure	MeRes 100	Mirage	Magnitude	NeoVas	Magmaris
Manufacturer	Abbott Vascular	Elixir	Reva Medical	ART	Meril LifeSciences	Manli	Amaranth Medical	Lepu Medical	Biotronik
Design									
Strut material	PLLA	PLLA	Tyrosine polycarbonate	PDLLA	PLLA	PLLA	PLLA	PLLA	Mg
Strut thickness	156 μm	120 μm	125 μm	170 μm	100 μm	125 μm	98 μm	170 μm	150 μm
Eluted drug	Everolimus	Novolimus	Sirolimus	None	Sirolimus	Sirolimus	Sirolimus	Sirolimus	Sirolimus
Minimal resorption time	3 y	2 y	3 y	2 y	2 y	14 mo	N/A	2 y	1 y
Availability	CE mark, FDA approval, sales discontinued	CE mark	CE mark	CE mark	CE Mark	1 y RCT data vs Absorb available	FIM trial currently enrolling	1 y RCT data vs Xience available	CE mark

Abbreviations: CE, European Conformity; FDA, Food and Drug Administration; FIM, first in man; Mg, magnesium; PDLLA, poly-D,L-lactic acid; PLLA, poly-L-lactic acid; RCT, randomized clinical trial.

Table 2
Randomized clinical trials comparing ABSORB BVS with DES

Study	ABSORB China	ABSORB II	ABSORB III	ABSORB IV	ABSORB Japan	AIDA	Compare ABSORB	EVERBIO II	TROFI II	ISAR-Absorb MI
BVS (n)	ABSORB (241)	ABSORB (335)	ABSORB (1322)	ABSORB (1300)	ABSORB (266)	ABSORB (924)	ABSORB (822)	ABSORB (78)	ABSORB (95)	ABSORB (173)
DES (n)	XIENCE (239)	XIENCE (166)	XIENCE (686)	XIENCE (1300)	XIENCE Prime (134)	XIENCE (921)	XIENCE (800)	Promus Element or Biomatrix Flex (160)	XIENCE (96)	EES (89)
Follow-up (years)	4	5	5	1	4	2	1	2	3	1
Primary end point	In-segment late loss at 1 y	Vasomotion and minimum lumen diameter at 3 y	TLF at 1 y	TLF at 30 d	TLF	TVF at 2 y	TLF at 1 y	Late lumen loss at 9 mo	Optical frequency domain imaging-derived healing score at 6 mo	1 y in-segment lumen loss
Clinical setting	Stable CAD	Stable CAD	Stable CAD	Stable CAD and ACS (including STEMI >72 h)	Stable CAD	Stable CAD and ACS (including STEMI and Cardiogenic Shock)	Stable CAD and ACS (including STEMI)	Stable CAD and ACS (including STEMI)	STEMI (no cardiogenic shock)	ACS (including STEMI)
Lesion characteristics	Up to 2 lesions De novo LL <28 mm	Up to 2 lesions De novo Overlapping allowed in lesions <48 mm	Up to 2 lesions De novo LL <28 mm	Up to 3 lesions De novo LL <24 mm	Up to 2 lesions De novo LL <28 mm	De novo LL <70 mm.	De novo Complex lesions (total occlusion, LL >28 mm, bifurcation with single stent strategy included)	No limits for lesion length, number of target lesions or vessels	No limits for lesion length, number of target lesions or vessels	De novo lesions in native vessels or coronary bypass grafts

Mandatory PSP	No	No	No	Yes	No	No	Yes	No	No	No
Mandatory Use of Intravascular Imaging	No	No	No	No	Yes (IVUS or OCT)	No	No	OCT in first 30 willing patients	Follow-up only	No
TVF RR/HR [95% CI]	1.00 [0.51–1.94] P = .99	2.11 [1.00–4.44] P = .0425	1.41 [1.10–1.81] P = .006	1.35 [0.93–1.97] P = .11	1.15 [0.48–2.72] P = .75	1.12 [0.85–1.48] P = .43	1.33 [0.88–2.02] P = .17	P = .12	P = .465	1.04 [0.39–2.78]
Ischemia-driven TLR RR/HR [95% CI]	1.66 [0.61–4.49] P = .31	1.65 [0.46–5.92] P = .56	1.23 [0.85–1.79] P = .27	2.28 [0.99–5.25] P = .0457	1.17 [0.31–4.46] P = 1.00	1.17 [0.86–1.68] P = .31	0.89 [0.48–1.62] P = .69	P = .23	P = .678	0.84 [0.27–2.57]
Cardiac death RR/HR [95% CI]	0.33 [0.03–3.17] P = .37	0.50 [0.10–2.43] P = .56	1.17 [0.51–2.69] P = .71	N/A	N/A	0.78 [0.42–1.44] P = .43	4.87 [0.57–41.7] P = .11	P = .55	N/A	1.02 [0.19–5.58]
TV MI RR/HR [95% CI]	2.99 [0.61–14.65] P = .28	5.70 [1.36–23.87] P = .0061	1.47 [1.02–2.11] P = .03	1.23 [0.84–1.81] P = .29	1.51 [0.41–5.47] P = .76	1.60 [1.01–2.53] P = .04	1.96 [1.10–3.51] P = .0204	P = .11	P = .327	0.51 [0.03–8.20]
Device thrombosis probable/definitive RR/HR [95% CI]	N/A P = .50	N/A P = .50	3.12 [1.21–8–05] P = .01	4.05 [0.86–19.06] P = .06	1.02 [0.19–5.47] P = 1.00	3.87 [1.78–8.42] P<.001	3.31 [1.22–9.98] P = .0123	N/A	P = .55	0.51 [0.07–3.62]

Abbreviations: ACS, acute coronary syndrome; CAD, coronary artery disease; CI, confidence interval; Co-Cr, cobalt-chrome; HR, hazard ratio; IVUS, intravascular ultrasound; LL, lesion length; OCT, optical coherence tomography; PSP, predilatation, sizing, post-dilatation; RR, risk ratio; STEMI, ST-elevation myocardial infarction; TLF, composite of cardiac death, target-vessel myocardial infarction; TV, target vessel; TVF, target vessel revascularization (TLR).

Apart from the leading first-generation Absorb BVS technology, several pBRS devices are under clinical and preclinical investigation (see **Table 1**). These devices include, but are not limited to, DESolve (Elixir Medical, Sunnyvale, CA), Fantom (REVA Medical, San Diego, CA), ART Pure (ART, Paris, France), MeRes100 (Meril Life Sciences, Gujarat, India), Mirage (Manli Cardiology, Singapore), NeoVas (Lepu Medical Technology, Beijing, China), Renuvia (Boston Scientific, Marlborough, MA), Aptitude and Magnitude (Amaranth Medical, Mountain View, CA), Xinsorb (HuaAn Biotechnology, Hangzhou, China), Firesorb (MicroPort, Shanghai, China), Unity (QualiMed, Winsen, Germany), and Falcon (Abbott Vascular, Chicago, IL).

The DESolve scaffold is a novolimus-eluting BRS that received CE mark approval in May 2014. The first generation had 150-μm strut thickness, and the currently available second generation, DESolve Cx PLUS, has 120-μm struts. The DESolve scaffolds differ from the ABSORB stents owing to an intrinsic self-correcting deployment property that should decrease strut malapposition, a relative elasticity that provides a wide range of expansions without risk of strut fracture, and an early degradation and resorption profile.[17] However, this self-correcting feature is able to generate only small radial forces, so that it improves stent positioning with no relevant impact on the vessel wall.[17] Randomized clinical data on the comparison with other BRSs or metallic DES are not available to date.

The Fantom scaffold is a sirolimus-eluting BRS made principally from an iodinated polycarbonate copolymer of tyrosine analogues (desaminotyrosine) and biocompatible hydroxyesters which received CE mark approval in 2017. Despite a strut thickness of 125 μm, the design and structural properties of the polymer afford radial strength comparable to contemporary metallic DES, with low rates of recoil, allowing rapid inflation during deployment.[18] However, limited comparison data are available on clinical outcomes after Fantom scaffold implantation.

The ART BRS is made from a PDLLA amorphous polymer and received CE mark approval in May 2015. Notably, the device is free from antiproliferative drugs, which might be associated with early endothelial coverage. Moreover, it showed rapid degradation time, which might lead to a decreased risk of late device thrombosis. Nevertheless, this concept should be confirmed in further studies.[5]

The main feature of the Mirage BRS is its helicoidal structure, which allows enhanced flexibility and low crossing profile. The radial strength of the device is comparable to metallic stents. In addition, a better embedding into the vessel wall has been suggested for its monofiber circular struts than other BRS; this should cause less peristrut shear stress and disturbance in the coronary blood flow, but no comparison data have been presented yet.[5]

The MeRes100 BRS has a hybrid cell design (closed cells at the edges and open cells along the length), which allows optimal vessel wall conformability and high radial strength. The couplets of triaxial platinum radiopaque markers may facilitate the device positioning. Twelve-months randomized angiographic results showed comparable late luminal loss to Absorb BVS; however, no more clinical data are available.[19]

The Renuvia BRS uses a Synergy DES delivery system, which may allow for good deliverability and trackability of the device; it has thinner struts and increased overexpansion capability compared with Absorb BVS. However, given the discouraging results from Abbott's Absorb clinical trial program, the clinical development of this device has been stopped.[20]

Amaranth has introduced 3 different bioresorbable stents in the past decade: FORTITUDE, APTITUDE, and MAGNITUDE. The latest has a strut thickness of 98 μm with preserved radial strength and overexpansion capabilities. Interestingly, at the interim 9-month results of the first-in-man trial, no ScT was found. Nevertheless, larger clinical studies would be needed to confirm these findings.[20]

The NeoVas is a novel sirolimus-eluting PLLA-based BRS with acceptable in-scaffold late loss and a high percentage of scaffold strut coverage at 6 months without ScT cases. In the first reported randomized study it was noninferior to cobalt chrome EES with comparable in-segment late loss, clinical efficacy and safety outcomes, including recurrent angina.[20] However, longer term follow-up and larger trials are needed to determine the true impact of this device.

OVERVIEW OF MAGNESIUM SCAFFOLDS

The Magmaris (BIOTRONIK AG, Bülach, Switzerland) BRS, formerly known as DREAMS 2G, is the first sirolimus-eluting, biocorrodible metallic BRS with a bioresorbable PLLA coating. It gained CE mark approval in June 2016. It is the successor to the uncoated AMS and the paclitaxel-eluting DREAMS platforms.[21] Compared with previous generation devices, it was conceived to achieve sufficient radial support as well as the possibility of some expansion reserve, and a 12-month scaffolding time followed by resorption. Magnesium alloy resorption is a process starting at the backbone surface: the alloy reacts with water to create magnesium hydroxide that is slowly converted to an amorphous calcium phosphate phase, which is absorbed by the body. It has been speculated that the electronegative charge of magnesium during the degradation process might result in antithrombotic and antiarrhythmic properties.[21] The preclinical studies supported the safety profile of the Magmaris scaffold with a higher expansion capacity without scaffold fracture, advanced healing, and lower acute thrombogenicity compared with the pBRS, with the absence of excessive lumen loss up to 2 years.[22] The BIOSOLVE II and III RCTs demonstrated encouraging acute and long-term clinical outcomes in type A/B lesions in patients affected by stable or unstable angina. They showed a 6.8% 3-year TLF rate similar to outcomes of the Absorb BVS and the Xience DES.[23] Remarkably, no definite or probably stent thrombosis was reported at 3 years, which is in marked contrast with the 3-year ST rate of 2.4% with Absorb BVS.[13] Moreover, a serial optical coherence tomography observational substudy demonstrated at 6-month follow-up an excellent vessel healing consisting in reduction of incomplete scaffold apposition, dissections, intraluminal mass, and jailed side branch.[24] Further safety data continue to be collected in worldwide registries, including patients with ACS. The preliminary midterm outcomes showed low TV-MI, ischemia-driven TLR, or ScT rates.[25] Thus, so far, magnesium-based scaffolds fulfill the main assumptions of vascular restoration therapy: support, resorption, and restoration. However, no RCT results are available and, learning from the undesirable experience gained with the Absorb BVS, Magmaris implantation has been restricted to patients with a long life expectancy and no contraindications to DAPT, and to de novo lesions with high likelihood to regain vasomotion and no complex anatomy. Moreover, meticulous vessel preparation and image-guided implantation are highly recommended to optimize the deployment. Conversely, in a recent report the second-generation drug-eluting bioresorbable Magmaris was associated with lower angiography efficacy (ie, higher late lumen loss) and a higher rate of TLR without thrombotic safety concerns at 1 year.[26] The next-generation magnesium scaffold DREAMS 3-G with thinner struts (ranging from 99 microns for the 2.5 mm scaffold to 147 microns for the 4.0 mm scaffold), a longer targeted scaffolding time of at least 3 months, improved radial strength, and superior deliverability owing to a better crossing profile, has been recently released.[21] It will be under evaluation in large-scale clinical trials, including

randomized studies, where its efficacy will be compared against metallic DES to confirm further advancements in performance in terms of safety and efficacy.

MECHANISM OF FAILURE

Owing to the disappointing above-mentioned outcomes, the currently clinically available BRS were given a class III indication for clinical use outside of studies in current European Society of Cardiology guidelines.[1] Careful considerations should be given to the possible mechanism of such results, because the available BRS have different mechanical properties, footprints, and thicknesses, as well as a unique biodegradation profile. Reasonably, it can be speculated that the failure of pBRS, especially of the leading first-generation Absorb BVS, was caused by a combination of faulty device design and a far from optimal implantation technique.[27] As a matter of fact, differently from metal alloys that are used for permanent implants, BRS materials have insufficient ductility and limited elongation to break, which limit scaffold expansion during deployment, along with low tensile strength and stiffness, which require the struts to be thick to prevent recoil during vessel remodeling. Other disadvantages include lower crossing profiles owing to greater strut thickness, limited biocompatibility of PLLA, and an extensive and heterogeneous time until degradation.[2,4] Therefore, several mechanisms have been acknowledged to be involved in BRS failure (**Fig. 1**).

Device Related

First, bulkier struts can promote the formation of platelet aggregates owing to their protrusion into the lumen and interruption of the laminar blood flow, inducing flow disturbances and amplifying endothelial shear stress, especially in cases of suboptimal implantation. Additionally, the limited mechanical properties of the scaffold have been associated with a lower acute minimal lumen diameter, which results in a greater risk of recoil compared with metallic EES, along with greater late luminal loss and decreased mean lumen area.[3,4] Mentioned features, associated with a greater neointimal hyperplasia, led to greater coronary artery lumen narrowing and consequent device failure.[27] Also, specifically for BRS technologies, as a result of the bioresorption process, the loss of integrity of the scaffold backbone led to prolapse of the scaffold remnants into the vessel lumen, possibly affecting the coronary blood flow, especially in case of delayed endothelization owing to wider struts and polymer coverage. However, it remains unknown the level

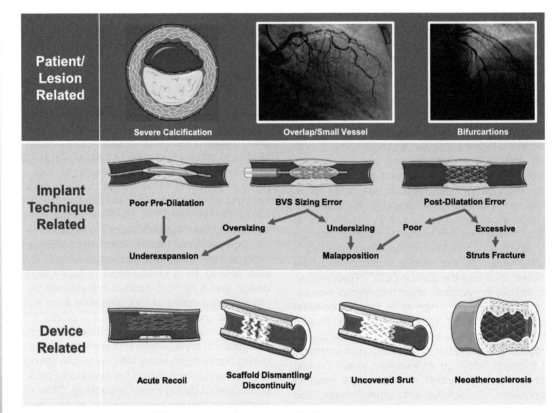

Fig. 1. Possible mechanism of BRS failure leading to clinical adverse events.

of thickness and maturity of the intimal layer required for the BRS structure to avoid losing mechanical integrity during bioresorption.[28] The finding of evagination and peristrut contrast staining in first-generation BRS is also linked to inflammatory reaction during polymer degrading process.[29] Last, the relatively long resorption, an excessively thin neointimal layer, and the endothelial dysfunction possibly accelerated by PLLA might allow the development of neoatherosclerosis.[3]

Implant Technique Related

As first reported by Puricel and associates, greater thrombogenicity might be associated with a suboptimal deployment technique. As a matter of fact, the thicker struts and larger footprint of pBRS require dedicated implantation protocol (prepare the lesion, size adequately, postdilate) to achieve the complete expansion of the backbone, avoiding malapposition.[30] A recent subanalysis of the available ABSORB RCTs showed that accurate adjustment of the scaffold and optimal postdilation correlate with a lower risk of TLF, whereas aggressive predilatation correlates with a lower risk of ST.[31]

Therefore, suboptimal implantation with incomplete lesion coverage, underexpansion, and malapposition would require a longer duration of DAPT to compensate for the much longer healing time and the higher risk of ScT.[32]

Patient or Lesion Related

Recent studies have identified several clinical scenarios associated with a greater risk of TLF than in use of DES. Owing to the pBRS design and possible failure of the recommended implantation protocol, the treatment of aorto-ostial lesions, bifurcations, small (reference vessel diameter of <2.40 mm) or calcified vessel is still discouraged.[5]

There have been limited reports of scaffold failure after metallic BRS implantation, some of them discovered in asymptomatic patients during planned staged procedures. Moreover, owing to the lack of systematic intracoronary imaging at the baseline procedure, it cannot be excluded the operator role rather than a scaffold failure. To date, the identified mechanisms of TLF included early focal recoil and collapse with scaffold dismantling and neointimal hyperplasia.[33]

BIORESORBABLE SCAFFOLDS PERSPECTIVES

Collectively, too many of the prophecies on pBRS technology remain unfulfilled and the available evidence on metallic BRS is currently limited to small observational studies. The Class IIIC recommendation in the latest European guidelines seems to be reasonable, because the current generation of BRS are not ready for clinical use outside of well-designed studies and should not be preferred over the current generation of DES in everyday clinical practice so far.[1,4] Nevertheless, all ongoing studies should be thoroughly monitored to understand the impact and possible mechanism of adverse events to guide the newer generation of scaffold improvements.[4] Regarding new studies, the preclinical testing should include mechanical and biocompatibility testing, and bench and in vivo examinations in animal models should evaluate luminal dimensions during degradation, acute and chronic inflammation, drug concentration, change in tissue composition, and the essential features of degradation products. Importantly, the duration of follow-up should be sufficient to capture all relevant biological processes pertaining to stent safety. The clinical pre–CE-mark phase should include initial human feasibility studies with BRS based on intravascular imaging evaluation and angiographic follow-up (small sized, selected patients) and a subsequent randomized trial based on surrogate endpoints (medium sized, comparator device). The post–CE-mark phase should include a large-scale, clinical, randomized trial with long-term follow-up and should be powered to confirm superiority over the comparator.[4] The design of newer devices is aimed to producing thinner and more biocompatible struts, with a smaller crossing profile and a more optimized degradation profile to allow rapid and full neointimal coverage before biodegradation without inflammation, and all this by maintaining or even improving the radial force. Apart from device developments, a rigorous dedicated protocol implantation seems to be fundamental to achieve optimal results of BRS implantation, even if recent study suggest that even optimal postprocedural results by predilatation, sizing, and postdilatation may not guarantee freedom from undesirable dismantling.[30] Furthermore, proper lesion selection is crucial and the use of BRS is strongly discouraged in heavily calcified vessels and coronary arteries with an reference vessel diameter of less than 2.5 mm, and excessive scaffold overlap should be avoided and a device-to-device technique should be applied yet.[4] Moreover, operators should be strongly encouraged to use intracoronary imaging for lesion assessment during implantation and follow-up. Finally, because prolonged DAPT may limit the risk of ScT, BRS should not be recommended in patients who cannot tolerate prolonged DAPT or who require treatment with oral anticoagulants.[32]

SUMMARY

Despite some expected benefits of BRS, none of the available data have confirmed the advantage of the first-generation BRS over the metallic DES. Thus, the current generations of BRS, especially the Absorb BVS, should not be preferred to conventional DES in everyday clinical practice. To not leave behind the desirable vascular restoration therapy concept, the next generations of BRS should aim not only to improve the acute performance of the device but, above all, to improve long-term safety. Such developments might be achieved both by device improvement, but also with a proper technique of implantation, intravascular imaging guidance, as well as careful patient and lesion selection. Accordingly, new-generation devices have been developed with thinner struts, greater radial force and vessel wall coverage, less recoil and shorter resorption time with a lesser degree of inflammation secondary to polymer resorption. Reasonable long-term safety/efficacy evaluations are now recommended to establish comparable mid-term clinical outcomes and clear clinical advantages after complete resorption compared with currently available metallic DES.

CLINICS CARE POINTS

- Despite advanced iterations in metallic DES, there remains a 2% to 3% per year incidence of device-related adverse events, regardless of stent type.
- The BRS aims to provide early drug delivery and mechanical support similar to metallic DES followed by complete resorption.
- Available long-term evidence focused on the Absorb BVS showing higher adverse events compared with everolimus-eluting DES, with a substantial reduction of the BRS-relative hazard after 3-year follow-up (complete resorption time).
- Careful considerations should be given on the possible mechanism of such unsatisfactory results because the available BRS have different mechanical properties, footprint and thickness and a unique biodegradation profile.
- An improved scaffold design and deployment technique to mitigate early BRS risk may

enhance the late benefit of complete resorption.

DISCLOSURE

G. Masiero, G. Rodinò, and G. Tarantini declared no conflicts regarding this publication.

REFERENCES

1. Neumann FJ, Sousa-Uva M, Ahlsson A, et al. 2018 ESC/EACTS Guidelines on myocardial revascularization. Eur Heart J 2019;40:87–165.
2. Kereiakes DJ, Onuma Y, Serruys PW, et al. Bioresorbable vascular scaffolds for coronary revascularization. Circulation 2016;134(2):168–82.
3. Raber L, Ueki Y. Bioresorbable scaffolds: unfulfilled prophecies. Circulation 2019;140(23):1917–20.
4. Byrne RA, Stefanini GG, Capodanno D, et al. Report of an ESC-EAPCI Task Force on the evaluation and use of bioresorbable scaffolds for percutaneous coronary intervention: executive summary. Eurointervention 2018;13(13):1574–86.
5. Ang HY, Bulluck H, Wong P, et al. Bioresorbable stents: current and upcoming bioresorbable technologies. Int J Cardiol 2017;228:931–9.
6. Tarantini G, Masiero G, Granada JF, et al. The BVS concept. From the chemical structure to the vascular biology: the bases for a change in interventional cardiology. Minerva Cardioangiol 2016;64(4):419–41.
7. Tarantini G, Masiero G, Fovino LN, et al, all RAI investigators. "Full-plastic jacket" with everolimus-eluting Absorb bioresorbable vascular scaffolds: clinical outcomes in the multicenter prospective RAI registry (ClinicalTrials.gov Identifier: NCT02298413). Int J Cardiol 2018;266:67–74.
8. Tarantini G, Mojoli M, Masiero G, et al, all RAI investigators. Clinical outcomes of overlapping versus non-overlapping everolimus-eluting absorb bioresorbable vascular scaffolds: an analysis from the multicentre prospective RAI registry (ClinicalTrials.gov identifier: NCT02298413). Catheter Cardiovasc Interv 2018;91(1):E1–16.
9. Cassese S, Byrne RA, Ndrepepa G, et al. Everolimus-eluting bio- resorbable vascular scaffolds versus everolimus-eluting metallic stents: a meta-analysis of randomised controlled trials. Lancet 2016;387(10018):537–44.
10. Chang CC, Onuma Y, Achenbach S, et al. COMPARE ABSORB trial investigators. Absorb bioresorbable scaffold versus Xience metallic stent for prevention of restenosis following percutaneous coronary intervention in patients at high risk of restenosis: rationale and design of the COMPARE ABSORB trial. Cardiovasc Revasc Med 2019; 20(7):577–82.
11. Stone GW, Ellis SG, Gori T, et al. Blinded outcomes and angina assessment of coronary bioresorbable scaffolds: 30-day and 1-year results from the ABSORB IV randomised trial. Lancet 2018;392: 1530–40.
12. Ali ZA, Serruys PW, Kimura T, et al. 2-year outcomes with the Absorb bioresorbable scaffold for treatment of coronary artery disease: a systematic review and meta-analysis of seven randomised trials with an individual patient data substudy. Lancet 2017; 390(10096):760–72.
13. Ali ZA, Gao R, Kimura T, et al. Three-Year outcomes with the ab- sorb bioresorbable scaffold: individual-patient-data meta-analysis from the ABSORB randomized trials. Circulation 2018;137(5):464–79.
14. Cassese S, Byrne RA, Jüni P, et al. Midterm clinical outcomes with everolimus-eluting bioresorbable scaffolds versus everolimus-eluting metallic stents for percutaneous coronary interventions: a meta-analysis of randomised trials. Eurointervention 2018;13(13):1565–73.
15. Kereiakes DJ, Ellis SG, Metzger DC, et al. Clinical outcomes before and after complete everolimus-eluting bioresorbable scaffold resorption: five-year follow-up from the ABSORB III trial. Circulation 2019;140(23):1895–903.
16. Onuma Y, Honda Y, Asano T, et al. Randomized comparison between everolimus-eluting bioresorbable scaffold and metallic stent: multimodality imaging through 3 years. JACC Cardiovasc Interv 2020;13(1):116–27.
17. Mattesini A, Bartolini S, Dini CS, et al. The DESolve novolimus bioresorbable Scaffold: from bench to bedside. J Thorac Dis 2017;9(Suppl. S9):950–8.
18. Abizaid A, Carrie D, Frey N, et al. 6-month clinical and angiographic outcomes of a novel radiopaque sirolimus-eluting bioresorbable vascular scaffold: the FANTOM II study. JACC Cardiovasc Interv 2017;10(18):1832–8.
19. Tenekecioglu E, Serruys PW, Onuma Y, et al. Randomized comparison of absorb bioresorbable vascular scaffold and mirage microfiber sirolimus-eluting scaffold using multimodality imaging. JACC Cardiovasc Interv 2017;10(11):1115–30.
20. Regazzoli D, Leone PP, Colombo A, et al. New generation bioresorbable scaffold technologies: an update on novel devices and clinical results. J Thorac Dis 2017;9(Suppl 9):S979–85.
21. Bennett J, De Hemptinne Q, McCutcheon K. Magmaris resorbable magnesium scaffold for the treatment of coronary heart disease: overview of its safety and efficacy. Expert Rev Med Devices 2019; 16(9):757–69.
22. Barkholt TØ, Webber B, Holm NR, et al. Mechanical properties of the drug-eluting bioresorbable magnesium scaffold compared with polymeric scaffolds and a permanent metallic drug-eluting stent.

Catheter Cardiovasc Interv 2019 [Online ahead of print].

23. Haude M, Ince H, Tolg R, et al. Sustained safety and performance of the second-generation drug-eluting absorbable metal scaffold (DREAMS 2G) in patients with de novo coronary lesions: 3-year clinical results and angiographic findings of the BIOSOLVE-II first-in- man trial. Eurointervention 2020;15(15): e1375–82.

24. Ozaki Y, Garcia-Garcia HM, Hideo-Kajita A, et al. Impact of procedural characteristics on coronary vessel wall healing following implantation of second-generation drug-eluting absorbable metal scaffold in patients with de-novo coronary artery lesions: an optical coherence tomography analysis. Eur Heart J Cardiovasc Imaging 2019;20:916–24.

25. Verheye S, Wlodarczak A, Montorsi P, et al. Twelve-month outcomes of 400 patients treated with a resorbable metal scaffold: insights from the BIOSOLVE-IV registry. Eurointervention 2020; 15(15):e1383–6.

26. Sabaté M, Alfonso F, Cequier A, et al. Magnesium-based resorbable scaffold versus permanent metallic sirolimus-eluting stent in patients with ST-segment elevation myocardial infarction: the MAG-STEMI randomized clinical trial. Circulation 2019; 140(23):1904–16.

27. Katagiri Y, Serruys PW, Asano T, et al. How does the failure of Absorb apply to the other bioresorbable scaffolds? An expert review of first-in-man and pivotal trials. Eurointervention 2019;15(1):116–23.

28. Raber L, Ueki Y. Understanding the bioresorbable vascular scaffold Achilles heel: insights from ABSORB Japan Serial Intracoronary Imaging. JACC Cardiovasc Interv 2020;13(1):128–31.

29. Gori T, Jansen T, Weissner M, et al. Coronary evaginations and peri-scaffold aneurysms following implantation of bioresorbable scaffolds: incidence, outcome, and optical coherence tomography analysis of possible mechanisms. Eur Heart J 2016;37: 2040–9.

30. Puricel S, Cuculi F, Weissner M, et al. Bioresorbable coronary scaffold thrombosis: multicenter comprehensive analysis of clinical presentation, mechanisms, and predictors. J Am Coll Cardiol 2016; 67(8):921–31.

31. Stone GW, Abizaid A, Onuma Y, et al. Effect of technique on outcomes following bioresorbable vascular scaffold implantation: analysis from the ABSORB trials. J Am Coll Cardiol 2017;70:2863–74.

32. Capodanno D, Angiolillo DJ. Antiplatelet therapy after implantation of Bioresorbable vascular scaffolds: a review of the published data, practical recommendations, and future directions. JACC Cardiovasc Interv 2017;10(5):425–37.

33. Ozaki Y, Garcia-Garcia HM, Shlofmitz E, et al. Second-generation drug-eluting resorbable magnesium scaffold: review of the clinical evidence. Cardiovasc Revasc Med 2020;21(1):127–36.

MicroRNAs and Long Noncoding RNAs in Coronary Artery Disease
New and Potential Therapeutic Targets

Lukasz Zareba, MD[a], Alex Fitas, MD[a], Marta Wolska, MD[a], Eva Junger, MD[a],
Ceren Eyileten, MD, PhD[a], Zofia Wicik, MD[a,b], Salvatore De Rosa, MD, PhD[c],
Jolanta M. Siller-Matula, MD, PhD[a,d], Marek Postula, MD, PhD[a,e],*

KEYWORDS

- Atherosclerosis • miRNAs • microRNA • lncRNAs • Long noncoding RNA • miR-155 • miR-33
- miR-92a

KEY POINTS

- Noncoding RNAs (ncRNAs) including long noncoding RNAs (lncRNAs) and microRNAs (miRNAs) play an important role in CAD onset and progression.
- The ability of ncRNAs to simultaneously regulate many target genes allows them to modulate various key processes involved in AS, including lipid metabolism, smooth muscle cell proliferation, autophagy, and foam cell formation.
- Both lncRNAs and miRNAs may have potential as novel therapeutics in CAD.

INTRODUCTION

Atherosclerosis (AS), the major underlying cause of coronary artery disease (CAD), is a chronic progressive inflammatory state that leads to plaque buildup inside arteries. An important trigger in AS is hypercholesterolemia, which induces endothelial injury allowing entry of lipids, such as low-density lipoprotein (LDL) particles, into the subendothelial space of the intimal layer of arteries, where they are then oxidized and act as strong chemoattractants. Macrophages also play a key role in AS; they engulf oxidized LDL (ox-LDL) and transform into foam cells, the prototypical cells in atherosclerotic plaques. Macrophages additionally increase proinflammatory cytokines, which induce the recruitment and proliferation of smooth muscle cells (SMCs). Vulnerable plaques are the leading cause of coronary thrombosis and are usually characterized by thin fibrous caps, few or absent SMCs, and increased number of inflammatory cells.[1] These processes are of particular importance in the pathology of AS and are often targeted in AS therapy.

The incidence and progression of CAD are closely linked with modulatory noncoding RNAs (ncRNAs), such as microRNAs (miRNAs) and

Funding: The work was supported financially as part of the internal funding of the Department of Experimental and Clinical Pharmacology, Medical University of Warsaw, Centre for Preclinical Research and Technology CEPT, Warsaw, Poland.
[a] Department of Experimental and Clinical Pharmacology, Medical University of Warsaw, Center for Preclinical Research and Technology CEPT, Banacha 1B Str., Warsaw 02-097, Poland; [b] Centro de Matemática, Computação e Cognição, Universidade Federal do ABC, Alameda da Universidade, s/n-Anchieta, São Paulo 09606-045, Brazil; [c] Division of Cardiology, Department of Medical and Surgical Sciences, "Magna Graecia" University, Viale Europa, Catanzaro 88100, Italy; [d] Department of Internal Medicine II, Division of Cardiology, Medical University of Vienna, Spitalgasse 23, Vienna 1090, Austria; [e] Longevity Center, Warsaw, Poland
* Corresponding author. Department of Experimental and Clinical Pharmacology, Medical University of Warsaw, Center for Preclinical Research and Technology CEPT, Banacha 1B Str., Warsaw 02-097, Poland.
E-mail address: mpostula@wum.edu.pl

long noncoding RNAs (lncRNAs).[2] miRNAs regulate gene expression at the post-transcriptional level by inhibiting gene translation or promoting messenger RNA degradation.[3–6] lncRNAs, however, are relevant in fundamental processes of gene regulation, such as chromatin modification and transcriptional regulation.[7]

The role of miRNAs in the pathophysiology of various diseases, especially cardiovascular diseases, was broadly reported.[4–6] They are involved in lipid metabolism, inflammation processes, SMCs proliferation, and foam cell formation, which demonstrates their importance in AS development. Nowadays, there is growing evidence that lncRNAs affect the onset and progression of cardiovascular diseases. lncRNAs have been identified as important regulators of complex biologic processes linked to the proper functioning of the cardiovascular system, including cardiac muscle development and in case of disrupted regulatory functions also multiple cardiovascular pathologies.[7] The multistage involvement of lncRNAs and miRNAs in the development of cardiovascular diseases makes them promising therapeutic targets.

We review current literature knowledge about miRNAs and lncRNAs involvement in CAD progression and their potential as novel therapeutic approach.

MicroRNA-155

miR-155 is coded by *BIC* gene and expressed in hematopoietic stem-progenitor and mature hematopoietic cells. It is known to be elevated during monocytic cell differentiation toward macrophages. miR-155 can target *SOCS1*, and *TNF-α*, related to inflammatory processes and pathogenesis of AS.[8] Various inflammatory mediators, such as tumor necrosis factor (TNF)-α, may enhance miR-155 expression in monocytes and macrophages.[9] miR-155 stimulates inflammatory gene expression through inhibition of *BCL6* gene, which is a negative regulator of nuclear factor (NF)-κB, thus its suppression leads to enhanced expression of NF-κB. As a result, miR-155 causes overexpression of NF-κB and plays a key role in inflammatory responses and regulates expression of proinflammatory cytokines, leukocytes recruitment, and cell survival.[8,10,11] However, miR-155 may alleviate inflammation by targeting *CARHSP1*, which impacts the stability of TNF-α. TNF-α directly activates NF-κB in response to injury and inflammation. The loss of its stability leads to decreased levels of TNF-α causing less activation of NF-κB pathway. Consequently, miR-155 may have a protective role in AS-associated foam cell formation via miR-155-*CARHSP1*-TNF-α pathway.[9]

Under physiologic conditions macrophages express scavenger receptors (SR), including SR-A1, CD36, and LOX-1. All the of listed SR present affinity to ox-LDL, which causes the transformation of macrophages to the foam cells. Increased levels of ox-LDL along with proinflammatory cytokines results in upregulation of LOX-1 expression. This process leads to lipid accumulation and foam cell formation.[12] Additionally, ox-LDL is responsible for enhanced miR-155 expression in macrophages. Surprisingly, miR-155 may alleviate inflammation and foam cells formation acting through *CARHSP1*.[9] However, several studies documented that miR-155 is associated with proinflammatory processes.[13,14] lncRNA, MALAT1, is known to sponge miR-155. MALAT1 can elevate the proliferation and repress the proinflammatory cytokine secretion and cell apoptosis via sponging miR-155 and increasing the antiinflammatory protein SOCS1 concentration.[13] Additionally, miR-155 directly inhibits SOCS1 expression and enhances p-STAT3 and PDCD4 expression. PDCD4 improves inflammatory response through the activation of NF-κB and inhibition of anti-inflammatory interleukin (IL)-10.[14]

Ox-LDL not only initiates inflammation but also stimulates apoptosis of macrophages. It acts through different pathways; among them p85α/*AKT* pathway was identified. miR-155 directly targets p85α gene, which leads to p85α suppression. This action results in inhibition of *AKT* activation and antiapoptotic effect.[15] Moreover, miR-155 is also involved in macrophage differentiation; it promotes macrophage transition into M1 phenotype and increases proinflammatory cytokines and chemokine secretion.[16] There is evidence of miR-155 involvement in foam cell formation by targeting *HBP1*.[17] Furthermore, upregulated miR-155 sensitized macrophages to inflammatory activation by abrogating *BCL6*-mediated inhibition of NF-κB signaling.[10] In contrary, miR-155 can inhibit the transformation of macrophages into foam cells by enhancing *CEH* signaling pathway in macrophages.[18]

miR-155 also contributes to the autophagy process, which is important for regeneration of vascular intimal wall injury. It promotes autophagy in vascular endothelial cells (VECs) by suppressing phosphorylated *PI3K/Akt/mTOR* pathway. *PI3K/Akt/mTOR* pathway plays an important role in the regulation of autophagy in AS. The activation of this pathway resulted in autophagy inhibition.[19] Moreover, in vitro analysis showed that miR-155 enhances ox-LDL-induced autophagy.[20] It indicates that miR-155 upregulation may have a protective effect in atherosclerotic lesions by promoting autophagy.

The role of miR-155 in AS development is ambiguous. Upregulation of miR-155 might contribute to the prevention of AS by inhibiting apoptosis and altering the inflammation process in atherosclerotic lesions.[9,15] However, downregulation of miR-155 shows a therapeutic effect by attenuating ox-LDL-mediated inflammation signaling, stimulating M2 macrophage phenotype and decreasing foam cell formation.[10,11,13,14,17] Furthermore, animal studies showed that antagomir-155 (miR-155 inhibitor) attenuated AS development and progression in mice.[10,17,21] Therefore, antagomir-155 should be considered as a potential therapeutic agent against AS. Several clinical trials are testing antagomir-155 safety and tolerability; however, none of them are registered for AS treatment. MRG-106 is a locked nucleic acid–modified oligonucleotide inhibitor of miR-155, which had promising preliminary results in a phase 1 clinical trial with cutaneous T-cell lymphoma.[22,23] Further investigations are needed to elucidate clinical effect of antagomir-155 in AS treatment.

MicroRNA-33

miR-33 family consists of miR-33a and miR-33b, which are encoded within the introns of the *SREBP2* and *SREBP1* genes, respectively. miR-33a and its host gene are transcriptionally upregulated under conditions of low sterol concentration. SREBP2 protein induces the expression of genes involved in cholesterol synthesis, whereas miR-33a inhibits genes involved in hydrolysis and export of cholesterol from the cell, including intracellular trafficking and cholesterol efflux.[24] miR-33 targets *ABCA1*, *ABCG1*, *CPT1A*, *IRS2*, *AMPK*, and *CROT* in hepatic cells and *ABCA1* and *ABCG1* in macrophages.[16,25] These genes are involved in glucose and lipid metabolism, both of which are impaired during AS development.

miR-33 has been shown to modulate *ABCA1* and *ABCG1* expression in macrophages.[26,27] These proteins mediate cholesterol efflux, and they are responsible for decreasing cholesterol concentration in many types of cells including macrophages. In AS, proinflammatory stimulation induces deposition of cholesterol in macrophages, triggering the formation of foam cells.[28] Several studies showed that downregulation of miR-33 in vivo increased cholesterol efflux in peripheral macrophages including arterial macrophages in atherosclerotic lesions.[26,29–31] Moreover, miR-33 modulates target genes *PDK4* and *PGC-1α*.[32] PDK4 is responsible for regulation of mitochondrial

respiration, whereas PGC-1α participates in mitochondrial biogenesis and regulation of carbohydrate and lipid metabolism.[33] miR-33 inhibition increased the expression of PDK4 and PGC-1α proteins, which resulted in boosted mitochondrial respiration and production of ATP in macrophages. This effect in combination with increased *ABCA1* expression resulted in promoting macrophage cholesterol efflux.[32]

Proinflammatory phenotype of macrophages in arterial wall lesions contributes to the formation of foam cells and atherosclerotic plaque development. miR-33 plays an important role in macrophage activation by promoting phenotype shift into proinflammatory M1. Inhibition of miR-33 expression resulted in an increased level of anti-inflammatory M2 markers (Arginase-1, IL-10) and reduced expression of proinflammatory M1 markers (inducible nitric oxide synthase and TNF-α).[30] Moreover, miR-33 modulates an expression of proinflammatory cytokines. The deficiency of miR-33 suppressed the secretion of IL-1β, IL-6, and TNF-α in ox-LDL-treated THP-1 macrophages.[34] Moreover, lack of miR-33 expression leads to the inhibition of NF-κB and TLR4 mediated pathways resulting in a reduction in arterial macrophage activation and polarization in vivo.[31] In contrast, miR-33 inhibition resulted in the elevation of M2 markers, such as anti-inflammatory IL-10, and M1 markers, such as IL-6. These results indicate a more complex role of miR-33 in the inflammatory regulation.[26]

miR-33 is involved in the regulation of autophagy by targeting genes engaged in autophagy pathways including *LAMP1*, *ATG5*, and *ATG12*. Moreover, it modulates AMPK-dependent activation of *TFEB* and *FOXO3*.[24,35] FOXO3 promotes autophagy, whereas TFEB is involved in the regulation of autophagy and lysosome biogenesis.[36] Inhibition of miR-33 resulted in increased expression of *LAMP1*, *ATG5*, and *ATG12*, and promoted AMPK-dependent activation of the *TFEB* and *FOXO3* in macrophage foam cells, and thus enhanced the autophagy process.[24,35]

Additionally, miR-33 contributes to the overall number of macrophages within the arterial wall. The inhibition of miR-33 expression results in decreased arterial macrophage content and decrease in atherosclerotic plaque size.[31]

miR-33 inhibition was shown to increase *ABCA1* expression. *ABCA1* has a role in mediating cholesterol efflux and transports it to lipid-poor apolipoproteins that consequently form nascent high-density lipoproteins (HDL). Activation of miR-33 was shown to inhibit the expression of *ABCA1* in mouse and human cells limiting cholesterol efflux to ApoA1 and therefore reducing lipid molecules accepted by nascent HDL.[37] The relationship between miR-33 inhibition and increased plasma HDL levels was also demonstrated in two nonhuman primate studies.[38] Furthermore, another study revealed that the difference in measured HDL cholesterol (HDL-C) levels in plasma was only significant in mice fed a chow diet receiving anti-miR-33 oligonucleotides therapy compared with control mice. In contrast, anti-miR-33 oligonucleotides-treated mice fed a western diet did not show a significant change in HDL-C plasma levels compared with control mice.[25] Therefore, the efficacy of miR-33 therapy in HDL elevation is controversial and must be further investigated to determine its true effect.

However, long-term inhibition of miR-33 by using anti-miR-33 oligonucleotides increased the expression of genes involved in fatty acid synthesis, such as ACC and FAS in the liver. Anti-miR-33 therapy resulted in elevated circulating triglyceride levels and caused lipid accumulation in the liver of mice fed with a high-fat diet.[39]

Taken together, miR-33 inhibition has been demonstrated as a promising therapeutic approach for delaying the development and enhancing the regression of AS. miR-33 inhibition achieves these effects by inducing cholesterol efflux from macrophages, decreasing the proinflammatory macrophage phenotype, inducing autophagy, and reducing macrophage content in atherosclerotic plaques. Rayner and colleagues[30] reported that anti-miR-33-treated mice showed reductions in plaque size and lipid content; increased markers of plaque stability; and decreased inflammatory genes expression, such as TNF-α, TLR6, and TLR13. However, the effects of miR-33 inhibition on HDL-C levels are still debated. The influence of miR-33 on glucose and lipid metabolism is important to recognize because it may contribute to complications and adverse effects of the treatment. miR-33 inhibition in LDL receptor–deficient mice promoted obesity, insulin-resistance, and hyperlipidemia.[31] Currently, no clinical trials on miR-33 are being conducted but effects and safety of antagomiR-33 treatment should be assed in the future.

MicroRNA-92A

The miR-92a family consists of miRNAs including miR-25, miR-92a, and miR-363 and is a part of the miR-17~19 cluster.[40] miR-17~9 cluster is involved in heart development and has numerous effects on the cardiovascular system. miR-92a-3p, a component of miR-17~19 cluster, stimulates cardiomyocytes metabolism through targeting the fatty acid translocase CD36 and ABCA8b genes.

CD36 is a transporter of fatty acids in the heart.[41] Its upregulation is mainly associated with increased free fatty acid uptake from cardiomyocytes that leads to enhanced β-oxidation process of free fatty acids, which is a process responsible for cellular energy production.[42] In contrast, ABCA8b main role is to transport HDL in cardiac cells. Depletion of miR-92a in myocardial infarction (MI) leads to enhanced activity of CD36, which maintains proper energy homeostasis of the heart under pathologic conditions.[41]

miR-92a is involved in vascular pathologies, including AS. Overexpression of miR-92a promotes macrophage participation in AS formation and atherosusceptibility through targeting KLF4.[43] KLF4 can promote macrophages differentiation into anti-inflammatory M2 type, and increase the expression of Ch25h and LXR, which causes cholesterol transport back to the liver and regulates vascular smooth muscle cell (VSMC).[44] Thus, miR-92a-induced downregulation of KLF4 leads to ECs injury, PDGF-BB-mediated proliferation, and migration of VSMCs and atherosclerotic plaque formation.[45] Additionally, overexpression of miR-92a enhances LDL uptake and proinflammatory cytokines expression in ECs, which enhances the plaque buildup.[43]

In contrary, overexpression of miR-92a downregulates ITAG5 gene expression. ITAG5 is responsible for the accumulation of proangiogenic factors, including vascular endothelial growth factor or endothelial nitric oxide synthase, and thus has influence on vascular tone and platelet aggregation. Moreover, ITAG5 is able to activate ERK1/2 and PI3K/AKT signaling pathways.[46] Both ERK1/2 and PI3K/AKT are involved in angiogenesis by promoting EC survival and migration. PI3K/AKT axis is also involved in MI progression and regulation of oxidative stress in CAD.[47] Thus, both can influence the progression of CAD and its long-term complications.

Consequently, miR-92a acts as a proatherogenic through targeting KLF4 and antiatherogenic via ITAG5. Moreover, miR-92a downregulation acts cardioprotectively via CD36, ABCA8b on post-MI heart.[41,43,46]

miR-92a shows the highest expression among all members of the miR-17~92 cluster in human ECs. Its overexpression causes inhibition of proangiogenic factor expression, such as ITGA5, impairment of ECs, and promotion of AS lesions. Inhibition of miR-92a expression may lead to increased angiogenesis and revascularization in injured hearts and reduction in AS severity. Moreover, in vivo study has shown the therapeutic effect of miR-92a downregulation in AS mice by preventing AS development.[48] Altogether, inhibition of miR-92a is a promising approach in CAD treatment. Currently, no clinical trials with miR-92a in CAD are being conducted. However, MRG-110 (a locked nucleic acid modified oligonucleotide inhibitor of miR-92), is currently being tested for angiogenesis induction to improve healing of chronic cutaneous wounds.[49,50] Positive results of that trial would pave the way to further applications of miR-92a inhibition in patients with ischemic heart disease or peripheral artery disease.

OTHER microRNAs AS A POTENTIAL THERAPEUTIC TARGET

VSMCs are the main source of plaque cells and extracellular matrix in all stages of AS. Inflammation enhances the proliferation of VSMCs and stimulates production of dense extracellular matrix, which leads to the development of more advanced atherosclerotic lesions. One of the genes responsible for regulation of the proliferation and migration of VSMC is *HMGB1*. This gene also enhances inflammation in atherosclerotic plaques via stimulation of expression of proinflammatory IL-1β in VSMCs.[51] miR-126-5p targets *HMGB1* and inhibits its expression, which causes the alleviation of AS. In patients with AS significant downregulation of miR-126-5p was observed.[52]

AS initiation and its severity is highly dependent on vascular inflammatory response, including proinflammatory cytokines and signaling pathways. Also, inflammatory macrophages play a crucial role in formation of atherosclerotic plaque. One of the genes responsible for inflammation regulation is *PDCD4*. It plays a role in regulation of apoptosis in VSMCs, promotion of inflammation by activation of NF-κB signaling pathway and inhibition of IL-10. miR-16 targets *PDCD4* expression and through downregulation decreases levels of proinflammatory cytokines, increases levels of anti-inflammatory factors, and reduces the *NF-KB* signaling pathway. Moreover, through targeting *PDCD4*, miR-16 can also reduce the activity of *MAPK* axis, which activates inflammatory macrophages.[53] In addition, miR-16 is released by ischemic peripheral muscle and exerts a proinflammatory action on remote vascular beds, increasing the expression of TNF-α and reducing the production of endothelial nitric oxide synthase and vascular endothelial growth factor.[54] Hence, blocking blood-borne miR-16 might reveal an easy and useful strategy to prevent endothelial dysfunction especially in patients with severe multibed AS.

Foam cells have great contribution to an atherosclerotic plaque formation. Development of those cells is caused by excessive lipid uptake by macrophages via SR receptors.[12] LOX-1 is one of the glycoproteins responsible of ox-LDL uptake in macrophages, which results in foam cells formation and plays a role in the development of AS. miR-98 directly targets and inhibits LOX-1 messenger RNA expression in macrophages. In the macrophages treated with ox-LDL, miR-98 expression is decreased, and LOX-1 synthesis is increased. Thus, miR-98 could repress the AS development acting through LOX-1.[55]

The activity of macrophages in formation of atherosclerotic plaque is also regulated by *MAML1*. *MAML1* is a component of Notch axis, which contributes to progression of AS mainly via regulation of inflammation. miR-133b can regulate Notch signaling pathway via targeting *MAML1*. Inhibition of either miR-133b or Notch axis can reduce plaque size, reduce macrophages proliferation and migration, and enhance their apoptosis. Moreover, Zheng and colleagues[56] reported that mice with AS treated with miR-133b antagomir showed wider lumen of the vessels, more stable plaque shape, smaller lipid core, and thicker fibrous cap of the plaque compared with those treated with miR-133b antagomir.

Impairment of autophagy plays a key role in the AS development. Both autophagy and AS are triggered by a few common factors, such as inflammation, reactive oxygen species, and shear stress. Impairment of autophagy leads to greater accumulation of lipids, increased death of VSMC, and, as a consequence, increased vulnerability of atherosclerotic plaque and AS progression.[1,12] ox-LDL, an important factor in foam cells formation, increases the levels of LC3, Beclin 1, and P63, markers of autophagy in human umbilical vascular endothelial cells (HUVECs). Additionally, ox-LDL upregulated the expression of *PI3K*, *Akt*, and *mTOR*. *PI3K/Akt/mTOR* pathway was proved to block autophagy in AS. miR-126 is a molecule specific for ECs. Its levels are reduced in ECs treated with ox-LDL. Upregulation of miR-126 expression in HUVECs leads to inhibition of ox-LDL activated *PI3K/Akt/mTOR* pathway and improvement of the autophagy. Thus, miR-126 can serve as a potential target in AS treatment.[57]

Not only inflammation and macrophages activity are promising targets in CAD treatment, but also EC pathologies and apoptosis. XIAP can inhibit apoptosis by binding to caspase-3. *XIAP* is a target of miR-122, which is able to suppress its expression. It was reported that the expression of miR-122 was upregulated in ox-LDL-induced apoptotic human aortic ECs. Thus, overexpression of miR-122 promotes apoptosis via *XIAP* suppression.[58]

Additionally, *Ets-1* gene and its downstream target p21 are responsible for angiogenesis and vascular remodeling and inflammation. *Ets-1* is a target gene of miR-221/222, which can suppress its expression. Even though miR-221/222 have antiapoptotic effect on ECs with excessive accumulation of ox-LDL, its expression in those cells is reduced. Thus, upregulation of miR-221/222 can potentially reduce the ox-LDL-induced cell death via inhibition of *Ets-1*.[59]

miR-29 is involved in vascular remodeling and aneurysm formation.[60,61] In this regard, a trial is already ongoing to test MRG-201, a miR-29 mimic to prevent keloid formation in individuals with predisposition to develop keloid scars.[62] Positive results of this trial might anticipate further therapeutic applications, including vascular remodeling to counteract AS or aneurysm formation and inhibition of myocardial fibrosis with heart failure (**Table 1**).

The prevalence of CAD in modern society constitutes a growing challenge for medical professionals. miRNAs offer a wide range of potential treatment approaches. Consequently, drugs acting on miRNAs could influence the processes crucial for the development and progression of AS and CAD (**Figs. 1** and **2**).

LONG NONCODING RNAs

lncRNAs have been demonstrated to play a key role in the pathogenesis of AS, by regulating the functions of ECs, inflammation, and cholesterol accumulation. lncRNAs can act as miRNA sponges, meaning that they prevent the regulatory functions of miRNAs by binding to them and hindering interactions with their target.[7]

lncRNA GAS5 is a 5′-terminal oligopyrimidine class of genes that control cell growth, proliferation, and survival. Notably, GAS5 knockdown in THP-1 cells alleviated apoptosis of ECs, an important factor in preventing atherosclerotic plaque necrosis, which could lead to plaque instability.[63] Silencing of GAS5 was shown to attenuate inflammation in atherosclerotic mice by first upregulating miR-135a, which increased the alleviating effects of GAS5 silencing, and second by reducing proinflammatory cytokines including IL-1β, IL-6, and TNF-α in macrophages through sponging miR-221.[64,65] lncRNA GAS5 was also identified to restrain the reverse-transportation of cholesterol, a key process in the progression of AS, by binding to EZH2, which inhibits the expression of ABCA1.[66] Collectively, lncRNA GAS5 inhibition

could alleviate apoptosis of ECs, inflammation, and increase reverse transportation of cholesterol, making it a potential therapeutic approach for AS.

The lncRNA MALAT1 was initially found in non–small cell lung cancer but has now been proven to be an important factor in AS.[67] The protective effect of MALAT1 in inflammation was demonstrated in knockout animal models, which showed increased adhesion to ECs and elevated levels of proinflammatory mediators partly by the reduction of miR-503.[68] Similarly, MALAT1 decreased ox-LDL-induced proinflammatory cytokines via regulating miR-155/SOCS1 pathway.[13] MALAT1 promoted autophagy, a protective mechanism in AS, in HUVECs by sponging miR-216a-5p and consequently upregulating Beclin-1 expression, and by inhibiting the PI3K/AKT pathway.[69,70] However, another study found that MALAT1 inhibited autophagy in endothelial progenitor cells.[71] Altogether, MALAT1 may be a useful target in AS treatment because it has been demonstrated to inhibit ox-LDL-induced inflammation and potentially induce autophagy.

lncRNA H19 regulates lipid metabolism, inflammation, apoptosis, and autophagy during development of AS. It was shown that H19 knockdown resulted in decreased WNT1 expression, which led to suppressed proliferation and increased apoptosis of VSMCs.[72] Moreover, H19 upregulation promoted the expression of ERK1/2 and mTOR proteins and inhibited the expression of autophagy-related proteins, such as LC3, p62, and Beclin1 in VSMCs.[73] ERK1/2 is responsible for increased proliferation and migration of VSMCs, whereas mTOR mediates hypoxia-induced proliferation of VSMCs.[74,75] Furthermore, H19 overexpression resulted in increased ACP5 protein expression in VECs, which promoted cell proliferation and suppressed apoptosis.[76] Additionally, H19 knockdown effectively decreased lipid accumulation and expression of proinflammatory factors, such as TNF-α and IL-1, by promoting the expression of miR-130b in ox-LDL-treated macrophage cells.[77] These findings indicate that lncRNA H19 contributes in the progression of AS by stimulating an excessive activation of VSMCs and VECs and promoting the lipid accumulation in macrophages. The ultimate effects of H19 on AS are still not fully understood. Nevertheless, the inhibitor of lncRNA H19 may help to attenuate AS and should be considered as a target for future animal and clinical studies.

lncRNA MIAT was found to activate PI3K/Akt signaling pathway and STAT3 in mice aortic cells and human aortic VSMCs, respectively.[78,79] PI3K/Akt regulates VSMCs proliferation and induces inflammatory response, whereas STAT3

Table 1
Role of miRNA in CAD development

miRNA	Upregulation/Downregulation of the miRNAs	Target/Signaling Pathway	Effect	Data Source (Reference Number)
miR-155	↑	BCL6	Proinflammatory effect by activating NF-κB signaling pathway and macrophages.	10
	↑		Anti-inflammatory effect by impairing TNF-α stability and thus NF-κB inhibition.	11
	↑	CARHSP1		9
	↓	SOCS1	Repression of ox-LDL-mediated inflammation and apoptosis in ECs.	13
	↑		Enhancement of STAT3 and NF-κB signaling. Promotion of inflammatory cytokine and chemokine production and atherosclerosis progression.	21
	↑		Increase of the expression of p-STAT and PDCD4, and the production of proinflammation mediators IL-6 and TNF-α.	14
	↑	$p85\alpha$	Antiapoptotic effect by AKT inhibiting.	15
	↓	HBP1	Decrease of lipid accumulation in macrophages and reduction of atherosclerotic plaques.	17
	↑	CEH	Inhibition of foam cell formation.	18
	↓	PI3K/Akt/mTOR	Induction of autophagy.	19
miR-33	↓	ABCA1, ABCG1	Induction of cholesterol efflux.	26,37
	↓	ABCA1	Induction of cholesterol efflux.	30
	↓	ABCA1	Induction of cholesterol efflux.	29
	↓	PDK4, PGC-1α	Induction of mitochondrial respiration and production of ATP.	32
	↓	Tnfa, Tlr6, Tlr13	Promotion of anti-inflammatory M2 phenotype in lesional macrophages.	30
	↓		Decrease of IL-1β, IL-6, and TNF-α secretion in ox-LDL-induced macrophages.	34
	↓		Restoration of autophagy function in atherosclerotic plaques.	24
	↓	ATG5, ATG12, LAMP1, FOXO3, TFEB	Enhanced autophagy.	35
	↓	ACC, FAS	Modulation of lipid accumulation in the liver.	39

(continued on next page)

Table 1
(continued)

miRNA	Upregulation/ Downregulation of the miRNAs	Target/Signaling Pathway	Effect	Data Source (Reference Number)
miR-92a	↓	CD36	FFA uptake to cardiomyocytes.	41
	↓	ABCA8B	Transport of HDL to cardiomyocytes.	41
	↑	ITAG5	Accumulation of proangiogenic factors, activation of proangiogenic ERK1/2 and PI3K/AKT signaling pathways.	46
	↑	KLF4	Promotion of macrophage participation in AS formation, enhancement of LDL uptake and proinflammatory cytokines expression in ECs.	43
	↑	KLF4	Promotion of PDGF-BB-mediated proliferation and migration of VSMCs.	45
↑ miR-34		PNUTS	Favors vascular aging.	91
		SIRT-1	Favors vascular aging.	92
↑ miR-23b		FoxO4, SIRT1	Induced differentiation of VSMCs, prevented from neointimal hyperplasia and adverse vascular remodeling.	93
miR-29		ADAM12, ADAMTS9, COL1A1/2, COL2A1, COL3A1, COL4A1/2, COL5A1/3, COL6A2, COL7A1, COL15A1, COL21A1, ELN, FBN1, FN1, MCL1, MMP2, MMP9, MMP15, MMP-24, TGFB1-3	Inhibited collagen synthesis and prevented from fibrosis.	60,61
↑ miR-126-5p		HMGB1	Reduced proliferation and migration of VSMC. Reduced expression of proinflammatory cytokine IL-1β in VSMCs.	52
↑ miR-98		LOX-1	Reduced uptake of ox-LDL in macrophages.	55
↑ miR-126		PI3K/Akt/mTOR	Inhibition of ox-LDL activated PI3K/Akt/mTOR pathway and improvement of the autophagy.	57
↑ miR-125a		ETS-1 PinX1	Inhibits proliferation and migration of VSMCs by inhibition of the PDGF-BB pathway.	94 95
↑ miR-122		XIAP	Promoted apoptosis in ox-LDL ECs.	58

↑ miR-221/222	Ets-1	Reduced ox-LDL-induced apoptosis in ECs.	59
↓ miR-133b	MAML1	Downregulation of Notch signaling pathway can reduce plaque size, macrophages proliferation, and migration.	56
↑ miR-16	PDCD4	Decreased proinflammatory cytokines levels, increased levels of anti-inflammatory factors, and reduced NF-κB and MAPK signaling pathways.	53
	RhoA/RhoGDIα	Increased activation of RhoA by targeting RhoGDIα reduced eNOS and VEGF expression and increases TNF-α in endothelial cells.	54

Abbreviations: ABCA1, adenosine triphosphate binding cassette subfamily A member 1; ABCA8b, ATP-binding cassette subfamily A member 8-B; ABCG1, ATP binding cassette subfamily G member 1; ACC, Acetyl-CoA carboxylase; Akt, protein kinase B; ATG, autophagy related gene; BCL6, B-cell lymphoma 6; CARHSP1, calcium-regulated heat stable protein 1; Ch25h, cholesterol-25-hydroxylase; ECM, extracellular matrix; ECs, endothelial cells; eNOS, endothelial nitric oxide synthase; ERK1/2, extracellular signal-regulated protein kinases 1 and 2; Ets-1, ETS proto-oncogene 1; FAS, fatty acid synthase; FFA, free fatty acid; FOXO3, forkhead box O3; HBP1, high-mobility group box-transcription protein 1; HMGB1, high mobility group box 1; ITAG5, integrin subunit alpha 5; KLF, Krüppel-like factor; LAMP1, lysosomal associated membrane protein 1; LOX-1, lectin-like ox-LDL receptor-1; LXR, liver X receptor; MAML1, mastermind-like protein 1; MAPK, mitogen-activated protein kinase; MLCK, myosin light-chain kinase; mTOR, mammalian target of rapamycin; PDCD4, programmed cell death protein 4; PDK4, pyruvate dehydrogenase kinase 4; PGC-1α, peroxisome proliferator-activated receptor gamma coactivator 1-alpha; PI3K, phosphorylated phosphoinositide 3-kinase; SOCS1, suppressor of cytokine signaling 1; STAT3, signal transducer and activator of transcription 3; TFEB, transcription factor EB; Tsp-1, antiangiogenic trombospondin-1; XIAP, X chromosome-linked inhibitor of apoptosis.

Data from Refs.[9–19,21,24,26,27,29,30,32,34,35,39,41,43,45,46,52–61,91–95]

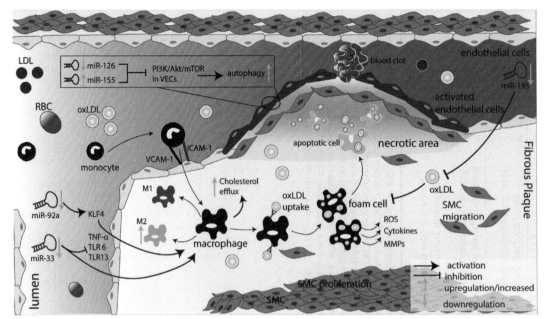

Fig. 1. MicroRNAs in atherosclerotic plaque initiation, progression, and rupture. (*Data from* Refs.[1,2,18–20,30,43,57])

promotes VSMCs proliferation.[80] Overexpression of MIAT facilitated proliferation, accelerated cell cycle progression, and hindered apoptosis in ox-LDL-induced VSMCs.[78] Moreover, MIAT upregulation promoted atherosclerotic plaque formation in mice models.[79] These findings indicate a potential role of MIAT as a therapeutic

approach in AS. lncRNA MIAT inhibitor should be considered in AS treatment and needs to be further investigated.

lncRNA XIST was shown to simulate *PTEN* and *NOD2* signaling by sponging miR-30a-5p and miR-320, respectively, in HUVECs.[81,82] The knockdown of XIST suppressed cell apoptosis,

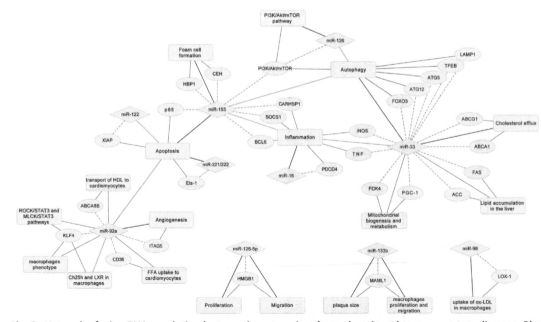

Fig. 2. Network of microRNA regulation by targeting genes in atherosclerosis and coronary artery diseases. *Blue, green,* and *red edges* represent modulation, activation, and inhibition, respectively. (*Data from* Refs.[9–19,21,26,29,30,32,35,37,39,41,43,45,46,52,53,55–59])

Table 2
Role of lncRNAs in CAD development

lncRNA	Target	miRNA Sponging	Effect	Data Source (Reference Number)
GAS5 ↓		miR-135a ↑	Alleviated apoptosis	63
		miR-221 ↓	Decreased inflammation	64
			Reduced the expression of proinflammatory cytokines	65
	EZH2 ↓		Increased reverse-transportation of cholesterol	66
MALAT1 ↓		miR-503 ↓	Increased adhesion to ECs and elevated expression of proinflammatory mediators	68
MALAT1 ↑	SOCS1 ↑	miR-155 ↓	Decreased ox-LDL induced proinflammatory cytokines	13
	Beclin 1 ↑	miR-216a-5p ↓	Promoted autophagy	69
	PI3K/AKT pathway		Promoted autophagy	70
			Inhibition of autophagy	71
H19 ↑	WNT1	miR-148b (competition to target binding)	Promoted proliferation and suppressed apoptosis of VSMCs	72
	ERK1/2, mTOR			73
	ACP5		Promoted proliferation and suppressed apoptosis of VECs	76
H19 ↓		miR-130b ↑	Increased expression of anti-inflammatory factors in macrophage	77
MIAT ↑	PI3K/Akt, STAT3	miR-181b ↓	Promoted proliferation, accelerated cell cycle progression, and suppressed apoptosis of VSMCs	79 78
XIST ↑	PTEN	miR-30a-5p ↓	Promoted cell apoptosis and inflammation response in HUVECs	81
	NOD2	miR-320 ↓		82
HOTAIR ↑			Promoted proliferation and migration of ECs	83
RNCR3 ↓	KLF2	miR-185-5p ↑	Reduced proliferation and migration of ECs and VSMCs	85
CASC11 ↑	IL-9 ↓		Supressed proliferation and induced apoptosis of VSMCs	96

(continued on next page)

Table 2 *(continued)*

lncRNA	Target	miRNA Sponging	Effect	Data Source (Reference Number)
ENST00113 ↓	PI3K/Akt/mTOR		Decreased proliferation, survival, and migration of VSMCs and HUVECs	86
lncRNA 430945 ↑	ROR2/RhoA		Promoted proliferation and migration of VSMCs	87
RAPIA ↑		miR-183-5p ↓	Promoted proliferation and suppressed apoptosis of macrophages	97
AF131217.1 ↓	KLF4	miR-128-3p–target competition	Regulation of HUVECs under shear stress	98
ATB ↑			Promoted apoptosis and inhibited proliferation of HUVECs	88
TUG1 ↑	FGF1	miR-133a ↓	Improved inflammatory factor expression and inhibited apoptosis in macrophages	90
LINC00657 ↑		miR-590-3p ↓	Promotes angiogenesis	99
AC096664.3 ↓	PPAR-γ/ABCG1		Induced cholesterol accumulation in VSMCs	100
SNHG16 ↑	Smad2	miR-205–target competition	Regulation of HSMCs migration and proliferation	89
OIP5-AS1 ↓		miR-320a ↑	Enhanced cell viability and repressed apoptosis of HUVECs	84

Abbreviations: ABCG1, ATP binding cassette subfamily G member 1; ACP5, acid phosphatase 5 protein; AKT, protein kinase B; ATB, long noncoding RNA activated by TGF-Beta; CASC11, cancer susceptibility 11 gene; ECs, endothelial cells; ERK1/2, extracellular signal-regulated protein kinases 1 and 2; EZH2, enhancer of zeste homolog 2; FGF1, fibroblast growth factor 1; GAS5, growth-arrest specific transcript 5; HOTAIR, HOX transcript antisense RNA; HSMCs, human mesenchymal stem cells; KLF, Krüppel-like factor; MALAT1, metastasis associated lung adenocarcinoma transcript 1; mTOR, mammalian target of rapamycin; NOD2, nucleotide-binding oligomerization domain 2; OIP5-AS1, OIP5 antisense RNA 1; PI3K, phosphorylated phosphoinositide 3-kinase; PPAR-γ, peroxisome proliferator-activated receptor gamma; PTEN, phosphatase and tensin homolog; RAPIA, lncRNA associated with the progression and intervention of atherosclerosis; RhoA, Ras homolog family member A; RNCR3, retinal noncoding RNA; ROR2, receptor tyrosine kinase like orphan receptor 2; Smad2, SMAD family member 2; SNHG16, small nucleolar RNA host gene 16; SOCS1, suppressor of cytokine signaling 1; STAT3, signal transducer and activator of transcription 3; TUG1, taurine-upregulated gene 1; VECs, vascular endothelial cells; WNT1, Wnt family member 1.
Data from Refs.13,63–66,68–73,76–78,81–90,96–100

increased cell viability, and decreased inflammatory response in HUVECs under ox-LDL stimuli. Endothelial cell proliferation and viability are highly impaired during AS development, thus inhibition of XIST may act protectively and should be considered as a therapeutic strategy in AS.

Several different lncRNAs may participate in the development of AS. lncRNAs HOTAIR, RNCR3, ENST00113, lncRNA 430945, ATB, SNHG16, and OIP5-AS1 are involved in the regulation of VSMC or VEC viability, proliferation, and migration.[83–89] Moreover, lncRNAs RAPIA and TUG1 enhance macrophage viability and reduce apoptosis.[87,90]

An increasing number of studies show lncRNAs as emerging important modulators of AS, making them promising targets for drug development. Further studies are needed to elucidate the mechanisms of their action and estimate their potential benefits and risks in clinical application (**Table 2**).

SUMMARY

Numerous studies have shown that miRNAs and lncRNAs might be promising therapeutic targets in CAD. miR-155 inhibitor has been described to be the most promising novel therapeutic strategy against progression of CAD. Moreover, inhibition of miR-33 and miR-92a has also been demonstrated as a promising therapeutic approach by delaying the development and enhancing the regression of CAD. No data about their safety in clinical trials have been available so far. In addition, lncRNAs, such as GAS5 and H19, were shown to have a relevant impact on CAD progression, thus their inhibition could be a potential therapeutic approach for CAD. Various limitations of ncRNAs used for CAD exist, including the lack of registered clinical trials and the incomplete understanding of the specific mechanism by which ncRNAs modulate CAD development on a molecular level. In addition, many ncRNAs have yet to be studied. Recent studies are promising, but further research is required to investigate ncRNA potential in clinical application.

HIGHLIGHTS OF THE ARTICLE

1. MiRNAs and lncRNAs could be a target of novel treatment as many studies showed promising results.
2. MiRNAs and lncRNAs have an important role both in regulation and pathophysiology of atherosclerosis in coronary artery disease.

CONTRIBUTORS

L. Zareba, C. Eyileten, and M. Postula contributed to the data collection and elaboration, writing, and approval of article; and is guarantor of the article. Z. Fitas, M. Wolska, and E. Junger contributed writing, editing, discussion, and approval of article. S. De Rosa and J.M. Siller-Matula contributed to revising and approval of the article. C. Eyileten and Z. Wicik contributed valuable graphical designs. The corresponding author attests that all listed authors meet authorship criteria and that no others meeting the criteria have been omitted.

CONFLICTS OF INTEREST

The authors state there are no conflicts of interest.

ACKNOWLEDGMENTS

The article was published as a result of the collaboration within the I-COMET team.

REFERENCES

1. Yang H, Mohamed AS, Zhou SH. Oxidized low density lipoprotein, stem cells, and atherosclerosis. Lipids Health Dis 2012;11:85.
2. Zhang Y, Zhang L, Wang Y, et al. MicroRNAs or long noncoding RNAs in diagnosis and prognosis of coronary artery disease. Aging Dis 2019;10(2):353–66.
3. Eyileten C, Wicik Z, De Rosa S, et al. MicroRNAs as diagnostic and prognostic biomarkers in ischemic stroke: a comprehensive review and bioinformatic analysis. Cells 2018;7(12):249.
4. Pordzik J, Jakubik D, Jarosz-Popek J, et al. Significance of circulating microRNAs in diabetes mellitus type 2 and platelet reactivity: bioinformatic analysis and review. Cardiovasc Diabetol 2019;18(1):113.
5. Pordzik J, Pisarz K, De Rosa S, et al. The potential role of platelet-related microRNAs in the development of cardiovascular events in high-risk populations, including diabetic patients: a review. Front Endocrinol (Lausanne) 2018;9:74.
6. Sabatino J, Wicik Z, De Rosa S, et al. MicroRNAs fingerprint of bicuspid aortic valve. J Mol Cell Cardiol 2019;134:98–106.
7. Schonrock N, Harvey RP, Mattick JS. Long noncoding RNAs in cardiac development and pathophysiology. Circ Res 2012;111(10):1349–62.
8. O'Connell RM, Zhao JL, Rao DS. MicroRNA function in myeloid biology. Blood 2011;118(11):2960–9.
9. Li X, Kong D, Chen H, et al. miR-155 acts as an anti-inflammatory factor in atherosclerosis-associated foam cell formation by repressing calcium-regulated heat stable protein 1. Sci Rep 2016;6:21789.
10. Nazari-Jahantigh M, Wei Y, Noels H, et al. MicroRNA-155 promotes atherosclerosis by repressing

Bcl6 in macrophages. J Clin Invest 2012;122(11): 4190–202.

11. Gomez I, Ward B, Souilhol C, et al. Neutrophil microvesicles drive atherosclerosis by delivering miR-155 to atheroprone endothelium. Nat Commun 2020;11(1):214.

12. Chistiakov DA, Bobryshev YV, Orekhov AN. Macrophage-mediated cholesterol handling in atherosclerosis. J Cell Mol Med 2016;20(1):17–28.

13. Li S, Sun Y, Zhong L, et al. The suppression of ox-LDL-induced inflammatory cytokine release and apoptosis of HCAECs by long non-coding RNA-MALAT1 via regulating microRNA-155/SOCS1 pathway. Nutr Metab Cardiovasc Dis 2018;28(11): 1175–87.

14. Ye J, Guo R, Shi Y, et al. miR-155 regulated inflammation response by the SOCS1-STAT3-PDCD4 axis in atherogenesis. Mediators Inflamm 2016;2016: 8060182.

15. Ruan Z, Chu T, Wu L, et al. miR-155 inhibits oxidized low-density lipoprotein-induced apoptosis in different cell models by targeting the p85alpha/AKT pathway. J Physiol Biochem 2020;76(2): 329–43.

16. Curtale G, Rubino M, Locati M. MicroRNAs as molecular switches in macrophage activation. Front Immunol 2019;10:799.

17. Tian FJ, An LN, Wang GK, et al. Elevated microRNA-155 promotes foam cell formation by targeting HBP1 in atherogenesis. Cardiovasc Res 2014;103(1):100–10.

18. Zhang F, Zhao J, Sun D, et al. MiR-155 inhibits transformation of macrophages into foam cells via regulating CEH expression. Biomed Pharmacother 2018;104:645–51.

19. Yin S, Yang S, Pan X, et al. MicroRNA155 promotes oxLDL induced autophagy in human umbilical vein endothelial cells by targeting the PI3K/Akt/mTOR pathway. Mol Med Rep 2018;18(3):2798–806.

20. Zhang Z, Pan X, Yang S, et al. miR-155 promotes ox-LDL-induced autophagy in human umbilical vein endothelial cells. Mediators Inflamm 2017; 2017:9174801.

21. Yang Y, Yang L, Liang X, et al. MicroRNA-155 promotes atherosclerosis inflammation via targeting SOCS1. Cell Physiol Biochem 2015;36(4):1371–81.

22. Querfeld C, Pacheco T, Foss F, et al. Preliminary results of a phase 1 trial evaluating MRG-106, a synthetic microRNA antagonist (LNA antimiR) of microRNA-155, in patients with CTCL. Blood 2016;128:1829.

23. NLM NLoM. Safety, tolerability and pharmacokinetics of MRG-106 in patients with mycosis fungoides (MF), CLL, DLBCL or ATLL. Available at: https://clinicaltrials.gov/ct2/show/NCT02580552? term=MRG-106&draw=2&rank=3. Accessed May 4, 2020.

24. Ouimet M, Ediriweera H, Afonso MS, et al. microRNA-33 regulates macrophage autophagy in atherosclerosis. Arterioscler Thromb Vasc Biol 2017;37(6):1058–67.

25. Rotllan N, Ramirez CM, Aryal B, et al. Therapeutic silencing of microRNA-33 inhibits the progression of atherosclerosis in Ldlr-/- mice–brief report. Arterioscler Thromb Vasc Biol 2013;33(8):1973–7.

26. Horie T, Baba O, Kuwabara Y, et al. MicroRNA-33 deficiency reduces the progression of atherosclerotic plaque in ApoE-/- mice. J Am Heart Assoc 2012;1(6):e003376.

27. Canfran-Duque A, Ramirez CM, Goedeke L, et al. microRNAs and HDL life cycle. Cardiovasc Res 2014;103(3):414–22.

28. Chistiakov DA, Melnichenko AA, Myasoedova VA, et al. Mechanisms of foam cell formation in atherosclerosis. J Mol Med (Berl) 2017;95(11): 1153–65.

29. Price NL, Rotllan N, Zhang X, et al. Specific disruption of Abca1 targeting largely mimics the effects of miR-33 knockout on macrophage cholesterol efflux and atherosclerotic plaque development. Circ Res 2019;124(6):874–80.

30. Rayner KJ, Sheedy FJ, Esau CC, et al. Antagonism of miR-33 in mice promotes reverse cholesterol transport and regression of atherosclerosis. J Clin Invest 2011;121(7):2921–31.

31. Price NL, Rotllan N, Canfran-Duque A, et al. Genetic dissection of the impact of miR-33a and miR-33b during the progression of atherosclerosis. Cell Rep 2017;21(5):1317–30.

32. Karunakaran D, Thrush AB, Nguyen MA, et al. Macrophage mitochondrial energy status regulates cholesterol efflux and is enhanced by anti-miR33 in atherosclerosis. Circ Res 2015;117(3):266–78.

33. Wende AR, Huss JM, Schaeffer PJ, et al. PGC-1alpha coactivates PDK4 gene expression via the orphan nuclear receptor ERRalpha: a mechanism for transcriptional control of muscle glucose metabolism. Mol Cell Biol 2005;25(24):10684–94.

34. Yang C, Lei X, Li J. Tanshinone IIA reduces oxidized low-density lipoprotein-induced inflammatory responses by downregulating microRNA-33 in THP-1 macrophages. Int J Clin Exp Pathol 2019; 12(10):3791–8.

35. Ouimet M, Koster S, Sakowski E, et al. Mycobacterium tuberculosis induces the miR-33 locus to reprogram autophagy and host lipid metabolism. Nat Immunol 2016;17(6):677–86.

36. Zhou H, Wang X, Ma L, et al. FoxO3 transcription factor promotes autophagy after transient cerebral ischemia/reperfusion. Int J Neurosci 2019;129(8): 738–45.

37. Rayner KJ, Suarez Y, Davalos A, et al. MiR-33 contributes to the regulation of cholesterol homeostasis. Science 2010;328(5985):1570–3.

38. Rayner KJ, Esau CC, Hussain FN, et al. Inhibition of miR-33a/b in non-human primates raises plasma HDL and lowers VLDL triglycerides. Nature 2011; 478(7369):404–7.

39. Goedeke L, Salerno A, Ramirez CM, et al. Long-term therapeutic silencing of miR-33 increases circulating triglyceride levels and hepatic lipid accumulation in mice. EMBO Mol Med 2014;6(9): 1133–41.

40. Li M, Guan X, Sun Y, et al. miR-92a family and their target genes in tumorigenesis and metastasis. Exp Cell Res 2014;323(1):1–6.

41. Rogg EM, Abplanalp WT, Bischof C, et al. Analysis of cell type-specific effects of MicroRNA-92a provides novel insights into target regulation and mechanism of action. Circulation 2018;138(22): 2545–58.

42. Samovski D, Sun J, Pietka T, et al. Regulation of AMPK activation by CD36 links fatty acid uptake to beta-oxidation. Diabetes 2015;64(2):353–9.

43. Chang YJ, Li YS, Wu CC, et al. Extracellular microRNA-92a mediates endothelial cell-macrophage communication. Arterioscler Thromb Vasc Biol 2019;39(12):2492–504.

44. Li Z, Martin M, Zhang J, et al. Kruppel-like factor 4 regulation of cholesterol-25-hydroxylase and liver X receptor mitigates atherosclerosis susceptibility. Circulation 2017;136(14):1315–30.

45. Wang J, Zhang C, Li C, et al. MicroRNA-92a promotes vascular smooth muscle cell proliferation and migration through the ROCK/MLCK signalling pathway. J Cell Mol Med 2019;23(5): 3696–710.

46. Xu X, Tian L, Zhang Z. Triptolide inhibits angiogenesis in microvascular endothelial cells through regulation of miR-92a. J Physiol Biochem 2019; 75(4):573–83.

47. Amin MA, Volpert OV, Woods JM, et al. Migration inhibitory factor mediates angiogenesis via mitogen-activated protein kinase and phosphatidylinositol kinase. Circ Res 2003;93(4):321–9.

48. Loyer X, Potteaux S, Vion AC, et al. Inhibition of microRNA-92a prevents endothelial dysfunction and atherosclerosis in mice. Circ Res 2014; 114(3):434–43.

49. Gallant-Behm CL, Piper J, Dickinson BA, et al. A synthetic microRNA-92a inhibitor (MRG-110) accelerates angiogenesis and wound healing in diabetic and nondiabetic wounds. Wound Repair Regen 2018;26(4):311–23.

50. NLM NLoM. Safety, tolerability, pharmacokinetics, and pharmacodynamics of MRG-110 following intradermal injection in healthy volunteers. Available at: https://clinicaltrials.gov/ct2/show/NCT03603431? term=NCT03603431&draw=2&rank=1. Accessed May 4, 2020.

51. Chistiakov DA, Orekhov AN, Bobryshev YV. Vascular smooth muscle cell in atherosclerosis. Acta Physiol (Oxf) 2015;214(1):33–50.

52. Chen Z, Pan X, Sheng Z, et al. Baicalin suppresses the proliferation and migration of ox-LDL-VSMCs in atherosclerosis through upregulating miR-126-5p. Biol Pharm Bull 2019;42(9): 1517–23.

53. Liang X, Xu Z, Yuan M, et al. MicroRNA-16 suppresses the activation of inflammatory macrophages in atherosclerosis by targeting PDCD4. Int J Mol Med 2016;37(4):967–75.

54. Sorrentino S, Iaconetti C, De Rosa S, et al. Hindlimb ischemia impairs endothelial recovery and increases neointimal proliferation in the carotid artery. Sci Rep 2018;8(1):761.

55. Dai Y, Wu X, Dai D, et al. MicroRNA-98 regulates foam cell formation and lipid accumulation through repression of LOX-1. Redox Biol 2018;16:255–62.

56. Zheng CG, Chen BY, Sun RH, et al. miR-133b downregulation reduces vulnerable plaque formation in mice with AS through inhibiting macrophage immune responses. Mol Ther Nucleic Acids 2019; 16:745–57.

57. Tang F, Yang TL. MicroRNA-126 alleviates endothelial cells injury in atherosclerosis by restoring autophagic flux via inhibiting of PI3K/Akt/mTOR pathway. Biochem Biophys Res Commun 2018; 495(1):1482–9.

58. Li Y, Yang N, Dong B, et al. MicroRNA-122 promotes endothelial cell apoptosis by targeting XIAP: therapeutic implication for atherosclerosis. Life Sci 2019;232:116590.

59. Qin B, Cao Y, Yang H, et al. MicroRNA-221/222 regulate ox-LDL-induced endothelial apoptosis via Ets-1/p21 inhibition. Mol Cell Biochem 2015; 405(1–2):115–24.

60. Boon RA, Seeger T, Heydt S, et al. MicroRNA-29 in aortic dilation: implications for aneurysm formation. Circ Res 2011;109(10):1115–9.

61. Maegdefessel L, Azuma J, Toh R, et al. Inhibition of microRNA-29b reduces murine abdominal aortic aneurysm development. J Clin Invest 2012; 122(2):497–506.

62. NLM NLoM. Efficacy, safety, and tolerability of remlarsen (MRG-201) following intradermal injection in subjects with a history of keloids. Available at: https://clinicaltrials.gov/ct2/show/NCT03601052? term=NCT03601052&draw=2&rank=1. Accessed May 4, 2020.

63. Chen L, Yang W, Guo Y, et al. Exosomal lncRNA GAS5 regulates the apoptosis of macrophages and vascular endothelial cells in atherosclerosis. PLoS One 2017;12(9):e0185406.

64. Shen S, Zheng X, Zhu Z, et al. Silencing of GAS5 represses the malignant progression of

atherosclerosis through upregulation of miR-135a. Biomed Pharmacother 2019;118:109302.

65. Ye J, Wang C, Wang D, et al. LncRBA GSA5, up-regulated by ox-LDL, aggravates inflammatory response and MMP expression in THP-1 macro-phages by acting like a sponge for miR-221. Exp Cell Res 2018;369(2):348–55.

66. Meng XD, Yao HH, Wang LM, et al. Knockdown of GAS5 inhibits atherosclerosis progression via reducing EZH2-mediated ABCA1 transcription in ApoE(-/-) mice. Mol Ther Nucleic Acids 2020;19: 84–96.

67. Ji P, Diederichs S, Wang W, et al. MALAT-1, a novel noncoding RNA, and thymosin beta4 predict metastasis and survival in early-stage non-small cell lung cancer. Oncogene 2003;22(39):8031–41.

68. Cremer S, Michalik KM, Fischer A, et al. Hemato-poietic deficiency of the long noncoding RNA MA-LAT1 promotes atherosclerosis and plaque inflammation. Circulation 2019;139(10):1320–34.

69. Wang K, Yang C, Shi J, et al. Ox-LDL-induced lncRNA MALAT1 promotes autophagy in human umbilical vein endothelial cells by sponging miR-216a-5p and regulating Beclin-1 expression. Eur J Pharmacol 2019;858:172338.

70. Li S, Pan X, Yang S, et al. LncRNA MALAT1 pro-motes oxidized low-density lipoprotein-induced autophagy in HUVECs by inhibiting the PI3K/AKT pathway. J Cell Biochem 2019;120(3): 4092–101.

71. Zhu Y, Yang T, Duan J, et al. MALAT1/miR-15b-5p/MAPK1 mediates endothelial progenitor cells auto-phagy and affects coronary atherosclerotic heart disease via mTOR signaling pathway. Aging (Al-bany NY) 2019;11(4):1089–109.

72. Zhang L, Cheng H, Yue Y, et al. H19 knockdown suppresses proliferation and induces apoptosis by regulating miR-148b/WNT/beta-catenin in ox-LDL-stimulated vascular smooth muscle cells. J Biomed Sci 2018;25(1):11.

73. Song Z, Wei D, Chen Y, et al. Association of astra-galoside IV-inhibited autophagy and mineralization in vascular smooth muscle cells with lncRNA H19 and DUSP5-mediated ERK signaling. Toxicol Appl Pharmacol 2019;364:45–54.

74. Shi L, Ji Y, Jiang X, et al. Liraglutide attenuates high glucose-induced abnormal cell migration, prolifer-ation, and apoptosis of vascular smooth muscle cells by activating the GLP-1 receptor, and inhibit-ing ERK1/2 and PI3K/Akt signaling pathways. Car-diovasc Diabetol 2015;14:18.

75. Lee J, Heo J, Kang H. miR-92b-3p-TSC1 axis is critical for mTOR signaling-mediated vascular smooth muscle cell proliferation induced by hypox-ia. Cell Death Differ 2019;26(9):1782–95.

76. Huang Y, Wang L, Mao Y, et al. Long noncoding RNA-H19 contributes to atherosclerosis and

77. Han Y, Ma J, Wang J, et al. Silencing of H19 inhibits the adipogenesis and inflammation response in ox-LDL-treated Raw264.7 cells by up-regulating miR-130b. Mol Immunol 2018;93:107–14.

78. Zhong X, Ma X, Zhang L, et al. MIAT promotes pro-liferation and hinders apoptosis by modulating miR-181b/STAT3 axis in ox-LDL-induced athero-sclerosis cell models. Biomed Pharmacother 2018;97:1078–85.

79. Sun G, Li Y, Ji Z. Up-regulation of MIAT aggravates the atherosclerotic damage in atherosclerosis mice through the activation of PI3K/Akt signaling pathway. Drug Deliv 2019;26(1):641–9.

80. Liao XH, Wang N, Zhao DW, et al. STAT3 protein regulates vascular smooth muscle cell phenotypic switch by interaction with myocardin. J Biol Chem 2015;290(32):19641–52.

81. Hu WN, Duan ZY, Wang Q, et al. The suppres-sion of ox-LDL-induced inflammatory response and apoptosis of HUVEC by lncRNA XIAT knockdown via regulating miR-30c-5p/PTEN axis. Eur Rev Med Pharmacol Sci 2019;23(17): 7628–38.

82. Xu X, Ma C, Liu C, et al. Knockdown of long non-coding RNA XIST alleviates oxidative low-density li-poprotein-mediated endothelial cells injury through modulation of miR-320/NOD2 axis. Biochem Bio-phys Res Commun 2018;503(2):586–92.

83. Peng Y, Meng K, Jiang L, et al. Thymic stromal lymphopoietin-induced HOTAIR activation pro-motes endothelial cell proliferation and migration in atherosclerosis. Biosci Rep 2017;37(4). BSR20170351.

84. Zhang C, Yang H, Li Y, et al. LNCRNA OIP5-AS1 regulates oxidative low-density lipoprotein-mediated endothelial cell injury via miR-320a/LOX1 axis. Mol Cell Biochem 2020;467(1–2): 15–25.

85. Shan K, Jiang Q, Wang XQ, et al. Role of long non-coding RNA-RNCR3 in atherosclerosis-related vascular dysfunction. Cell Death Dis 2016;7(6): e2248.

86. Yao X, Yan C, Zhang L, et al. LncRNA ENST00113 promotes proliferation, survival, and migration by activating PI3K/Akt/mTOR signaling pathway in atherosclerosis. Medicine (Baltimore) 2018;97(16): e0473.

87. Cui C, Wang X, Shang XM, et al. lncRNA 430945 promotes the proliferation and migration of vascular smooth muscle cells via the ROR2/RhoA signaling pathway in atherosclerosis. Mol Med Rep 2019;19(6):4663–72.

88. Yu H, Ma S, Sun L, et al. TGFbeta1 upregulates the expression of lncRNAAATB to promote atheroscle-rosis. Mol Med Rep 2019;19(5):4222–8.

89. Lin Y, Tian G, Zhang H, et al. Long non-coding RNA SNHG16 regulates human aortic smooth muscle cell proliferation and migration via sponging miR-205 and modulating Smad2. J Cell Mol Med 2019;23(10):6919–29.

90. Zhang L, Cheng H, Yue Y, et al. TUG1 knockdown ameliorates atherosclerosis via up-regulating the expression of miR-133a target gene FGF1. Cardiovasc Pathol 2018;33:6–15.

91. Boon RA, Iekushi K, Lechner S, et al. MicroRNA-34a regulates cardiac ageing and function. Nature 2013;495(7439):107–10.

92. Guo Y, Li P, Gao L, et al. Kallistatin reduces vascular senescence and aging by regulating microRNA-34a-SIRT1 pathway. Aging Cell 2017;16(4):837–46.

93. Iaconetti C, De Rosa S, Polimeni A, et al. Downregulation of miR-23b induces phenotypic switching of vascular smooth muscle cells in vitro and in vivo. Cardiovasc Res 2015;107(4):522–33.

94. Gareri C, Iaconetti C, Sorrentino S, et al. miR-125a-5p modulates phenotypic switch of vascular smooth muscle cells by targeting ETS-1. J Mol Biol 2017;429(12):1817–28.

95. Hou P, Li H, Yong H, et al. PinX1 represses renal cancer angiogenesis via the mir-125a-3p/VEGF signaling pathway. Angiogenesis 2019;22(4):507–19.

96. Tao K, Hu Z, Zhang Y, et al. LncRNA CASC11 improves atherosclerosis by downregulating IL-9 and regulating vascular smooth muscle cell apoptosis and proliferation. Biosci Biotechnol Biochem 2019;83(7):1284–8.

97. Sun C, Fu Y, Gu X, et al. Macrophage-enriched lncRNA RAPIA: a novel therapeutic target for atherosclerosis. Arterioscler Thromb Vasc Biol 2020;40(6):1464–78.

98. Lu Q, Meng Q, Qi M, et al. Shear-sensitive lncRNA AF131217.1 inhibits inflammation in HUVECs via regulation of KLF4. Hypertension 2019;73(5):e25–34.

99. Bao MH, Li GY, Huang XS, et al. Long noncoding RNA LINC00657 acting as a miR-590-3p sponge to facilitate low concentration oxidized low-density lipoprotein-induced angiogenesis. Mol Pharmacol 2018;93(4):368–75.

100. Xu BM, Xiao L, Kang CM, et al. LncRNA AC096664.3/PPAR-gamma/ABCG1-dependent signal transduction pathway contributes to the regulation of cholesterol homeostasis. J Cell Biochem 2019;120(8):13775–82.

New Advances in the Treatment of Severe Coronary Artery Calcifications

Pierluigi Demola, MD, Francesca Ristalli, MD, Brunilda Hamiti, CRN,
Francesco Meucci, MD, Carlo Di Mario, MD, PhD, FRCP, FSCAI, FESC,
Alessio Mattesini, MD*

KEYWORDS

- Coronary artery calcification calcific lesion • IVUS • OCT • Coronary atherectomy
- Intravascular lithotripsy

KEY POINTS

- Coronary artery calcifications challenging scenarios.
- Intracoronary imaging is necessary to understand calcific lesion features.
- Accurate evaluation of lesion characteristics is crucial.
- Evaluate calcific arc, length and thickness before percutaneous coronary intervention.
- Plaque modification can be achieved with different devices before stent and optimization.

INTRODUCTION

Coronary artery calcification (CAC) is associated with adverse cardiovascular events. It is part of 2 distinct processes: calcific atherosclerosis and medial artery calcification, etymologically the word atherosclerosis derives from the Greek word for gruel (ἀθήρα, atèra) and hardening (σκλήρωσις, sklèrosis).

Calcific atherosclerosis occurs in the intima and is inflammatory-dependent. Medial artery calcification is related primarily to age, male sex, Caucasian ethnicity, diabetes mellitus and chronic kidney disease (CKD).

Vascular calcification is remarkably accelerated and contributes to a higher risk of cardiovascular morbidity and mortality.[1,2]

Coronary calcification is localized within intimal plaque except in patients with CKD who develop principally medial and intimal calcific layer.[3]

Constant healings and modifications of plaques after ruptures or hemorrhages lead to development of obstructive fibro-calcific lesions, common in patients with chronic angina and sudden cardiac death.[4,5]

Understanding plaque characteristics and distribution is crucial to select a "plaque modification strategy" before stent implantation to minimize malapposition.[6]

CALCIFIC LESIONS PHONOTYPES

Calcium regulatory mechanisms that affect bone formation influence coronary artery calcification, made by hydroxyapatite, carbonate apatite, and calcium-deficient apatite. "Eccentric calcium" occurs involving less than 270° of lumen perimeter. "Concentric calcium" is a cross-section involvement of lumen with greater than 270° of calcium.

High-pressure ballooning can achieve calcium fracture in the thinner areas. Atherectomy based

Financial support and sponsorship: A. Mattesini, C. Di Mario and B. Hamiti are Investigators and Study Coordinator in the coronary trial Disrupt CAD II, supported by Shockwave Medical and have received institutional grants for that study.
Structural Interventional Cardiology, Department of Clinical and Experimental Medicine, Careggi University Hospital, Largo Brambilla, 3, Florence 50134, Italy
* Corresponding author.
E-mail address: amattesini@gmail.com

cardiology.theclinics.com

procedures aim to partially ablate the calcium allowing the fracture of calcified structures and permitting further luminal gain.

IMAGING OF CORONARY CALCIFIC LESION

Accurate evaluation of coronary lesions is crucial to perform perfectly planned percutaneous coronary intervention (PCI). Particularly rich mineral content CAC are detected by fluoroscopic methods; calcium creates radio-opacities noted before contrast injection. Intravascular ultrasound (IVUS) is more accurate than angiography for detection of calcific lesions, with sensitivity of 90% to 100% and specificity of 99% to 100%.[3,7] Clinical data demonstrate the enhanced sensitivity of IVUS in detecting coronary calcium compared with angiography (73% of cases vs 38%; $P<.001$).[4]

Calcium reflects ultrasound, recognized as a bright echo with acoustic shadowing.[5] Moreover IVUS provides discrimination of deep versus superficial calcium, thickness cannot be evaluated using IVUS. The calcium arc is classified as follows: none or involving 1 quadrant (0° to 90°), 2 quadrants (91° to 180°), 3 quadrants (181° to 270°), or 4 quadrants (271° to 360°). Calcium location is superficial if present in the intimal-luminal interface, or deep if within the medial-adventitial border or closer to the adventitia than the lumen, or even both superficial and deep.[6] Calcium thickness cannot be determined directly with IVUS and volume cannot be calculated with the same accuracy of optical coherence tomography (OCT).

For this reason, historically calcific arc circumference detected by IVUS was considered a very important parameter, an arc greater than 180° could predict a probable risk of stent underexpansion.[8]

In the PROSPECT study (Providing Regional Observations to Study Predictors of Events in the Coronary Tree) patients with higher dense calcium volumes were more likely to have higher rates of major adverse cardiovascular events (MACE) at 3 years.[9–11]

OCT offers high spatial resolution imaging (10–20 mm), better than IVUS (150–200 mm). Intravascular frequency domain OCT is the finest modality for the assessment of coronary calcium distribution.

Definition of calcific arc degree detected with IVUS is well integrated with OCT parameters such as calcium thickness, calcium length, and calcium 3-dimensional volume that correlate negatively with stent expansion and correct response to balloon dilation. Particularly, Fujino and colleagues[12] combined calcific arch greater than 180° (2 points), calcific thickness greater than

0.5 mm (1 point), and calcific longitudinal length greater than 5 mm (1 point) to create a scoring system that can predict higher risk of stent underexpansion, more observed in calcific lesions reaching score of 4. The interaction between calcium arc and thickness is important to predict the success of cracking the calcific layer with a conventional balloon. As shown by Maejima and colleagues[13] calcium cracks after balloon angioplasty were associated with a greater arc and a thinner minimal thickness of the calcium component.

NEW TREATMENT ERA OF CORONARY CALCIFIC LESIONS

Calcification makes difficult to deliver devices and increases the risk of PCI failure.

One in 4 patients undergoing PCI presents a calcific lesion. Heavily calcified lesions are a particular threat for drug-eluting stents, damaging the polymer/drug coating during tough advancement and subsequently allowing only poor diffusion of the drug to the subintima.[14–16]

Calcified lesions are associated with increased intraprocedural complications such as underexpansion, asymmetrical expansion, malapposition and postprocedural risk of in-stent restenosis and thrombosis.[17–20] Asymmetrical calcific lesions predispose to coronary dissection or perforation.[21,22]

Calcified lesions can be approached with success and procedural good accomplishment.[23]

WIRE SELECTION

Frequently "workhorse" guidewires are adequate for most CAC, but in cases with significant angulation or tortuosity, hydrophilic coating guidewires may facilitate manipulation. If this option is not successful, "buddy" guidewire or deep coronary intubation with a child-in-mother catheter could be an easy solution.

In case of severe CAC also microcatheters for lesion crossing so that the operator can exchange finer wires required for atheroablative devices.

If microcatheter does not cross, an 0.009-inch RotaWire (for rotational atherectomy; Boston Scientific, Natick, MA) or 0.012-inch ViperWire (for orbital atherectomy; Cardiovascular Systems, Inc., St. Paul, MN) and directly proceed to atheroablation.

BALLOON ANGIOPLASTY FOR CORONARY ARTERY CALCIFICATIONS: NOT JUST UNDER PRESSURE

With common balloon for angioplasty, the forces privilege less hard parts, preferentially not involved by CAC. Resistances to radial forces may bring to several complications. Noncompliant balloon (NCB) can tolerate high inflating pressures without increasing too much in diameter, uniformly expanding the coronary segment.

OPN NC balloon (SIS Medical, Frauenfeld, Switzerland) is a rapid exchange percutaneous transluminal coronary angioplasty device, with its unique twin-layer technology can allow super high pressure (to 4560 kPa) with very poor diameter expansion, dedicated especially for in-stent restenosis (ISR), it has nominal pressure at 10 atm and a rated burst pressure of 35 atm. It available in various diameters ranging from 1.5 to 4.5 mm and 3 lengths: 10, 15, 20 mm. The limitation of the OPN balloon is the high profile that undermines any attempt to recross when inflated.[24]

OPN NC high-pressure balloon can be easily used in case of the failure of conventional balloons, providing a safe and easy alternative strategy in case of failure of conventional NC balloon dilatation.[25]

However, CAC may become resistant to further high-pressure dilatation after compression.

In 1990s, medical technology brings to light a new modified noncompliant balloon provided of sharp microblades ($\sim$0.25 mm in height) settled longitudinally on the surface, called Flextome Cutting Balloon, as a newborn called Wolverine balloon, with a cutting functional height of 0.005 foot, available in monorail and over-the-wire, with 3 different blade lengths: 6, 10, 15 mm. When inflated the cutting balloon creates radial incision on the fibrocalcific plaque, allowing expansion with conventional balloon minimizing elastic recoil of vessel. Cutting balloon angioplasty (CBA) is used to treat mainly fibro-calcific plaque or in ISR.[26]

For dilatation of various kind of hard lesions, it was designed the AngioSculpt scoring balloon (AngioScore, Fremont, CA), an innovative device consisting of a double lumen catheter with a semi-compliant, nylon balloon surrounded by an external nitinol-based helical scoring edge, thought to be more flexible and manageable. This technology decreased incidence of balloon slippage, a more uniform balloon expansion, reducing elastic recoil and an optimal postinflation minimal lumen diameter.

AngioSculpt is available in 3 different lengths of 10, 15, and 20 mm and balloon diameters from 2.0 to 3.5 mm. Radiopaque markers demarcate the proximal and distal edge of the balloon for fluoroscopic visualization. During balloon deflation, the nitinol cage has an active role in the device deflation.

The indications of scoring balloons are growing with operators experience, but nowadays this technique is meant for lesion preparation before stenting: complex vessels or in select cases of ISR and bifurcation lesions, promising are its adapted uses in valvuloplasty and drug-covered balloon technologies.

ATHERECTOMY TECHNIQUES
Rotational Atherectomy

In the past 3 decades rotational atherectomy (RA) has represented the main atheroablative technique for high calcium content coronary lesions. Few modifications to its essential mechanics have been imported, but significant incremental improvement in technique has been introduced. The current RA system available is the *Rotablator System* (Boston Scientific, Natick, MA). RA has recently evolved as a unique tool for calcified coronary lesions, with a new entity called RotaPro system.

This unique device is composed of a diamond-encrusted elliptical burr on the top that rotates at high speeds. The burr is tracked over a 0.009-inch guidewire, placed across the lesion, it crosses many times the calcified lesions with rotational speeds of 140,000 to 150,000 rpm.

Rotational atherectomy bases its functional principle on the concept that different components (such as for example, fibro-calcific lesion and calcium deposits) have an altered elasticity.[27] The burr prefers to ablate inelastic materials, sparing healthy part.[27,28] Thus, hard and inelastic plaques are rigid and can be pulverized preferentially. Its main and primary use is to facilitate balloon angioplasty and correct stent deployment. The STRATAS study (Study to Determine Rotablator and Transluminal Angioplasty Strategy) compared outcomes of an aggressive versus routine strategy (maximum burr:artery ratio >0.70 alone or with adjunctive balloon inflation ≤1 atm vs maximum burr:artery ratio ≤0.70 with routine balloon inflation ≥4 atm). There were no advantages for clinical success, final minimum lumen diameter, or residual stenosis, and there were higher rates of periprocedural creatine kinase-myocardial band release and target lesion revascularization (TLR) at 6 months.[29]

The CARAT (Coronary Angioplasty and Rotablator Atherectomy Trial) was on the same line, aggressive strategy does not pay back.[30]

RA stepped away from aggressive debulking permitting development of smaller burrs, sheaths, and guide catheters with much more safety and efficiency, moving toward a "modification approach of CAC."

Rotational modification of calcium and preparation of lesion is meant to enable drug-eluting stent delivery therefore reducing ISR, but in several trials the beneficial effect is not well established.

ROTAXUS trial did not show a benefit of routinely using rotational atherectomy in patients with moderately or severely calcified obstructive coronary artery disease: 240 patients with complex calcified coronary lesions were randomly assigned to rotational atherectomy followed by stenting versus no rotational atherectomy stenting. The atherectomy group had higher levels of late in-stent lumen loss at 9 months. In follow-up at 9 months postprocedure, rates of restenosis, TLR, definite stent thrombosis, and major adverse cardiac events were similar between the 2 groups before paclitaxel-eluting stent implantation.[16] In current clinical practice RA use is mainly reserved to uncrossable CAC stenosis or for bailout lesion preparation in case of incomplete balloon expansion.

Orbital Atherectomy

The orbital atherectomy (OA) system was first described in 2008 and its use was meant for peripheral arteries.[31] This technique was transported in coronary field. The OA system is composed of a diamond-encrusted eccentric crown at the distal end of a drive shaft, powered by a pneumatic console. The operator can directly control anterograde and retrograde movement of the crown and orbit speed (from 80,000–120,000 rpm). The crown is continuously infused by a lubricant solution (ViperSlide).

Unlike the RA burr, the OA crown has diamond chips on front and back, thus permitting anterograde and retrograde atheroablation, OA is capable of treating different CAC scenarios, unlike to RA that needs different burrs to obtain larger cross-sectional areas, OA enlarging orbit of crown movement at faster speed reaches the same target. With single OA 1.25-mm crown through a 6-Fr guiding catheter the operator can be effective on reference vessels up to 3.5 mm in diameter. The movement is slow and poking; it permits intermittent coronary blood flow around the burr and reduces the risk stalling/entrapment. Conversely, in OA, the motion is uniform, gradual and continuous, pausing in interest segments to enable atheroablation. In expert operators, tactile and also audible changes could be felt. We report in **Figs. 1-3** an OCT guided PCI of LAD treated by OA.

The treatment time should not pass 30 seconds, in fact a sound alert can be heard after 25 seconds of nonstop treatment; the safety is guaranteed as shown in ORBIT I trial by rapid and continuous infusion of ViperSlide. In the ORBIT I trial we have 94% procedural success rate in 50 patients, on the other hand clinical complications included 2 in hospital myocardial infarctions (4%) and cumulative rates of MACE: 6 coronary dissections (12%) and 1 perforation, with no slow-flow/no-reflow.[32,33] ORBIT II study with 443 patients presenting de novo calcified plaque to treatment with OA, OA was associated with a 97.7% rate of successful stent delivery, a 98.8% rate of less

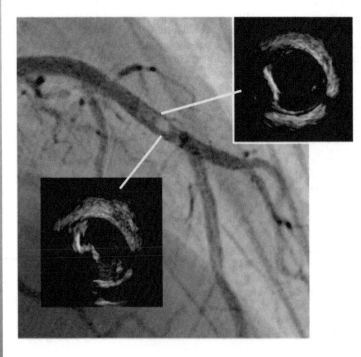

Fig. 1. Calcific nodule in mid LAD at coronary angiography and IVUS imaging.

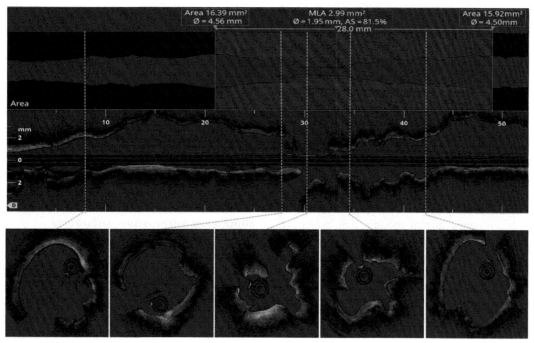

Fig. 2. OCT before OA.

than 50% stenosis post-PCI, and low rates of in-hospital Q-wave myocardial infarction (0.7%).[34–36]

Yamamoto and colleagues[37] found that in larger luminal area, OA led to a more radical plaque modification compared with RA, but in lesions with smaller lumen area, a similar degree of plaque modification occurred. Final stent expansion was similar, however Kini and colleagues[38] show a

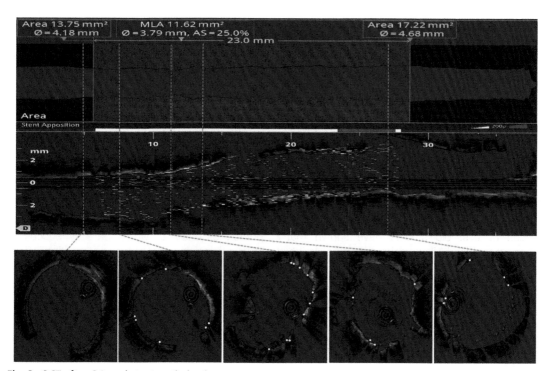

Fig. 3. OCT after OA and stent optimization.

better final stent apposition after OA. Orbital versus Rotational Atherectomy Effects On Coronary Microcirculation in PCI known as ORACLE (NCT03021577) will clarify another issue: the effect on microcirculation.

Excimer Laser Coronary Atherectomy

Laser was introduced for treatment of limbs ischemia[39] in 1980s, and was later supported for the use in coronary circulation.[40–43] Thanks to development of modern catheter and safe lasing techniques,[44,45] ELCA reached satisfying clinical outcomes.[46] The mechanics of ELCA are based on pulsed gas lasers, a mix of rare gas and a halogen element to generate short wavelength ultraviolet light (UVL): shorter is the wavelength, less deeper the penetration, less heat is produced and thus less traumatic for tissues. The principles of ELCA are 3: photochemical, photo-thermal, and photomechanical. UVL breaks carbon–carbon bonds, photochemical principle, elevating temperature of intracellular water and lead to rupture of cellular membrane and generating a bubble of vapor on the catheter tip, photothermal principle. At last, continuous formation and implosion of bubbles fragments the intravascular in a particulate of less than 10 μm diameter. The CVX-300 cardiovascular laser Excimer system (by Spectranetics, Colorado Springs, CO) uses Xenon chloride (XeCl) as the active medium. Operator personal safety devices should be carefully observed.

ELCA catheters are compatible with any standard 0.014-inch guidewire. Coronary catheters are available in four diameters (0.9, 1.4, 1.7, 2.0 mm) and those most commonly used have a concentric array of laser fibers at the tip.

Usually 0.9-mm × 80 catheter is used in fibrocalcific lesions thanks to its enhanced delivery and ability to emit laser energy at high power (80 mJ/mm^2) at the highest repletion rate (80 Hz). This is a situation where ELCA may be used, unless there are very significant calcification.[47,48] In highly fibrocalcific lesions, even for ELCA PCI more expert operators, the default choices remain RA or OA.

Efficacy of ELCA in PCI was achieved in 96.4% in ELLEMENT registry,[49] but careful case selection is mandatory successful procedures.

Shockwave Intravascular Lithotripsy

High-pressure balloon dilation and atherectomy may result inadequate to modify deeper calcium.

Coronary intravascular lithotripsy (IVL) with the Shockwave device (Shockwave Medical Inc., Santa Clara, CA), CE marked in 2017, is an innovative technique that can affect deeper calcium layer and alters calcium structure of plaque before stenting the lesion. Ali and colleagues[50] who studied 31 patients using OCT after IVL, firstly described this mechanism. The practice is borrowed on the well-known treatment strategy for renal calculi, used for decades to fragment kidney stones sparing soft tissues.

The Shockwave Medical coronary catheter is composed of a single-use catheter that contains multiple sonic emitters in a unique balloon, producing approximately 3 kV energy. The emitters create sonic pressure waves that spread uniformly and circumferentially. These waves can physically

---

Table 1
Treatment indications of coronary lesions with high calcium content before stenting and optimization

TECHNIQUES	NC BALLOON				CUTTING/SCORING BALLOON				ROTATIONAL ATHERECTOMY				ORBITAL ATHERECTOMY				ELCA				LITHOPLASTY BALLOON			
Lesion Types / Characteristics	Cr	UncL	OL	ULM	Cr	UncL	OL	ULM	Cr	UncL	OL	ULM	Cr	UncL	OL	ULM	Cr	UncL	OL	ULM	Cr	UncL	OL	ULM
Calcium Arc < 180° / Calcium Lenght < 5 mm / Calcium Thickness < 0.5 mm																								
Calcium Arc ≥ 180° / Calcium Lenght < 5 mm / Calcium Thickness < 0.5 mm																								
Calcium Arc ≥ 180° / Calcium Lenght ≥ 5 mm / Calcium Thickness < 0.5 mm																								
Calcium Arc ≥ 180° / Calcium Lenght ≥ 5 mm / Calcium Thickness ≥ 0.5 mm																								
Calcium Arc < 180° / Calcium Lenght ≥ 5 mm / Calcium Thickness ≥ 0.5 mm																								

Red: Generally not to be used; Yellow: To use after careful evaluation; Green: First line choice.

This table shows the technical advices to better face each calcific lesion type in different anatomical and pathological settings.

Abbreviations: Cr, Crossable lesion not involving ostium and with protected left main; OL, Ostial Lesions; ULM, Unprotected Left Main; UncL, Uncrossable Lesions.

fracture calcium, minimizing barotrauma attributable to low inflation pressure (4 atm).

Catheters available for this technique vary from 2.5 to 4.0 mm diameter and 12 mm in length, the generator delivers 10 pulses in sequence (1 pulse/s) till a maximum of 80 pulses per catheter.

Lithotripsy balloon is inflated to 405 kPa during, following pulsatile energy erogation.

Feasibility of intravascular lithotripsy for modification of severe coronary artery calcification was demonstrated in the Disrupt CAD I study (Disrupt Coronary Artery Disease).[51] After this, Disrupt CAD II was a prospective multicenter, single-arm post-approval study designed to assess the safety and performance of the Coronary IVL System to treat calcified stenotic coronary lesions.[52]

Patients had silent ischemia, unstable or stable angina with myocardial ischemia, or stabilized acute coronary syndrome without elevation in cardiac biomarkers, presenting a single target lesion requiring PCI with a diameter stenosis ≥50% and length ≤32 mm, in native coronary arteries.

The post-IVL luminal gain was 0.8 ± 0.5 mm and residual stenosis was 29% ± 12% with further decrease to 12% ± 5% following drug-eluting stent implantation.

No comparison data are available between atherectomy techniques and IVL, a retrospective review of 54 patients treated with IVL reported a higher incidence of isolated ventricular beats or asynchronous cardiac pacing during shockwave, not associated with clinical adverse events.[53]

WHAT'S NEXT TO HANDLE?

Lately technological advancements in PCI CAC equipment are consistent: resistant balloons that can reach very high pressures, sharp cutting and scoring devices, formidable burrs in RA and OA, modern balloon producing intense waves like in IVL and futuristic lasers. We can see even hybrid promising approaches to these lesions (Rota-Tripsy).[54] Particularly, IVL has a huge potential in concentric calcifications for its 3 main characteristics: safety, efficacy, and short learning curve.

We recently proposed a newer PCI algorithm based on imaging techniques, such as OCT and IVUS.[55] Based on our experience, calcium spread deeply but also longitudinally through the vessel wall, thus deeper calcified lesions should correspond to longer and more concentric involvement. This rationale permits to add an adjunctive point to the Fujino score for an arc greater than 270° and a length greater than 5 mm, thus directing the expert operator to the best procedure.

However, it is important to stay grounded in our everyday practice: coronaries anatomic and pathologic characteristics deeply impact on PCI planning, incomplete expansion and poor stent apposition, more frequent in calcified lesions, are predictive of target lesion failure and late stent thrombosis: calcium is a predictor of interventional treatment failure.[56]

We summarize in **Table 1** our PCI strategy in CAC.

Concluding, we always need to evaluate the stability of other vessels, even if they are not the principal aim of our work, evaluating completely the coronary tree and its balance. As is well known, each treatment should be tailored for patient and lesion characteristics.

REFERENCES

1. Yu SY. Calcification processes in atherosclerosis. Adv Exp Med Biol 1974;43:403–25.
2. Schmid K, McSharry WO, Pameijer CH, et al. Chemical and physicochemical studies on the mineral deposits of the human atherosclerotic aorta. Atherosclerosis 1980;37:199–210.
3. Friedrich GJ, Moes NY, Muhlberger VA, et al. Detection of intralesional calcium by intracoronary ultrasound depends on the histologic pattern. Am Heart J 1994;128:435–41.
4. Mintz GS, Popma JJ, Pichard AD, et al. Patterns of calcification in coronary artery disease. A statistical analysis of intravascular ultrasound and coronary angiography in 1155 lesions. Circulation 1995;91: 1959–65.
5. Mintz GS, Nissen SE, Anderson WD, et al. American College of Cardiology clinical expert consensus document on standards for acquisition, measurement and reporting of intravascular ultrasound studies (IVUS). J Am Coll Cardiol 2001;37:1478–92.
6. Madhavan MV, Madhusudhan T, Mintz GS, et al. Coronary artery calcification. J Am Coll Cardiol 2014; 63(No. 17):1703–12.
7. Kawasaki M, Bouma BE, Bressner J, et al. Diagnostic accuracy of optical coherence tomography and integrated backscatter intravascular ultrasound images for tissue characterization of human coronary plaques. J Am Coll Cardiol 2006;48:81–8.
8. Hoffmann R, Mintz GS, Popma JJ, et al. Treatment of calcified coronary lesions with Palmaz-Schatz stents. An intravascular ultrasound study. Eur Heart J 1998;19:1224–31.
9. Xu Y, Mintz GS, Tam A, et al. Prevalence, distribution, predictors, and outcomes of patients with calcified nodules in native coronary arteries: a 3-vessel intravascular ultrasound analysis from Providing Regional Observations to Study Predictors of Events in the Coronary Tree (PROSPECT). Circulation 2012; 126:537–45.

10. Stone GW, Maehara A, Lansky AJ, et al. A prospective natural history study of coronary atherosclerosis. N Engl J Med 2011;364:226–35.

11. Shimizu T, Maehara A, Farah T, et al. Relationship between coronary artery calcification, high-risk "vulnerable plaque" characteristics, and future adverse events: the PROSPECT study. J Am Coll Cardiol 2012;59(13 Supplement):E2102.

12. Fujino A, Mintz GS, Matsumura M, et al. A new optical coherence tomography-based calcium scoring system to predict stent underexpansion. EuroIntervention 2018;13:e2182–9.

13. Maejima N, Hibi K, Saka K, et al. Relationship between thickness of calcium on optical coherence tomography and crack formation after balloon dilatation in calcified plaque requiring rotational atherectomy. Circ J 2016;80(6):1413–9.

14. Frink RJ, Achor RW, Brown AL Jr, et al. Significance of calcification of the coronary arteries. Am J Cardiol 1970;26:241–7.

15. Moussa I, Ellis SG, Jones M, et al. Impact of coronary culprit lesion calcium in patients undergoing paclitaxel- eluting stent implantation (a TAXUS-IV sub study). Am J Cardiol 2005;96:1242–7.

16. Abdel-Wahab M, Richardt G, Joachim Büttner H, et al. High-speed rotational atherectomy before paclitaxel- eluting stent implantation in complex calcified coronary lesions: the randomized RO-TAXUS (Rotational Atherectomy Prior to Taxus Stent Treatment for Complex Native Coronary Artery Disease) trial. JACC Cardiovasc Interv 2013;6:10–9.

17. Fujimoto H, Nakamura M, Yokoi H. Impact of calcification on the long-term outcomes of sirolimus-eluting stent implantation: subanalysis of the Cypher Post-Marketing Surveillance Registry. Circ J 2012; 76(1):57–64.

18. Fujii K, Carlier SG, Mintz GS, et al. Stent underexpansion and residual reference segment stenosis are related to stent thrombosis after sirolimus-eluting stent implantation: an intravascular ultrasound study. J Am Coll Cardiol 2005;45(7):995–8.

19. Kawaguchi R, Tsurugaya H, Hoshizaki H, et al. Impact of lesion calcification on clinical and angiographic outcome after sirolimus-eluting stent implantation in real-world patients. Cardiovasc Revasc Med 2008;9(1):2–8.

20. Mosseri M, Satler LF, Pichard AD, et al. Impact of vessel calcification on outcomes after coronary stenting. Cardiovasc Revasc Med 2005;6(4): 147–53.

21. Fitzgerald PJ, Ports TA, Yock PG. Contribution of localized calcium deposits to dissection after angioplasty. An observational study using intravascular ultrasound. Circulation 1992;86:64–70.

22. Shimony A, Zahger D, Van Straten M, et al. Incidence, risk factors, management and outcomes of coronary artery perforation during percutaneous coronary intervention. Am J Cardiol 2009;104: 1674–7.

23. Bangalore S, Vlachos HA, Selzer F, et al. Percutaneous coronary intervention of moderate to severe calcified coronary lesions: insights from the National Heart, Lung, and Blood Institute Dynamic Registry. Catheter Cardiovasc Interv 2011;77:22–8.

24. Secco GG, Buettner A, Parisi R, et al. Clinical experience with very high-pressure dilatation for resistant coronary lesions. Cardiovasc Revasc Med 2019; 20(12):1083–7.

25. Secco GG, Ghione M, Mattesini A, et al. Very high-pressure dilatation for undilatable coronary lesions: indications and results with a new dedicated balloon. EuroIntervention 2016;12:359–65.

26. Barbato E, Shlofmitz E, Milkas A, et al. State of the art: evolving concepts in the treatment of heavily calcified and undilatable coronary stenoses - from debulking to plaque modification, a 40-year-long journey. EuroIntervention 2017;13(6):696–705.

27. Levin TN, Holloway S, Feldman T. Acute and late clinical outcome after rotational atherectomy for complex coronary disease. Cathet Cardiovasc Diagn 1998;45(2):122–30.

28. Reifart N, Vandormae IM, Krajcar M, et al. Randomized comparison of angioplasty of complex coronary lesions at a single center. Excimer laser, rotational atherectomy, and balloon angioplasty comparison (ERBAC) study. Circulation 1997;96(1):91–8.

29. Whitlow PL, Bass TA, Kipperman RM, et al. Results of the study to determine rotablator and transluminal angioplasty strategy (STRATAS). Am J Cardiol 2001; 87:699–705.

30. Safian RD, Feldman T, Muller DWM, et al. Coronary angioplasty and rotablator atherectomy trial (CARAT): immediate and late results of a prospective multicenter randomized trial. Catheter Cardiovasc Interv 2001;53(2):213–20.

31. Heuser RR. Treatment of lower extremity vascular disease: the diamondback 360 degrees orbital atherectomy system. Expert Rev Med Devices 2008;5: 279–86.

32. Parikh K, Chandra P, Choksi N, et al. Safety and feasibility of orbital atherectomy for the treatment of calcified coronary lesions: the ORBIT I trial. Catheter Cardiovasc Interv 2013;81:1134–9.

33. Bhatt P, Parikh P, Patel A, et al. Orbital atherectomy system in treating calcified coronary lesions: 3-year follow-up in first human use study (ORBIT I trial). Cardiovasc Revasc Med 2014;15(4):204–8.

34. Chambers JW, Feldman RL, Himmelstein SI, et al. Pivotal trial to evaluate the safety and efficacy of the orbital atherectomy system in treating de novo, severely calcified coronary lesions (ORBIT II). JACC Cardiovasc Interv 2014;7:510–8.

35. Lee M, Généreux P, Shlofmitz R. Orbital atherectomy for treating de novo, severely calcified coronary

lesions: 3-year results of the pivotal ORBIT II trial. Cardiovasc Revasc Med 2017;18(4):261–4.

36. Généreux P, Lee AC, Kim CY, et al. Orbital atherectomyfor treating de novo severely calcified coronary narrowing (1-year results from the pivotal ORBIT II trial). Am J Cardiol 2015;115(12):1685–90.

37. Yamamoto MH, Maehara A, Karimi Galougahi K, et al. Mechanisms of orbital versus rotational atherectomy plaque modification in severely calcified lesions assessed by optical coherence tomography. JACC Cardiovasc Interv 2017;10(24):2584–6.

38. Kini AS, Vengrenyuk Y, Pena J, et al. Optical coherence tomography assessment of the mechanistic effects of rotational and orbital atherectomy in severely calcified coronary lesions. Catheter Cardiovasc Interv 2015;86(6):1024–32.

39. Choy DSJ, Choy DSJ. History and State-of-the-Art of Lasers in Cardiovascular Disease. Laser Medicine and Surgery News and Advances 1988;6(3):34–8.

40. Cook SI, Eigler NL, Shefer A, et al. Percutaneous excimer laser coronary angioplasty of lesions not ideal for balloon angioplasty. Circulation 1991;84:632–3.

41. Koster R, Kahler J, Brockhoff C, et al. Laser coronary angioplasty: history, present and future. Am J Cardiovasc Drugs 2002;2:197–207.

42. Bittl JA, Sanborn TA, Tcheng JE. Clinical success, complications and restenosis rates with excimer laser coronary angioplasty. Am J Cardiol 1992;70:1553–9.

43. Geschwind HJ, Dubois-Rande JL, Zelinsky R, et al. Percutaneous coronary mid-infrared laser angioplasty. Am Heart J 1991;122:552–8.

44. Tcheng JE. Saline infusion in excimer laser coronary angioplasty. Semin Interv Cardiol 1996;1:135–41.

45. Topaz O. A new safer lasing technique for laser facilitated coronary angioplasty. J Intervent Cardiol 1993;6:297–306.

46. Topaz O. Coronary laser angioplasty. In: Topol EJ, editor. Textbook of interventional cardiology. Philadelphia: WB Saunders; 1995. p. 235–55.

47. Bittl JA. Clinical results with excimer laser coronary angioplasty. Semin Interv Cardiol 1996;1:129–34.

48. Bilodeau L, Fretz EB, Taeymans Y, et al. Novel use of a high energy excimer laser catheter for calcified and complex coronary artery lesions. Catheter Cardiovasc Interv 2004;62:155–61.

49. Latib A, Takagi K, Chizzola G, et al. Excimer Laser LEsion modification to expand non-dilatable stents: the ELLEMENT registry. Cardiovasc Revasc Med 2014;15:8–12.

50. Ali ZA, Brinton TJ, Hill JM, et al. Optical coherence tomography characterization of coronary lithoplasty for treatment of calcified lesions: first description. JACC Cardiovasc Imaging 2017;10:897–906.

51. Brinton TJ, Ali ZA, Hill JM, et al. Feasibility of shockwave coronary intravascular lithotripsy for the treatment of calcified coronary stenoses (Disrupt CAD I study). Circulation 2019;139:834–6.

52. Ali ZA, Nef H, Escaned J, et al. Safety and effectiveness of coronary intravascular lithotripsy for treatment of severely calcified coronary stenoses: the disrupt CAD II study. Circ Cardiovasc Interv 2019;12:e008434.

53. Wilson SJ, Spratt JC, Hill J, et al. Coronary intravascular lithotripsy is associated with a high incidence of 'shocktopics' and asynchronous cardiac pacing. EuroIntervention 2020;15(16):1429–35.

54. Jurado-Román A, Gonzálvez A, Galeote G, et al. Combination of rotational atherectomy and intravascular lithotripsy for the treatment of severely calcified lesions. JACC Cardiovasc Interv 2019;12(Issue 15):e127–9.

55. Sorini Dini C, Nardi G, Ristalli F, et al. Contemporary approach to heavily calcified coronary lesions. Interv Cardiol 2019;14(3):154–63.

56. Mattesini A, Di Mario C. Calcium: a predictor of interventional treatment failure across all fields of cardiovascular medicine. Int J Cardiol 2017;231:97–9.

Refractory Angina—Unsolved Problem

Marcin Makowski, MD, PhDa,*, Joanna Samanta Makowska, MD, PhDb,
Marzenna Zielińska, MD, PhDa

KEYWORDS

- Refractory angina pectoris • Neuromodulation • Spinal cord stimulation • Coronary sinus reducer
- Enhanced external counter-pulsation

KEY POINTS

- Refractory angina affects up to 5% to 10% of patients with coronary artery disease and is a lingering problem in everyday clinical practice.
- The recommendations for management are based on registries, not on randomized clinical trials, which are restricted to small groups of patients.
- Management of patients with refractory angina should be carried out in or supervised by experienced centers with access to multiple pharmacologic and interventional options. Decisions to disqualify patients from coronary revascularization should be made by the heart team individually and should consider patients' needs and expectations.
- Introduction of new drug compounds and new interventional methods increases therapeutic options for this difficult-to-treat group of patients.

EPIDEMIOLOGY

Based on European Society of Cardiology (ESC) Joint Study Group on the Treatment of Refractory Angina estimation, the incidence of refractory angina ranges from 5% to 10% of patients with coronary artery disease.[1] In the Andrell and colleagues[2] study, refractory angina affects 2% of patients with stable angina pectoris who were referred to coronary angiography. Refractory angina pectoris (RAP) decreases the quality of life, increases the number of hospitalizations, and is linked to increased cost for health care systems.[2] The mortality rate in this subgroup of patients differs significantly among studies, ranging from 1% to 22%.[3–8] According to centers specialized in RAP treatment, 1-year mortality is 3.9%, and up to 29.4% after 9 years of follow-up.[9]

PATHOPHYSIOLOGY

Traditionally, the pathomechanism of angina pain in coronary artery disease is attributed to oxygen supply-demand imbalance. Ischemia of cardiomyocytes leads to the release of the compounds stimulating nerve endings (substance P, adenosine, histamine, bradykinin, and lactic acid). Stimulation of nociceptive fibers in heart muscle leads to the conducting of the impulses to the central nervous system, thereby creating ischemic pain. The mechanism of the transmission of pain signals from the cell to nerve fibers is not fully elucidated. It is proposed that changes in potentials of membrane receptors are caused by neurotransmitter release.[10–12] It is stated that the chemosensitivity of receptors and their voltage changes, which could be translated to pain stimuli.[10,12]

Nociceptive endings are located in myelinated (A) and unmyelinated (C) fibers, forming cardiac visceral sensory nerves creating sympathetic and vagal systems.[13,14] Sympathetic fibers travel via dorsal root ganglion to posterior thalamus. Vagal afferents fibers also reach posterior thalamus via the nucleus of tractus solitarius. Based on PET, several cortical structures from posterior thalamus

a Department of Interventional Cardiology, Medical University of Lodz, Central Clinical Hospital, ul. Pomorska 251, Lodz 92-213, Poland; b Department of Rheumatology, Medical University of Lodz, Pieniny 30, Lodz 92-113, Poland
* Corresponding author.
E-mail address: drmarmak@gmail.com

Cardiol Clin 38 (2020) 629–637
https://doi.org/10.1016/j.ccl.2020.07.009
0733-8651/20/© 2020 Elsevier Inc. All rights reserved.

are activated during anginal pain.[15] Little or even no peripheral stimulus could provoke severe cardiac pain.[16] Some observations in patients with microvascular angina show enhanced activation in the area connected with pain perception on brain level, which suggests central abnormalities in pain mechanism.

There is evidence that peripheral neuropathy can impair pain signaling; classic examples are diabetic patients who can experience silent ischemic episodes.[17,18] There is no straightforward correlation between the intensity of pain sensation and the severity of ischemia.[19] The intervention method depends on the pain source and its transmission.

PHARMACOLOGIC TREATMENT

The aim of the optimal medical treatment of refractory angina is symptom reduction, an increase of exercise tolerance, and prevention of further cardiovascular events. The group of patients with refractory angina presents various comorbidities that also should be taken into consideration while choosing the most appropriate treatment method.[20,21] β-Blockers, calcium channel blockers, and long-acting and short-acting nitrates are traditional antianginal first-line drugs recommended by guidelines.[22] Patients after myocardial infarction, especially those with reduced ejection fraction, benefit from β-blockers,[23] whereas nondihydropyridine calcium channel blockers are associated with increased mortality in this particular group.[23]

Drugs that improve prognosis in coronary artery disease are acetylsalicylic acid (ASA), 75 mg daily; or in cases of contraindications, clopidogrel, 75 mg daily; and statins. Statin dose should be adjusted to achieve treatment goal, which is low-density lipoprotein cholesterol levels below 1.8 mmol/L (70 mg/dL).[22]

Prasugrel and ticagrelor are given together with ASA (if not contraindicated), in the long term, secondary prevention in following doses (prasugrel, 10 mg daily, or 5 mg daily in cases of body mass 75 years old; ticagrelor, 60 mg twice a day). Also 2.5 mg of rivaroxaban, twice a day, can be administered to lower mortality.[24]

In cases of a combination of ASA with clopidogrel, prasugrel, ticagrelor, or rivaroxaban, the risk of hemorrhagic complications should be assessed. Drug combination increases anticoagulant effect in patients with refractory angina (patients with type 2 diabetes mellitus, renal insufficiency, or atherosclerosis–peripheral artery disease) decrease rate of ischemic events.[25–27] In cases of hypersensitivity to ASA, drug desensitization

should be taken into consideration because ASA is a treatment of choice and patients require life-long treatment with the compound.[28]

In 1 small randomized controlled trial, the beneficial effect of the uric acid–lowering compound, allopurinol (600 mg daily), was found. Allopurinol treatment increased the time to the ischemic event and the appearance of angina during exertion.[29] In a study by Singh and Yu,[30] a reduction of myocardial infarction rate was found, especially in the elderly and especially if allopurinol was given for longer than for 2 years.

In large clinical trials, the percentage of patients adherent to prescribed treatment (including β-blockers) varies between 50% and 90%. An increase in the heart rate above 70 beats per minute at rest in a group of patients with decreased ejection fraction was linked to increased risk of death due to cardiovascular events.[31] The most frequent contraindications to β-blockers include bradycardia, conduction disorders, and bronchial spasm (both asthma and chronic obstructive pulmonary disease). In cases of induction of bronchoconstriction after this class of drugs, a switch to calcium blockers is indicated. Calcium blockers do not lead to proper control of the heart rate; in that case, ivabradine may be helpful.[22] In cases of atrial fibrillation and poor rate control, addition of digoxin is recommended. In critical cases, when the control rate in atrial fibrillation is difficult or impossible despite pharmacologic therapy, ablation of an atrioventricular node with pacemaker (optimal His bundle stimulation or resynchronization therapy) implantation is an option.[32]

Long-acting and short-acting nitrates are basal antianginal therapy. The problems appearing during nitrate treatment are tachyphylaxis and drug tolerance. In some cases, it is useful to combine nitrates, once daily, with molsidomine. Sometimes, a useful method is temporarily withdrawing nitrates with an exchange, for example, to nicorandil. Nicorandil is a nitrate-like drug that vasodilates coronary arteries and has cardioprotective potentials.[33] Efficacy of nicorandil was demonstrated in the Impact Of Nicorandil in Angina (IONA) trial, with major cardiovascular events (MACEs) reduction compared with the placebo group.[34]

Ivabradine blocks If channels, which regulate sinoatrial node chronotropic function. This drug is ideal for patients in whom β-blockers or calcium channels blockers are contraindicated. Ivabradine decreases heart rate, not affecting the systemic pressure; it also can be used together with a β-blocker to achieve a pulse rate below 70 beats per minute[35] or with a calcium channel blockers in cases of contraindications to β-blockers. The drugs are effective compared with β-blockers in angina reduction[36] and increase free of angina time during exercise.[35]

The anti-ischemic mechanism action of ranolazine is not fully understood. Probably, the drug affects channels similarly to amiodarone mainly via inhibition of late sodium currents.[37] In a few trials in patients with stable angina, ranolazine increases exercise time and ischemic threshold.[38–40] It is supposed that ranolazine improves coronary flow in areas of myocardial ischemia.[41]

Trimetazidine is a metabolic drug that acts on the cellular level by blocking thiolase (an enzyme involved in the β-oxidation of fatty acids) and increases glucose oxidation.[42,43] In the cells in ischemic conditions, in which oxygen supply is not sufficient, oxidation of glucose requires 10% to 15% less oxygen than β-oxidation of fatty acid to create the same amount of energy (adenosine triphosphate). In this way, the drug helps the cell to maintain basic functions in ischemic cells. There is evidence that trimetazidine improves exercise time to ischemia occurrence and decreases angina frequency.[44] In a meta-analysis of 23 randomized trials with trimetazidine, however, this anti-ischemic effect and reduction of MACEs were not confirmed.[45] In cases of comorbid hypertension, heart failure, and type 2 diabetes mellitus, the addition of angiotensin-converting enzyme I inhibitors or angiotensin receptor II blockers is recommended.[22]

Other drugs, like perhexiline, L-arginine, testosterone, thrombolytic agents (urokinase), and chelation therapy, are available; however, their efficacy and safety in refractory angina have not been confirmed.

ROLE OF THE HEART TEAM

Patients with refractory angina should be treated in specialized centers, where wide spectrum of treatment methods are available. Detailed analysis of each case allows personalizing the treatment and increasing its efficacy. Proper assessment of the pathogenesis of pain in individual patients plays a pivotal role in the choice of the optimal management plan.

The first step to be taken is coronary angiography. Cardiologists performing coronarography, in cases of advanced lesions in coronary arteries, should refer patients to a heart team consultation, to make a shared decision on further steps. In each case, better control of concomitant diseases is recommended (ie, glycemia, blood pressure, lipids, and body weight). Patients are obliged to cease smoking, control body weight, and adjust their diet. Each patient disqualified from the revascularization procedure should be supplied with

psychological help and should be included in a cardiac rehabilitation program. The Hospital Anxiety and Depression Scale can be useful to screen patients.[46] Complex analysis of each case, adjustment to patient expectations, and psychological support are crucial components of patients' management.[47]

Reevaluation of contraindications for revascularization also is pivotal. The center for treatment of refractory angina should have available various modalities of percutaneous coronary intervention (including chronic total occlusion atherectomy and shockwave balloon) and coronary artery bypass graft (especially minimally invasive procedure on heart beating). The heart team, with experienced surgeons and interventional cardiologists, should decide, based on current angiogram and patient clinic, on referral or exclusion from further revascularization. In selected cases (after risk assessment), it even is possible to perform not complete revascularization. Next, based on careful examination, concomitant abnormalities that could mimic angina, like anemia, chronic obstructive pulmonary disease, and hyperthyroidism, should be excluded.

CARDIAC REHABILITATION

Changes in lifestyle and cardiac rehabilitation reduce cardiac mortality.[48,49] Physical training adjusted to patients' state, brings effects in long-term observation, improves quality of life, and should be implemented in each patient ok the program or the treatment program.[50–52] In elderly and disabled patients, musculoskeletal disorders can hamper rehabilitation and rehabilitation programme should be adjusted to a patient's disability level.

In cases of a lack of efficacy of pharmacologic treatment, some invasive techniques can be implemented (**Table 1**).[22]

Enhanced external counter-pulsation (EECP) is a noninvasive method using 3 sets of pneumatic cuffs around the lower extremities, which work in a coordinated manner with the heart pump. In diastole, they fill, increasing vein backflow, imitating muscle pump; in systole, they deflate and therefore decrease afterload.[53,54]

The benefits of this method include not only mechanical support but also the proangiogenic effect, with an increase of the growth factors levels and circulating CD34+ cells that can stimulate the growth of the collateral circulation.[55–58] Also, some beneficial effects on the factors regulating vessel tonus were observed, that is, increase in the concentration of nitric oxide and decrease in the endothelin levels.[59] Reduction of the vasoconstriction increases control of blood pressure and

Table 1
Nonpharmacologic treatment options in refractory angina

Therapy	Mechanism of Action	Strength of Evidence
Coronary sinus reducer	Coronary flow redistribution	ESC: IIb/B ACC/AHA: NA
SCS	Pain termination	ESC: IIb/B ACC/AHA: IIb/B
EECP	Mechanic support, vascular relaxation	ESC: IIb/B ACC/AHA: IIB/B
Transmyocardial laser revascularization (surgical or percutaneous)	Angiogenesis, myocardial denervation	ESC: III/A ACC/AHA: IIb/B

Abbreviation: AHA, American Heart Association.
Data from Knuuti, J., et al., 2019 ESC Guidelines for the diagnosis and management of chronic coronary syndromes. Eur Heart J, 2020. 41(3): p. 407-477.

reduces angina.[60] In the multicenter study of enhanced external counterpulsation, the improvement of ischemia-induced pain by physical exercise was observed.[61]

EXTRACORPOREAL SHOCKWAVE THERAPY

Low-energy extracorporeal shockwave therapy (ESWT) is similar to lithotripsy but with lower energy. It is possible to stimulate in situ expression of proangiogenic vascular endothelial growth factor and nitric oxide.[62,63] In a few small randomized trials, ESWT confirmed positive results in increasing exercise time and reduction of angina.[64,65]

NEUROMODULATION

Neuromodulation is a method using chemical or electrical stimuli to break the pain signal pathway from heart to brain. The reduction of sympathetic afference stimulation, besides termination or alleviation of pain sensation, also decreases vasoconstriction.[66,67]

Spinal cord stimulation (SCS) is an invasive method used by neurosurgeons for treating patients with persistent pain that is refractory to medical therapy. This method is wildly available in many countries. For angina pain treatment, surgically epidural space is reached and a multipolar electrode is positioned between the C7 and T4 vertebrae. In this position, electrical stimulation has an impact on afferent sympathetic fibers and affects regional neurochemistry changes, which finally leads to pain elimination or reduction. There is evidence of the increase in γ-aminobutyric acid, that limits nociceptive afference.[68] The electrode is connected with a device that is placed subcutaneously. The therapy requires stimulation for 1 hour, 2 times per day, and on patient demand. Based on the results of several trials, the method reduces angina and nitrate consumption and improves exercise capacity and the quality of life.[69–72]

Other therapeutic options use neuromodulation: subcutaneous electrical nerve stimulation (SENS), thoracic epidural anesthesia, left stellate ganglion blockade (LSBG), and endoscopic thoracic sympathectomy are available. These methods are used successfully in specialized centers, but they still need validation in the randomized trials. The SENS method was tested in a small pilot study and demonstrated safety and feasibility using the same protocol as in SCS.[73] Reduction of angina and sublingual nitrate consumption was observed in all studied patients. The method seems safer in patients requiring anticoagulation or dual antiplatelet therapy compared with SCS, in which an electrode has to be positioned in epidural space. There are some concerns about safety in patients with other implantable electrical devices like implantable cardioverter defibrillators.

The methods of the left stellate ganglion blockade and endoscopic thoracic sympathectomy are feasible but data on its efficacy are scarce.[74,75] These methods require further randomized studies to confirm their usefulness and safety profiles.

CORONARY SINUS REDUCER

The idea of heart revascularization by grafting a systemic artery into coronary sinus was described by Beck and colleagues in 1948.[76] Nowadays, the possibility of narrowing coronary sinus by a special hourglass-shaped stent is a novel method of treating patients with refractory angina in a less traumatic way. The method was tested positively in a few studies.[77,78] The sinus reducer mechanism of action increases the trans-sinusal gradient pressure of blood and redistribution from less ischemic epicardium to the ischemic endocardium.[79–83] In the Coronary Sinus Reducer for Treatment of Refractory Angina (COSIRA) study, angina pain was decreased effectively by reducer compared with the control group.[84] An improvement in quality of life also was stated.[84] The efficacy of coronary sinus reducer therapy was confirmed in a group of patients with nonrevascularized chronic total occlusions. They had better outcomes than patients without chronic total occlusions (CTO);[85] higher efficacy in this subgroup may be the consequence of the better collateral flow.[86,87] Chronic ischemia may stimulate neoangiogenesis. Redistribution of coronary flow through increased resistance in sinus may be beneficial and may lead to the development of collateral flow by stimulation of neoangiogenesis.

Until now, an adequate response to RAP treatment has not been defined. In a study by Andrell and colleagues,[69] 18% of patients received adjunctive nonpharmacologic treatment, but, in more than 50% of patients, there was no method that used in monotherapy would be sufficient enough to reduce angina symptoms.[69] Nevertheless, safety and efficacy aspects of all invasive procedures should be evaluated carefully in prospective optimally randomized trials.

GENE THERAPY AND STEM CELLS

Stem cell treatment and gene therapy still are considered experimental treatments.

Improvement of systolic fraction of left ventricle and reduction of angina and mortality were observed in some studies using $CD34^+$ and $CD133^+$ cell therapy.[88–93] These changes were observed even 2 years after the procedure.[89] In the RENEW: Efficacy and Safety of Targeted Intramyocardial Delivery of Auto CD34+ Stem Cells for Improving Exercise Capacity in Subjects With Refractory Angina study, treatment with autologous stem cells also increased the pain-free exercise time.[94] The results of placebo-controlled trials, however, are less encouraging.[8,95,96]

TRANSMYOCARDIAL LASER REVASCULARIZATION

The idea of creating channels into ischemic myocardium to restore perfusion is based on an animal model of a reptile heart. In this method, using a surgical or percutaneous approach, 20 to 40 transmural 1-mm channels from epicardium to endocardium are created. An analysis of 7 trials conducted by the National Institute for Health and Care Excellence showed a statistically significant increase in mortality, heart attack rate, progression to heart failure, and thromboembolic complications.[97]

SUMMARY

Refractory angina increases mortality, impairs quality of life, and increases cost caused by repeated hospitalizations. The real number of patients with refractory angina is hard to assess. In Andrell and colleagues'[2] study, the prevalence of RAP was 2.1% but that seems underestimated because elderly and patients with comorbidities often are excluded from the studies.

In most patients, angina symptoms can be reduced by optimal pharmacologic treatment. Introduction of ivabradine, ranolazine, more efficient antiplatelet treatment, and anticoagulation increased angina treatment options. Only those in whom another alternative diagnosis was excluded, who did not respond to pharmacologic treatment (approximately 20%–30% of RAF), are qualified for intervention therapies. The term, untreatable angina, should be avoided because it suggests that there is no treatment option available for the patients. In recent years, novel intervention modalities were introduced and are included to present ESC and American College of Cardiology (ACC) recommendations. In RAP patients, the effect of a placebo cannot be neglected. In the TLRM study, a 30% improvement in exercise duration and a significant decrease in angina symptoms were reported in the control group. There is evidence that even placebo interventions alone could improve exercise duration and reduce angina. These strong placebo effects make the performance of reliable randomized interventional studies difficult.

A diagnostic and therapeutic process of patients with RAP should be conducted in specialized centers. Angina clinics should cover all diagnostic procedures and have a team experienced in percutaneous and surgical treatment and access to a full range of pharmacotherapy. A step-by-step process, starting from pharmacologic treatment, is pivotal. Each center performing revascularization procedures should be able to consult with a center specialized in RAP treatment. Because each case should be analyzed individually, a decision on further steps should be taken by a multidisciplinary heart team and should be accepted by the patient. The decision should be based on optimal benefit-risk balance. Despite a wide range of therapeutic options, elimination or reduction of angina sometimes is impossible; therefore, close cooperation with a psychologist also should be taken into consideration.

DISCLOSURE

The authors declare no conflicts of interest.

REFERENCES

1. Mannheimer C, Camici P, Chester MR, et al. The problem of chronic refractory angina; report from the ESC Joint study group on the treatment of refractory angina. Eur Heart J 2002;23(5):355–70.

2. Andrell P, Ekre O, Grip L, et al. Fatality, morbidity and quality of life in patients with refractory angina pectoris. Int J Cardiol 2011;147(3):377–82.

3. Allen KB, Dowling RD, Fudge TL, et al. Comparison of transmyocardial revascularization with medical therapy in patients with refractory angina. N Engl J Med 1999;341(14):1029–36.

4. Burkhoff D, Schmidt S, Schulman SP, et al. Transmyocardial laser revascularisation compared with continued medical therapy for treatment of refractory angina pectoris: a prospective randomised trial. ATLANTIC Investigators. Angina Treatments-Lasers and Normal Therapies in Comparison. Lancet 1999;354(9182):885–90.

5. Frazier OH, March RJ, Horvath KA. Transmyocardial revascularization with a carbon dioxide laser in patients with end-stage coronary artery disease. N Engl J Med 1999;341(14):1021–8.

6. Oesterle SN, Sanborn TA, Ali N, et al. Percutaneous transmyocardial laser revascularisation for severe angina: the PACIFIC randomised trial. Potential Class Improvement from Intramyocardial Channels. Lancet 2000;356(9243):1705–10.

7. Henry TD, Grines CL, Watkins MW, et al. Effects of Ad5FGF-4 in patients with angina: an analysis of pooled data from the AGENT-3 and AGENT-4 trials. J Am Coll Cardiol 2007;50(11):1038–46.

8. Kastrup J, Jorgensen E, Ruck A, et al. Direct intramyocardial plasmid vascular endothelial growth factor-A165 gene therapy in patients with stable severe angina pectoris A randomized double-blind placebo-controlled study: the Euroinject One trial. J Am Coll Cardiol 2005;45(7):982–8.

9. Henry TD, Satran D, Hodges JS, et al. Long-term survival in patients with refractory angina. Eur Heart J 2013;34(34):2683–8.

10. Fu LW, Longhurst JC. Regulation of cardiac afferent excitability in ischemia. Handb Exp Pharmacol 2009; 194:185–225.

11. Pan HL, Chen SR. Sensing tissue ischemia: another new function for capsaicin receptors? Circulation 2004;110(13):1826–31.

12. Gaspardone A, Crea F, Tomai F, et al. Substance P potentiates the algogenic effects of intraarterial infusion of adenosine. J Am Coll Cardiol 1994;24(2): 477–82.

13. Foreman RD, Garrett KM, Blair RW. Mechanisms of cardiac pain. Compr Physiol 2015;5(2):929–60.

14. Goldberger JJ, Arora R, Buckley U, et al. Autonomic nervous system dysfunction: JACC focus seminar. J Am Coll Cardiol 2019;73(10):1189–206.

15. Rosen SD, Paulesu E, Frith CD, et al. Central nervous pathways mediating angina pectoris. Lancet 1994;344(8916):147–50.

16. Rosen SD, Camici PG. The brain-heart axis in the perception of cardiac pain: the elusive link between ischaemia and pain. Ann Med 2000;32(5): 350–64.

17. Langer A, Freeman MR, Josse RG, et al. Detection of silent myocardial ischemia in diabetes mellitus. Am J Cardiol 1991;67(13):1073–8.

18. Shakespeare CF, Katritsis D, Crowther A, et al. Differences in autonomic nerve function in patients with silent and symptomatic myocardial ischaemia. Br Heart J 1994;71(1):22–9.

19. Klein J, Chao SY, Berman DS, et al. Is 'silent' myocardial ischemia really as severe as symptomatic ischemia? The analytical effect of patient selection biases. Circulation 1994;89(5):1958–66.

20. Camm AJ, Manolis A, Ambrosio G, et al. Unresolved issues in the management of chronic stable angina. Int J Cardiol 2015;201:200–7.

21. Ferrari R, Camici PG, Crea F, et al. Expert consensus document: a 'diamond' approach to personalized treatment of angina. Nat Rev Cardiol 2018;15(2): 120–32.

22. Knuuti J, Wijns W, Saraste A, et al. 2019 ESC Guidelines for the diagnosis and management of chronic coronary syndromes. Eur Heart J 2020;41(3): 407–77.

23. Fihn SD, Gardin JM, Abrams J, et al. 2012 ACCF/ AHA/ACP/AATS/PCNA/SCAI/STS Guideline for the diagnosis and management of patients with stable ischemic heart disease: a report of the American College of Cardiology Foundation/American Heart Association Task Force on Practice Guidelines, and the American College of Physicians, American Association for Thoracic Surgery, Preventive Cardiovascular Nurses Association, Society for Cardiovascular Angiography and Interventions, and Society of Thoracic Surgeons. J Am Coll Cardiol 2012;60(24): e44–164.

24. Mega JL, Braunwald E, Wiviott SD, et al. Rivaroxaban in patients with a recent acute coronary syndrome. N Engl J Med 2012;366(1):9–19.

25. Bhatt DL, Bonaca MP, Bansilal S, et al. Reduction in ischemic events with ticagrelor in diabetic patients with prior myocardial infarction in PEGASUS-TIMI 54. J Am Coll Cardiol 2016;67(23):2732–40.

26. Bansilal S, Bonaca MP, Cornel JH, et al. Ticagrelor for secondary prevention of atherothrombotic events in patients with multivessel coronary disease. J Am Coll Cardiol 2018;71(5):489–96.

27. Bonaca MP, Bhatt DL, Storey RF, et al. Ticagrelor for prevention of ischemic events after myocardial infarction in patients with peripheral artery disease. J Am Coll Cardiol 2016;67(23):2719–28.

28. Makowska JP, Makowski M, Kowalski ML. NSAIDs hypersensitivity: when and how to desensitize? Curr Treat Options Allergy 2015;2:124–40.

29. Noman A, Ang DS, Ogston S, et al. Effect of high-dose allopurinol on exercise in patients with chronic stable angina: a randomised, placebo controlled crossover trial. Lancet 2010;375(9732):2161–7.

30. Singh JA, Yu S. Allopurinol reduces the risk of myocardial infarction (MI) in the elderly: a study of Medicare claims. Arthritis Res Ther 2016; 18(1):209.

31. Beautiful Study G, Ferrari R, Ford I, et al. The BEAU-TIFUL study: randomized trial of ivabradine in patients with stable coronary artery disease and left ventricular systolic dysfunction - baseline characteristics of the study population. Cardiology 2008; 110(4):271–82.

32. Kirchhof P, Benussi S, Kotecha D, et al. 2016 ESC Guidelines for the management of atrial fibrillation developed in collaboration with EACTS. Eur Heart J 2016;37(38):2893–962.

33. Treese N, Erbel R, Meyer J. Acute hemodynamic effects of nicorandil in coronary artery disease. J Cardiovasc Pharmacol 1992;20(Suppl 3):S52–6.

34. Group IS. Effect of nicorandil on coronary events in patients with stable angina: the Impact of Nicorandil in Angina (IONA) randomised trial. Lancet 2002; 359(9314):1269–75.

35. Tardif JC, Ponikowski P, Kahan T, et al. Efficacy of the I(f) current inhibitor ivabradine in patients with chronic stable angina receiving beta-blocker therapy: a 4-month, randomized, placebo-controlled trial. Eur Heart J 2009;30(5):540–8.

36. Tardif JC, Ford I, Tendera M, et al. Efficacy of ivabradine, a new selective I(f) inhibitor, compared with atenolol in patients with chronic stable angina. Eur Heart J 2005;26(23):2529–36.

37. Antzelevitch C, Belardinelli L, Zygmunt AC, et al. Electrophysiological effects of ranolazine, a novel antianginal agent with antiarrhythmic properties. Circulation 2004;110(8):904–10.

38. Chaitman BR, Skettino SL, Parker JO, et al. Anti-ischemic effects and long-term survival during ranolazine monotherapy in patients with chronic severe angina. J Am Coll Cardiol 2004;43(8):1375–82.

39. Chaitman BR, Pepine CJ, Parker JO, et al. Effects of ranolazine with atenolol, amlodipine, or diltiazem on exercise tolerance and angina frequency in patients with severe chronic angina: a randomized controlled trial. JAMA 2004;291(3):309–16.

40. Stone PH, Gratsiansky NA, Blokhin A, et al. Antianginal efficacy of ranolazine when added to treatment with amlodipine: the ERICA (Efficacy of Ranolazine in Chronic Angina) trial. J Am Coll Cardiol 2006; 48(3):566–75.

41. Stone PH, Chaitman BR, Stocke K, et al. The anti-ischemic mechanism of action of ranolazine in stable ischemic heart disease. J Am Coll Cardiol 2010;56(12):934–42.

42. MacInnes A, Fairman DA, Binding P, et al. The antianginal agent trimetazidine does not exert its functional benefit via inhibition of mitochondrial long-chain 3-ketoacyl coenzyme A thiolase. Circ Res 2003;93(3):e26–32.

43. Kantor PF, Lucien A, Kozak R, et al. The antianginal drug trimetazidine shifts cardiac energy metabolism from fatty acid oxidation to glucose oxidation by inhibiting mitochondrial long-chain 3-ketoacyl coenzyme A thiolase. Circ Res 2000;86(5):580–8.

44. Szwed H, Sadowski Z, Elikowski W, et al. Combination treatment in stable effort angina using trimetazidine and metoprolol: results of a randomized, double-blind, multicentre study (TRIMPOL II). TRI-Metazidine in POLand. Eur Heart J 2001;22(24): 2267–74.

45. Ciapponi A, Pizarro R, Harrison J. Trimetazidine for stable angina. Cochrane Database Syst Rev 2005;(4):CD003614.

46. Spinhoven P, Ormel J, Sloekers PP, et al. A validation study of the Hospital Anxiety and Depression Scale (HADS) in different groups of Dutch subjects. Psychol Med 1997;27(2):363–70.

47. Payne TJ, Johnson CA, Penzien DB, et al. Chest pain self-management training for patients with coronary artery disease. J Psychosom Res 1994;38(5): 409–18.

48. O'Connor GT, Buring JE, Yusuf S, et al. An overview of randomized trials of rehabilitation with exercise after myocardial infarction. Circulation 1989;80(2): 234–44.

49. de Lorgeril M, Salen P, Martin JL, et al. Mediterranean diet, traditional risk factors, and the rate of cardiovascular complications after myocardial infarction: final report of the Lyon Diet Heart Study. Circulation 1999;99(6):779–85.

50. Leaf DA, Kleinman MT, Hamilton M, et al. The exercise-induced oxidative stress paradox: the effects of physical exercise training. Am J Med Sci 1999; 317(5):295–300.

51. Mittleman MA, Maclure M, Tofler GH, et al. Triggering of acute myocardial infarction by heavy physical exertion. Protection against triggering by regular exertion. Determinants of Myocardial Infarction Onset Study Investigators. N Engl J Med 1993; 329(23):1677–83.

52. Lewin RJ. Improving quality of life in patients with angina. Heart 1999;82(6):654–5.

53. Sinvhal RM, Gowda RM, Khan IA. Enhanced external counterpulsation for refractory angina pectoris. Heart 2003;89(8):830–3.

54. Michaels AD, McCullough PA, Soran OZ, et al. Primer: practical approach to the selection of patients for and application of EECP. Nat Clin Pract Cardiovasc Med 2006;3(11):623–32.

55. Kiernan TJ, Boilson BA, Tesmer L, et al. Effect of enhanced external counterpulsation on circulating CD34+ progenitor cell subsets. Int J Cardiol 2011; 153(2):202–6.

56. Braith RW, Conti CR, Nichols WW, et al. Enhanced external counterpulsation improves peripheral artery flow-mediated dilation in patients with chronic angina: a randomized sham-controlled study. Circulation 2010;122(16):1612–20.

57. Bonetti PO, Barsness GW, Keelan PC, et al. Enhanced external counterpulsation improves endothelial function in patients with symptomatic coronary artery disease. J Am Coll Cardiol 2003;41(10): 1761–8.

58. Michaels AD, Raisinghani A, Soran O, et al. The effects of enhanced external counterpulsation on myocardial perfusion in patients with stable angina: a multicenter radionuclide study. Am Heart J 2005; 150(5):1066–73.

59. Akhtar M, Wu GF, Du ZM, et al. Effect of external counterpulsation on plasma nitric oxide and endothelin-1 levels. Am J Cardiol 2006;98(1): 28–30.

60. Campbell AR, Satran D, Zenovich AG, et al. Enhanced external counterpulsation improves systolic blood pressure in patients with refractory angina. Am Heart J 2008;156(6):1217–22.

61. Arora RR, Chou TM, Jain D, et al. The multicenter study of enhanced external counterpulsation (MUST-EECP): effect of EECP on exercise-induced myocardial ischemia and anginal episodes. J Am Coll Cardiol 1999;33(7):1833–40.

62. Aicher A, Heeschen C, Sasaki K, et al. Low-energy shock wave for enhancing recruitment of endothelial progenitor cells: a new modality to increase efficacy of cell therapy in chronic hind limb ischemia. Circulation 2006;114(25):2823–30.

63. Mariotto S, Cavalieri E, Amelio E, et al. Extracorporeal shock waves: from lithotripsy to anti-inflammatory action by NO production. Nitric Oxide 2005; 12(2):89–96.

64. Wang Y, Guo T, Ma TK, et al. A modified regimen of extracorporeal cardiac shock wave therapy for treatment of coronary artery disease. Cardiovasc Ultrasound 2012;10:35.

65. Assmus B, Walter DH, Seeger FH, et al. Effect of shock wave-facilitated intracoronary cell therapy on LVEF in patients with chronic heart failure: the CELLWAVE randomized clinical trial. JAMA 2013; 309(15):1622–31.

66. Hautvast RW, Blanksma PK, DeJongste MJ, et al. Effect of spinal cord stimulation on myocardial blood flow assessed by positron emission tomography in patients with refractory angina pectoris. Am J Cardiol 1996;77(7):462–7.

67. de Jongste MJ, Haaksma J, Hautvast RW, et al. Effects of spinal cord stimulation on myocardial ischaemia during daily life in patients with severe coronary artery disease. A prospective ambulatory electrocardiographic study. Br Heart J 1994;71(5): 413–8.

68. Prager JP. What does the mechanism of spinal cord stimulation tell us about complex regional pain syndrome? Pain Med 2010;11(8):1278–83.

69. Andrell P, Yu W, Gersbach P, et al. Long-term effects of spinal cord stimulation on angina symptoms and quality of life in patients with refractory angina pectoris–results from the European Angina Registry Link Study (EARL). Heart 2010;96(14):1132–6.

70. Eddicks S, Maier-Hauff K, Schenk M, et al. Thoracic spinal cord stimulation improves functional status and relieves symptoms in patients with refractory angina pectoris: the first placebo-controlled randomised study. Heart 2007;93(5):585–90.

71. Lanza GA, Grimaldi R, Greco S, et al. Spinal cord stimulation for the treatment of refractory angina pectoris: a multicenter randomized single-blind study (the SCS-ITA trial). Pain 2011;152(1):45–52.

72. Zipes DP, Svorkdal N, Berman D, et al. Spinal cord stimulation therapy for patients with refractory angina who are not candidates for revascularization. Neuromodulation 2012;15(6):550–8 [discussion: 558–9].

73. Buiten MS, DeJongste MJ, Beese U, et al. Subcutaneous electrical nerve stimulation: a feasible and new method for the treatment of patients with refractory angina. Neuromodulation 2011;14(3):258–65 [discussion: 265].

74. Claes G, Drott C, Wettervik C, et al. Angina pectoris treated by thoracoscopic sympathecotomy. Cardiovasc Surg 1996;4(6):830–1.

75. Gramling-Babb P, Miller MJ, Reeves ST, et al. Treatment of medically and surgically refractory angina pectoris with high thoracic epidural analgesia: initial clinical experience. Am Heart J 1997;133(6):648–55.

76. Beck CS, Stanton E, et al. Revascularization of heart by graft of systemic artery into coronary sinus. J Am Med Assoc 1948;137(5):436–42.

77. Banai S, Ben Muvhar S, Parikh KH, et al. Coronary sinus reducer stent for the treatment of chronic refractory angina pectoris: a prospective, open-label, multicenter, safety feasibility first-in-man study. J Am Coll Cardiol 2007;49(17):1783–9.

78. Konigstein M, Meyten N, Verheye S, et al. Transcatheter treatment for refractory angina with the coronary sinus reducer. EuroIntervention 2014;9(10):1158–64.

79. Camici PG, Crea F. Coronary microvascular dysfunction. N Engl J Med 2007;356(8):830–40.

80. Ido A, Hasebe N, Matsuhashi H, et al. Coronary sinus occlusion enhances coronary collateral flow

and reduces subendocardial ischemia. Am J Physiol Heart Circ Physiol 2001;280(3):H1361–7.

81. Paz Y, Shinfeld A. Mild increase in coronary sinus pressure with coronary sinus reducer stent for treatment of refractory angina. Nat Clin Pract Cardiovasc Med 2009;6(3):E3.

82. Syeda B, Schukro C, Heinze G, et al. The salvage potential of coronary sinus interventions: meta-analysis and pathophysiologic consequences. J Thorac Cardiovasc Surg 2004;127(6):1703–12.

83. Mohl W, Kajgana I, Bergmeister H, et al. Intermittent pressure elevation of the coronary venous system as a method to protect ischemic myocardium. Interact Cardiovasc Thorac Surg 2005;4(1):66–9.

84. Verheye S, Jolicoeur EM, Behan MW, et al. Efficacy of a device to narrow the coronary sinus in refractory angina. N Engl J Med 2015;372(6):519–27.

85. Zivelonghi C, Verheye S, Timmers L, et al. Efficacy of coronary sinus reducer in patients with non-revascularized chronic total occlusions. Am J Cardiol 2020;126:1–7.

86. Fedele FA, Capone RJ, Most AS, et al. Effect of pressure-controlled intermittent coronary sinus occlusion on pacing-induced myocardial ischemia in domestic swine. Circulation 1988;77(6):1403–13.

87. Toggart EJ, Nellis SH, Liedtke AJ. The efficacy of intermittent coronary sinus occlusion in the absence of coronary artery collaterals. Circulation 1987;76(3):667–77.

88. Hartikainen J, Hassinen I, Hedman A, et al. Adenoviral intramyocardial VEGF-DDeltaNDeltaC gene transfer increases myocardial perfusion reserve in refractory angina patients: a phase I/IIa study with 1-year follow-up. Eur Heart J 2017;38(33):2547–55.

89. Henry TD, Losordo DW, Traverse JH, et al. Autologous CD34+ cell therapy improves exercise capacity, angina frequency and reduces mortality in no-option refractory angina: a patient-level pooled analysis of randomized double-blinded trials. Eur Heart J 2018;39(23):2208–16.

90. Henry TD, Schaer GL, Traverse JH, et al. Autologous CD34(+) Cell therapy for refractory angina: 2-year outcomes from the ACT34-CMI study. Cell Transplant 2016;25(9):1701–11.

91. Sung PH, Lee FY, Tong MS, et al. The five-year clinical and angiographic follow-up outcomes of intracoronary transfusion of circulation-derived CD34+ cells for patients with end-stage diffuse coronary artery disease unsuitable for coronary intervention-phase i clinical trial. Crit Care Med 2018;46(5):e411–8.

92. Jimenez-Quevedo P, Gonzalez-Ferrer JJ, Sabate M, et al. Selected CD133(+) progenitor cells to promote angiogenesis in patients with refractory angina: final results of the PROGENITOR randomized trial. Circ Res 2014;115(11):950–60.

93. Wojakowski W, Jadczyk T, Michalewska-Wludarczyk A, et al. Effects of transendocardial delivery of bone marrow-derived CD133(+) cells on left ventricle perfusion and function in patients with refractory angina: final results of randomized, double-blinded, placebo-controlled REGENT-VSEL trial. Circ Res 2017;120(4):670–80.

94. Povsic TJ, Henry TD, Traverse JH, et al. The RENEW trial: efficacy and safety of intramyocardial autologous CD34(+) cell administration in patients with refractory angina. JACC Cardiovasc Interv 2016;9(15):1576–85.

95. Rosengart TK, Lee LY, Patel SR, et al. Angiogenesis gene therapy: phase I assessment of direct intramyocardial administration of an adenovirus vector expressing VEGF121 cDNA to individuals with clinically significant severe coronary artery disease. Circulation 1999;100(5):468–74.

96. Vale PR, Losordo DW, Milliken CE, et al. Randomized, single-blind, placebo-controlled pilot study of catheter-based myocardial gene transfer for therapeutic angiogenesis using left ventricular electromechanical mapping in patients with chronic myocardial ischemia. Circulation 2001;103(17):2138–43.

97. Schofield PM, McNab D, National Institute for H, et al. NICE evaluation of transmyocardial laser revascularisation and percutaneous laser revascularisation for refractory angina. Heart 2010;96(4):312–3.

Stent Thrombosis After Percutaneous Coronary Intervention

From Bare-Metal to the Last Generation of Drug-Eluting Stents

Alberto Polimeni, MD, PhD[a,b,1], Sabato Sorrentino, MD, PhD[a,b,1], Carmen Spaccarotella, MD[a,b], Annalisa Mongiardo, MD[a], Jolanda Sabatino, MD, PhD[a,b], Salvatore De Rosa, MD, PhD[a,b], Tommaso Gori, MD, PhD[c], Ciro Indolfi, MD[a,b,d],*

KEYWORDS

• BMS • DES • BRS • Thrombosis • Stent

KEY POINTS

• Although rare, thrombosis still remains a major complication after coronary stent implantation.
• Although the causes of stent thrombosis are multifactorial, the device-related mechanism is a key factor.
• Knowing the different characteristics of the stents is of paramount importance for choosing the most suitable stent for the specific patient in clinical practice.

INTRODUCTION

The introduction in clinical practice of coronary stents has set a milestone in the history of interventional cardiology. Developed to overcome the limitation of plain old balloon angioplasty (POBA), this technology over the years has become a standard of care in the treatment of coronary artery disease. The continuous technical evolution has brought several types of stents to cope with the increasing complexity of the lesions that currently are accessible to the percutaneous approach. Accordingly, being familiar with the technical features of each platform and its related safety and efficacy profile is becoming of paramount importance. Stent thrombosis (ST) is an uncommon but harmful complication of percutaneous coronary implantation (PCI), causing myocardial infarction in approximately 60% to 70% of the cases, and leading to an increased risk of mortality (20%–25%).[1] The type of stent implanted is a major factor in determining the risk of coronary ST.[2] Therefore, this review article describes evidence from clinical trials or observational studies on the coronary stent types used most often (**Fig. 1**) and their related risk of ST in the modern era of interventional cardiology.

Conflict of interest statement: The authors have no conflicts of interest to declare.
[a] Division of Cardiology, Department of Medical and Surgical Sciences, "Magna Graecia" University, Viale Europa, Catanzaro 88100, Italy; [b] Research Center for Cardiovascular Diseases, "Magna Graecia" University, Viale Europa, Catanzaro 88100, Italy; [c] Kardiologie I, Zentrum für Kardiologie, University Medical Center Mainz, Deutsches Zentrum für Herz und Kreislauf Forschung, Langenbeckstraße 1, Standort Rhein-Main 55131, Germany; [d] Mediterranea Cardiocentro, Via Orazio, 2, Naples 80122, Italy
[1] These authors contributed equally to this work.
* Corresponding author. Division of Cardiology, Department of Medical and Surgical Sciences, "Magna Graecia" University, Viale Europa, Catanzaro 88100, Italy.
E-mail address: indolfi@unicz.it

Cardiol Clin 38 (2020) 639–647
https://doi.org/10.1016/j.ccl.2020.07.008

cardiology.theclinics.com

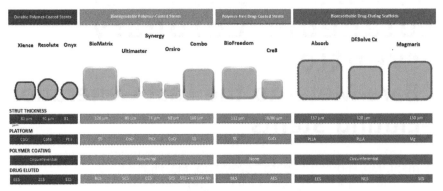

Fig. 1. Comparison of the main characteristics of different categories of coronary stent.

BARE-METAL STENT

Bare-metal stents (BMSs) have been developed to avoid elastic recoil and late vascular remodeling after POBA. Since their introduction in clinical practice in 1986 with the Wallstent (Schneider AG) and in 1987 with the first Food and Drug Administration–approved Palmaz-Schatz stent (Johnson & Johnson), BMSs progressively replaced POBA and became standard of care for PCI in the late 1990s. Despite the continuous improvement in stent technology, however, long-term follow-up revealed 20% to 30% incidence of in-stent restenosis (ISR).[3] The high rate of ISR observed with these platforms is caused by the proliferation and migration of vascular smooth muscle cells within stent struts, a phenomenon widely studied using in vitro and in vivo models.[4–7] The introduction in clinical practice of drug-eluting stents (DESs) to overcome this limitation led to progressive decline in the use of BMSs, with a significant reduction of ISR. Several studies and registries have shown that the rates of early ST between BMSs and first-generation DESs were quite similar[8]; the risk of very late ST (VLST) was surprisingly higher with DESs, thus becoming a concern for fast and generalized use of medicated platforms.[9] Characteristics and potential mechanisms underlying VLST differ significantly between BMS and DES platforms. In 61 patients with VLST, reported by Nakamura and colleagues,[10] using the optical coherence technique, the malapposed or uncovered strut and stent underexpansion were observed more frequently in DESs, whereas thin-cap fibroatheroma, neoatherosclerosis, and lipid neointima were observed more frequently in BMSs than in DESs.

Despite the improvement of implantation techniques and the introduction in clinical practice of the less thrombogenic second-generation DESs that ensure reasonable discontinuation of the dual antiplatelet therapy (DAPT),[11] the BMS has

continued to be used for a long time, for those patients in whom a prolonged antithrombotic therapy did not ensure a reasonable risk-benefit tradeoff. The recently published Italian Multicenter Registry of Bare Metal Stent Use in Modern Percutaneous Coronary Intervention Era (AMARCORD) registry, including 58,879 patients undergoing PCI and stent implantation in 18 Italian sites, reported a progressive decrease in BMS use, from 10.1% in 2013% to 0.3%, in 2017. The main reasons for BMS implantation were ST-elevation myocardial infarction (STEMI) (23.1%), advanced age (24.4%), and physician perception of high bleeding risk (HBR) (34.0%). At a mean follow-up of 2.2 years ± 1.5 years, the rates of definitive ST were 2.3% (1.2% at 30 days and 1.9% at 1 year).[12] Several clinical trials and prospective studies have shown superiority of second-generation DESs compared with BMSs.

DURABLE POLYMER DRUG-ELUTING STENT

Evidence from post mortem pathology and intra-coronary imaging supports the concept that the increased thrombosis observed in patients receiving first-generation DESs essentially was due to the fact that the cytotoxic drugs eluted by the stents inhibit not only the proliferation and migration of the vascular smooth muscle cells that are responsible for restenosis but also the growth and mobility of endothelial cells, fundamental for the healing of the vessel after the stent implantation.[13,14] Furthermore, first-generation DESs were coated with permanent polymers like methacrylate compounds that facilitate drug release but remain on the stent after drug elution, causing vascular inflammation, hypereosinophilia, and thrombogenic reactions.[15,16] The increased stent strut thickness that was necessary to warrant sufficient radial strength to first-generation DESs also has a major impact in thrombosis. Several studies demonstrated that thick-strutted stents are more thrombogenic than comparable thin-strutted devices.[17]

The second-generation DESs were designed to overcome these safety issues, employing new and more biocompatible polymer coatings, less toxic antiproliferative drugs and thin-strut metal alloys. The introduction of cobalt chromium (CoCr), a more biocompatible material, increasingly is used in new-generation coronary stents. In comparison with stainless steel, CoCr has a higher radiopacity and radial strength. This allows for the production of thinner struts with a similar radiological visibility and radial strength. For all these reasons, the zotarolimus-eluting stent (ZES) and everolimus-eluting stent (EES) have demonstrated a decreased risk of late ST and very-late ST in comparison with old-generation DESs.

In the COMPARE trial, the rates of definite and probable ST were reduced significantly among EES compared with paclitaxel-eluting stent-treated patients (0.7% vs 2.6%, respectively; P = .002) at 12 months.[18] In recent work published by Tada and colleagues,[19] in unselected patients in a large German cohort, the cumulative incidence of definite ST at 3 years was 1.5% with the BMS, 2.2% with the first-generation DESs, and 1.0% with the second-generation DESs. The consistent superiority of newer-generation DESs also is demonstrated in meta-analyses, showing odds ratios between 0.31 and 0.56 for ST in different DES types compared with BMSs.[20] Furthermore, much evidence also supports second-generation DESs for those patients who historically have been treated with BMSs, because of low risk of ISR or high risk of early coronary thrombotic events (such as STEMI patients) or because of not tolerating a prolonged DAPT (such as HBR patients). In regard to STEMI patients, several clinical trials and observational registries have shown superiority of DESs over BMSs.[21,22] In a large pooled analysis, including 2665 patients enrolled in the Clinical Evaluation of the Xience-V stent in Acute Myocardial Infarction) (EXAMINATION) and Comparison of Biolimus Eluted From an Erodible Stent Coating With Bare Metal Stents in Acute ST-Elevation Myocardial Infarction (COMFORTABLE-AMI) trials, newer-generation DESs were associated with a significant reduction of 1-year definite ST (relative risk 0.35; 95% CI, 0.16–0.75; P = .006) compared with BMSs.[22]

For patients with large vessel diameter, BMSs seemed a reasonable option, because of the theoretically lower risk of developing a clinical overt ISR. Despite a similar risk of ST compared with DESs, BMSs have shown higher rates of stent failure. In a recently published post hoc analysis from the EXAMINATION trial, including 1498 patients with ST-segment elevated myocardial infarction undergoing primary PCI, despite no differences in terms of ST between groups, DES implantation was associated with a trend toward a reduction of the target lesion (hazard ratio [HR] 0.53; 95% CI, 0.27–1.02; P = .05) and target vessel revascularization (HR 0.60; 95% CI, 0.34–1.03; P = .066) in patients with larger vessel diameter.[23]

Finally, the perception of HBR has become the most frequent reason supporting BMS implantation in these last years. The rationale underlying this choice is the possibility of avoiding the prolonged antithrombotic therapy required to prevent the mild and long-term risk of ST observed with DESs.[24–27] Improvement in stent technology and implantation technique, however, significantly decreased such risk, thus supporting early DAPT discontinuation after DES implantation even for this subgroup of patients.[25] Several trials and prospective registries have shown the superiority of the second-generation DESs over BMSs under a mandated short DAPT period.[28,29]

Recently, the ZEUS study[30] showed that a treatment strategy consisting of ZES implantation followed by a personalized course of DAPT, resulted in a lower risk of major adverse cardiac events (MACEs) and definite or probable ST compared with BMSs (ST, 2.0% vs 4.1%, respectively; P = .019) in patients at HBR or thrombosis or at low risk of restenosis (no planned stent <3.0 mm diameter was intended to be implanted) at 1-year follow-up. Several studies recently have been published, or are ongoing, aiming at generalizing this concept to an even more larger types of DESs in HBR population, including the Xience Short DAPT programs (NCT03218787), the EVOLVE Short DAPT[31] (NCT02605447), the ONYX ONE[32] (NCT03344653), the POEM (NCT03112707), and MASTER DAPT[33] (NCT03023020) studies. The ONYX trial, randomizing either Resolute Onyx (Medtronic, CA, USA) DES (durable polymer [DP] DES) (n = 1003) or Bio-Freedom polymer-free [PF]-drug-coated stent (DCS) (n = 993) with 1-month DAPT, documented noninferiority of the DP-ZES compared with the BioFreedom DCS in the primary endpoint, including death from cardiac causes, myocardial infarction, or ST, with no differences in the rate of ST between groups (1.3% for the Onyx DES and 2.1% for the BMS).

Looking at the long-term performances of second-generation DESs in this high-risk population, in a pooled analysis from 4 all-comer postapproval registries that included 10,502 HBR patients who underwent PCI with CoCr-EES implantation, the 4-year rate of probable or definite ST was 1.5%.[34] Rates were similar to the ones observed in other all-comers registries testing the long-term effectiveness of CoCr-EES. For example, the Randomized Comparison of a Zotarolimus-Eluting Stent With an Everolimus-Eluting Stent for Percutaneous Coronary Intervention (RESOLUTE) trial, randomizing patients to Resolute ZES (R-ZES) (n = 1140) or CoCr-EES (n = 1152), showed 1.6% and 2.3% of ST at 4 years of follow-up, respectively, in the EES and R-ZES groups.

BIORESORBABLE POLYMER DRUG-ELUTING STENT

Another direction to improve drug-carrier systems was the development of erodible polymers. Biodegradable polymers (BPs) remain temporary on the DES surface and have the potential to enhance biocompatibility and improve the delayed healing in the vessel. These stents use BPs that remain only temporarily on the DES surface and have the potential of less chronic vessel wall inflammation, similar to a BMS, as reported by Yin and colleagues.[35]

Long-term data, however, after implantation of newer generations of thin-strut BP-based DESs still are lacking. A meta-analysis by Cassese and colleagues[36] showed for the first time that the ultra–thin-strut BP–sirolimus-eluting stent (SES) displays a performance comparable to the DP-EES, the benchmark of contemporary DESs, also for ST (1.3% vs 1.9%; P = .45) at 1-year follow-up, and, more interestingly, there was no time-dependent risk of ST associated with BP-SES versus DP-EES.

Long-term data are available only for early-generation BP–biolimus eluting-stents (BESs). Lu and colleagues[37] showed that BP-BESs were associated with lower rates of MACEs, target lesion revascularization, and ST (2.6% vs 3.8%, respectively; P = .003) to the DP-DES of first and second generations at 5 years of follow-up. When BP-BES was compared with CoCr-EES, however, no differences in ST (BP-BES 0.4% vs CoCr-EES 0.7%) were observed at 2-year follow-up[38] and also at longer-term follow-up (5 years).[39] With the intention of improving the characteristics of the BP-DES, in terms of strut thickness, polymer biodegradation coating, and drug release kinetics, new devices were developed. The Synergy (Boston Scientific, Marlborough, USA) BP-DES, a novel thin-strut platinum/chromium alloy stent that elutes everolimus from a rapid BP matrix, was one of the most intensively studied. In the EVOLVE II trial, it was noninferior to the PROMUS (Boston Scientific, Marlborough, USA) Element Plus EES with respect to definite/probable ST (0.4% vs 0.6%, respectively; P = .50) at 1-year follow-up.[40]

The Orsiro coronary stent (Biotronik AG, Bülach, Switzerland) consists of an ultra–thin-strut CoCr design with a bioresorbable, poly-L lactic acid polymer coating that elutes the antiproliferative drug sirolimus. This bioresorbable polymer SES was evaluated in the BIOFLOW V trial. At 1-year follow-up, the number of patients with late ST was significantly lower in the bioresorbable polymer SES group than in the DP-EES group, despite similar rates of definite or probable ST between groups (<1% vs 1%, respectively; P = .694).[41]

POLYMER-FREE DRUG-ELUTING STENT

To overcome the limitations related to DPs and BPs, PF-DES platforms were introduced. Elimination of the polymer might lower the rates of late ST, as suggested by previous studies in comparison with first-generation DESs.[42] The attainment of optimal drug-release kinetics, however, is the real challenge of PF-DES technology. First-generation devices had the limit of a too rapid drug elution (90% within 2 days) and failed to achieve the desirable inhibition of neointima formation.[43] After that, several randomized controlled trials were performed to evaluate the clinical performance of different PF-DES platforms. Recently, the MiStent, a DES with a fully absorbable polymer coating containing and embedding a microcrystalline form of sirolimus into the vessel wall, was evaluated in the DESSOLVE III trial[44] At 1-year follow-up, the rate of definite/probable ST was similar in comparison with DP-EES (0.7% vs 0.9%, respectively; P = .76).

Despite their improvements, PF platforms showed clinical outcomes and rates of ST comparable with modern permanent or BP-based DES up to 5 years' follow-up[45] Recently, Torii and colleagues[46] tested the hypothesis that the fluoropolymer on EES (FP-EES) is the most important component of its design with respect to thromboresistance by comparing stents of similar design with and without coating in a swine ex vivo shunt model. They demonstrated that FP-EES has the lowest platelet adherence compared with BP-DES, PF-DES, and BMS, with the lowest inflammatory cell density. These results reflect the phenomenon of fluoropassivation, representing one proposed mechanism for clinically observed low ST rates in FP-EES.[46] Because of their supposed lower risk of VLST, PF-DESs have been tested in high-risk profile populations, such as patients at HBR or with diabetes. The LEADERS FREE trial randomized 2466 HBR patients to either the BioFreedom DCS (Biosensors

Europe, Morges, Switzerland) or a similar BMS undergoing PCI under a 1-month mandated DAPT therapy. DESs were noted to be superior to BMSs for the primary composite endpoint, including cardiac death, MI, or ST at 2 years of follow-up, with a similar 2-year rate of definite/probable ST between the groups (2.1% for the DCS and 2.3% for the BMS). The Cre8 stent (CID SpA, member of Alvimedica, Saluggia, Italy) is an 80-μm–strut thickness CoCr PF-DES, releasing sirolimus from reservoirs placed on the abluminal stent surface. In a recently published propensity match analysis pooling 2 recent multicenter, observational independent studies conducted at 22 Italian centers, such as the Amphilimus Italian Multicentre Registry (ASTUTE) and the Polymer Free Biolimus-Eluting Stent Implantation in All-Comers Population (RUDI-FREE), aimed at comparing the safety and efficacy profile of Cre8 stent and BioFreedom biolimus-eluting stent (BES) PF-DESs in real-world patients undergoing PCI. In a total population of 2320 patients, both BES and Cre8 stents had similar rates of 1-year target lesion failure (4.2% vs 4.0%, respectively; HR 0.98; 95% CI; 0.57–1.70) as well as low 1-year rate of definite or probable ST (0.9% and 0.8%, respectively; HR 1.17; 95% CI, 0.36–3.81). The subgroup analysis showed a potential benefit of Cre8 in patients with diabetes mellitus, while of BioFreedom BES in patients without diabetes mellitus (P for interaction = 0.002).[47] Randomized trials comparing PF-DES to the DP-DES, however, are warranted to establish the safety and efficacy profile of these platforms in dedicated subgroups of patients.

BIORESORBABLE VASCULAR SCAFFOLD

In order to overcome the limits of DESs, fully bioresorbable scaffolds (BRSs) were introduced in 2012. The most studied BRS was the Absorb BVS.[48] Despite promising results at short-term follow-up, the Absorb BVS showed an increase of in-scaffold thrombosis in comparison with EES at long-term follow-up.[49–53]

The negative results of ABSORB II and AIDA at 3 years' follow-up[54,55] confirmed by several meta-analyses (ST, BRS 2.4% vs EES 0.7%),[52,56–59] resulted in the end of Absorb BVS use and withdrawal from the market in September 2017.

The experience with Absorb BVS, however, provided some precious lessons, in particular about the paramount role of implantation techniques. Several studies[60–65] in different clinical settings showed that an optimal deployment technique—pre-dilation, proper sizing, and post-dilation[66,67]—significantly reduced the rates of scaffold thrombosis (ScT), the Achilles heel of Absorb BVS.[68] These results were contrasted across the studies and some doubt remained whether the risk of ScT is due to the Absorb BVS platform or the implantation technique.[69]

The initial assumption of BRSs was to provide temporary mechanical support to the vessel without compromising the restoration of vascular physiology with the potential of preventing late adverse events after the complete resorption.[70] The 5-year outcome data of ABSORB Japan[71] showed that there were no significant differences in the composite or individual endpoint outcomes between the Absorb BVS and Xience arms through 5 years or between 3 years and 5 years. Similar results were reported in a single-center study, where the incidence of very late adverse events in patients with a BRS implantation decreased over years (ScT was 3.6% in the first year, 2.2% in the second-third year, and 0.6% in the fourth to fifth years after implantation). Recently, a summary-level meta-analysis by Stone and colleagues[72] of 4 trials, reporting 5-year follow-up data, showed a ScT in 0.1% of BVS-treated patients versus 0.3% of EES-treated patients between 3 years and 5 years (HR 0.44; 95% CI, 0.07–2.70) (P for interaction = .03), suggesting that the period of ScT risk for the Absorb BVS ends at 3 years.

OTHER BIORESORBABLE PLATFORMS

In such a scenario, the Biotronik magnesium-based Magmaris, Fantom (Reva Medical, San Diego, California), poly-L lactide-based polymer scaffold (Elixir Medical Corporation, Sunnyvale, California), ART (Terumo, Tokyo, Japan), and several other ones, including materials, such as tyrosine polycarbonate, salicylic acid polymer, and iron, were introduced. Although promising, the use of these devices in clinical practice is currently limited for the lack of randomized clinical studies and the current guidelines that limit their use.[73]

Recently, despite initial success of first studies, the Reva Medical company filed for bankruptcy protection in early 2020, although the next-generation DREAMS 3G, the evolution of Magmaris, with thinner struts and prolonged scaffolding time while keeping a 12-month resorption time, is being tested in the First in Men Study (BIOMAG-I; NCT04157153) and will be available for clinical trials in the near future.

Finally, it is unclear if the material technology will allow in future to overcome the limitations of current BRSs.

REFERENCES

1. Cutlip DE, Baim DS, Ho KK, et al. Stent thrombosis in the modern era: a pooled analysis of multicenter coronary stent clinical trials. Circulation 2001; 103(15):1967–71.

2. D'Ascenzo F, Iannaccone M, Saint-Hilary G, et al. Impact of design of coronary stents and length of dual antiplatelet therapies on ischaemic and bleeding events: a network meta-analysis of 64 randomized controlled trials and 102 735 patients. Eur Heart J 2017;38(42):3160–72.

3. Kastrati A, Mehilli J, Pache J, et al. Analysis of 14 trials comparing sirolimus-eluting stents with bare-metal stents. N Engl J Med 2007;356(10):1030–9.

4. Iaconetti C, Polimeni A, Sorrentino S, et al. Inhibition of miR-92a increases endothelial proliferation and migration in vitro as well as reduces neointimal proliferation in vivo after vascular injury. Basic Res Cardiol 2012;107(5):296.

5. Iaconetti C, De Rosa S, Polimeni A, et al. Down-regulation of miR-23b induces phenotypic switching of vascular smooth muscle cells in vitro and in vivo. Cardiovasc Res 2015;107(4):522–33.

6. Gareri C, Iaconetti C, Sorrentino S, et al. miR-125a-5p modulates phenotypic switch of vascular smooth muscle cells by targeting ETS-1. J Mol Biol 2017; 429(12):1817–28.

7. Sorrentino S, Iaconetti C, De Rosa S, et al. Hindlimb ischemia impairs endothelial recovery and increases neointimal proliferation in the carotid artery. Sci Rep 2018;8(1):761.

8. Roukoz H, Bavry AA, Sarkees ML, et al. Comprehensive meta-analysis on drug-eluting stents versus bare-metal stents during extended follow-up. Am J Med 2009;122(6):581 e581–510.

9. Camenzind E, Steg PG, Wijns W. Stent thrombosis late after implantation of first-generation drug-eluting stents: a cause for concern. Circulation 2007; 115(11):1440–55 [discussion: 1455].

10. Nakamura D, Attizzani GF, Toma C, et al. Failure mechanisms and neoatherosclerosis patterns in very late drug-eluting and bare-metal stent thrombosis. Circ Cardiovasc Interv 2016;9(9):e003785.

11. Sorrentino S, Giustino G, Baber U, et al. Dual antiplatelet therapy cessation and adverse events after drug-eluting stent implantation in patients at high risk for atherothrombosis (from the PARIS Registry). Am J Cardiol 2018;122(10):1638–46.

12. Giannini F, Pagnesi M, Campo G, et al. Italian multicenter registry of bare metal stent use in modern percutaneous coronary intervention era (AMARCORD): a multicenter observational study. Catheter Cardiovasc Interv 2020. https://doi.org/10.1002/ccd.28798.

13. Curcio A, Torella D, Cuda G, et al. Effect of stent coating alone on in vitro vascular smooth muscle cell proliferation and apoptosis. Am J Physiol Heart Circ Physiol 2004;286(3):H902–8.

14. Joner M, Finn AV, Farb A, et al. Pathology of drug-eluting stents in humans: delayed healing and late thrombotic risk. J Am Coll Cardiol 2006;48(1): 193–202.

15. Virmani R, Guagliumi G, Farb A, et al. Localized hypersensitivity and late coronary thrombosis secondary to a sirolimus-eluting stent: should we be cautious? Circulation 2004;109(6):701–5.

16. Virmani R, Liistro F, Stankovic G, et al. Mechanism of late in-stent restenosis after implantation of a paclitaxel derivate-eluting polymer stent system in humans. Circulation 2002;106(21):2649–51.

17. Kolandaivelu K, Swaminathan R, Gibson WJ, et al. Stent thrombogenicity early in high-risk interventional settings is driven by stent design and deployment and protected by polymer-drug coatings. Circulation 2011;123(13):1400–9.

18. Kedhi E, Joesoef KS, McFadden E, et al. Second-generation everolimus-eluting and paclitaxel-eluting stents in real-life practice (COMPARE): a randomised trial. Lancet 2010;375(9710):201–9.

19. Tada T, Byrne RA, Simunovic I, et al. Risk of stent thrombosis among bare-metal stents, first-generation drug-eluting stents, and second-generation drug-eluting stents: results from a registry of 18,334 patients. JACC Cardiovasc Interv 2013;6(12):1267–74.

20. Kang SH, Park KW, Kang DY, et al. Biodegradable-polymer drug-eluting stents vs. bare metal stents vs. durable-polymer drug-eluting stents: a systematic review and Bayesian approach network meta-analysis. Eur Heart J 2014;35(17):1147–58.

21. Raber L, Kelbaek H, Ostojic M, et al. Effect of biolimus-eluting stents with biodegradable polymer vs bare-metal stents on cardiovascular events among patients with acute myocardial infarction: the COMFORTABLE AMI randomized trial. JAMA 2012;308(8):777–87.

22. Sabate M, Raber L, Heg D, et al. Comparison of newer-generation drug-eluting with bare-metal stents in patients with acute ST-segment elevation myocardial infarction: a pooled analysis of the EXAMINATION (clinical evaluation of the Xience-V stent in acute myocardial INfArcTION) and COMFORTABLE-AMI (comparison of biolimus eluted from an erodible stent coating with bare metal stents in acute ST-elevation myocardial infarction) trials. JACC Cardiovasc Interv 2014;7(1):55–63.

23. Costa F, Brugaletta S, Pernigotti A, et al. Does large vessel size justify use of bare-metal stents in primary percutaneous coronary intervention? Circ Cardiovasc Interv 2019;12(9):e007705.

24. Sorrentino S, Baber U, Claessen BE, et al. Determinants of significant out-of-hospital bleeding in patients undergoing percutaneous coronary

intervention. Thromb Haemost 2018;118(11): 1997–2005.

25. Sorrentino S, Sartori S, Baber U, et al. Bleeding risk, dual antiplatelet therapy cessation, and adverse events after percutaneous coronary intervention: the PARIS registry. Circ Cardiovasc Interv 2020; 13(4):e008226.

26. Faggioni M, Baber U, Sartori S, et al. Influence of baseline anemia on dual antiplatelet therapy cessation and risk of adverse events after percutaneous coronary intervention. Circ Cardiovasc Interv 2019; 12(4):e007133.

27. Schoos M, Chandrasekhar J, Baber U, et al. Causes, timing, and impact of dual antiplatelet therapy interruption for surgery (from the patterns of non-adherence to anti-platelet regimens in stented patients registry). Am J Cardiol 2017;120(6):904–10.

28. Ariotti S, Adamo M, Costa F, et al. Is bare-metal stent implantation still justifiable in high bleeding risk patients undergoing percutaneous coronary intervention?: a pre-specified analysis from the zeus trial. JACC Cardiovasc Interv 2016;9(5):426–36.

29. Urban P, Meredith IT, Abizaid A, et al. Polymer-free drug-coated coronary stents in patients at high bleeding risk. N Engl J Med 2015;373(21):2038–47.

30. Valgimigli M, Patialiakas A, Thury A, et al. Zotarolimus-eluting versus bare-metal stents in uncertain drug-eluting stent candidates. J Am Coll Cardiol 2015;65(8):805–15.

31. Mauri L, Kirtane AJ, Windecker S, et al. Rationale and design of the EVOLVE Short DAPT Study to assess 3-month dual antiplatelet therapy in subjects at high risk for bleeding undergoing percutaneous coronary intervention. Am Heart J 2018;205:110–7.

32. Kedhi E, Latib A, Abizaid A, et al. Rationale and design of the Onyx ONE global randomized trial: a randomized controlled trial of high-bleeding risk patients after stent placement with 1month of dual antiplatelet therapy. Am Heart J 2019;214:134–41.

33. Frigoli E, Smits P, Vranckx P, et al. Design and rationale of the management of high bleeding risk patients post bioresorbable polymer coated stent implantation with an abbreviated versus standard DAPT regimen (MASTER DAPT) study. Am Heart J 2019;209:97–105.

34. Sorrentino S, Claessen BE, Chandiramani R, et al. Long-term safety and efficacy of durable polymer cobalt-chromium everolimus-eluting stents in patients at high bleeding risk: a patient-level stratified analysis from four postapproval studies. Circulation 2020;141(11):891–901.

35. Yin Y, Zhang Y, Zhao X. Safety and efficacy of biodegradable drug-eluting vs. bare metal stents: a meta-analysis from randomized trials. PLoS One 2014; 9(6):e99648.

36. Cassese S, Ndrepepa G, Byrne RA, et al. Outcomes of patients treated with ultrathin strut biodegradable-polymer sirolimus-eluting stents versus fluoropolymer-based everolimus-eluting stents. A meta-analysis of randomized trials. EuroIntervention 2018;14(2):224–31.

37. Lu P, Lu S, Li Y, et al. A comparison of the main outcomes from BP-BES and DP-DES at five years of follow-up: a systematic review and meta-analysis. Sci Rep 2017;7(1):14997.

38. Kaiser C, Galatius S, Jeger R, et al. Long-term efficacy and safety of biodegradable-polymer biolimus-eluting stents: main results of the Basel Stent Kosten-Effektivitats Trial-PROspective Validation Examination II (BASKET-PROVE II), a randomized, controlled noninferiority 2-year outcome trial. Circulation 2015;131(1):74–81.

39. Vlachojannis GJ, Smits PC, Hofma SH, et al. Biodegradable polymer biolimus-eluting stents versus durable polymer everolimus-eluting stents in patients with coronary artery disease: Final 5-year report from the COMPARE II trial (abluminal biodegradable polymer biolimus-eluting stent versus durable polymer everolimus-eluting stent). JACC Cardiovasc Interv 2017;10(12):1215–21.

40. Kereiakes DJ, Meredith IT, Windecker S, et al. Efficacy and safety of a novel bioabsorbable polymer-coated, everolimus-eluting coronary stent: the EVOLVE II randomized trial. Circ Cardiovasc Interv 2015;8(4):e002372.

41. Kandzari DE, Mauri L, Koolen JJ, et al. Ultrathin, bioresorbable polymer sirolimus-eluting stents versus thin, durable polymer everolimus-eluting stents in patients undergoing coronary revascularisation (BIOFLOW V): a randomised trial. Lancet 2017; 390(10105):1843–52.

42. Urban P, Macaya C, Rupprecht HJ, et al. Randomized evaluation of anticoagulation versus antiplatelet therapy after coronary stent implantation in high-risk patients: the multicenter aspirin and ticlopidine trial after intracoronary stenting (MATTIS). Circulation 1998;98(20):2126–32.

43. Hausleiter J, Kastrati A, Wessely R, et al. Prevention of restenosis by a novel drug-eluting stent system with a dose-adjustable, polymer-free, onsite stent coating. Eur Heart J 2005;26(15): 1475–81.

44. de Winter RJ, Katagiri Y, Asano T, et al. A sirolimus-eluting bioabsorbable polymer-coated stent (MiStent) versus an everolimus-eluting durable polymer stent (Xience) after percutaneous coronary intervention (DESSOLVE III): a randomised, single-blind, multicentre, non-inferiority, phase 3 trial. Lancet 2018;391(10119):431–40.

45. Gao K, Sun Y, Yang M, et al. Efficacy and safety of polymer-free stent versus polymer-permanent drug-eluting stent in patients with acute coronary syndrome: a meta-analysis of randomized control trials. BMC Cardiovasc Disord 2017;17(1):194.

46. Torii S, Cheng Q, Mori H, et al. Acute thrombogenicity of fluoropolymer-coated versus biodegradable and polymer free stents. EuroIntervention 2018; 14(16):1685–93.

47. Chiarito M, Sardella G, Colombo A, et al. Safety and efficacy of polymer-free drug-eluting stents. Circ Cardiovasc Interv 2019;12(2):e007311.

48. Indolfi C, De Rosa S, Colombo A. Bioresorbable vascular scaffolds - basic concepts and clinical outcome. Nat Rev Cardiol 2016;13(12):719–29.

49. Ali ZA, Gao R, Kimura T, et al. Three-year outcomes with the absorb bioresorbable scaffold: individual-patient-data meta-analysis from the ABSORB randomized trials. Circulation 2018;137(5):464–79.

50. Ali ZA, Serruys PW, Kimura T, et al. 2-year outcomes with the Absorb bioresorbable scaffold for treatment of coronary artery disease: a systematic review and meta-analysis of seven randomised trials with an individual patient data substudy. Lancet 2017; 390(10096):760–72.

51. Kereiakes DJ, Ellis SG, Metzger C, et al. 3-year clinical outcomes with everolimus-eluting bioresorbable coronary scaffolds: the ABSORB III trial. J Am Coll Cardiol 2017;70(23):2852–62.

52. Stone GW, Gao R, Kimura T, et al. 1-year outcomes with the Absorb bioresorbable scaffold in patients with coronary artery disease: a patient-level, pooled meta-analysis. Lancet 2016; 387(10025):1277–89.

53. Chevalier B, Cequier A, Dudek D, et al. Four-year follow-up of the randomised comparison between an everolimus-eluting bioresorbable scaffold and an everolimus-eluting metallic stent for the treatment of coronary artery stenosis (ABSORB II Trial). EuroIntervention 2018;13(13):1561–4.

54. Serruys PW, Chevalier B, Sotomi Y, et al. Comparison of an everolimus-eluting bioresorbable scaffold with an everolimus-eluting metallic stent for the treatment of coronary artery stenosis (ABSORB II): a 3 year, randomised, controlled, single-blind, multicentre clinical trial. Lancet 2016;388(10059): 2479–91.

55. Wykrzykowska JJ, Kraak RP, Hofma SH, et al. Bioresorbable scaffolds versus metallic stents in routine PCI. N Engl J Med 2017;376(24):2319–28.

56. Polimeni A, Anadol R, Munzel T, et al. Long-term outcome of bioresorbable vascular scaffolds for the treatment of coronary artery disease: a meta-analysis of RCTs. BMC Cardiovasc Disord 2017; 17(1):147.

57. Sorrentino S, Giustino G, Mehran R, et al. Everolimus-eluting bioresorbable scaffolds versus everolimus-eluting metallic stents. J Am Coll Cardiol 2017;69(25):3055–66.

58. Collet C, Asano T, Sotomi Y, et al. Early, late and very late incidence of bioresorbable scaffold thrombosis: a systematic review and meta-analysis of randomized clinical trials and observational studies. Minerva Cardioangiol 2017;65(1):32–51.

59. Mukete BN, van der Heijden LC, Tandjung K, et al. Safety and efficacy of everolimus-eluting bioresorbable vascular scaffolds versus durable polymer everolimus-eluting metallic stents assessed at 1-year follow-up: a systematic review and meta-analysis of studies. Int J Cardiol 2016;221: 1087–94.

60. Polimeni A, Anadol R, Munzel T, et al. Bioresorbable vascular scaffolds for percutaneous treatment of chronic total coronary occlusions: a meta-analysis. BMC Cardiovasc Disord 2019;19(1):59.

61. Polimeni A, Weissner M, Schochlow K, et al. Incidence, clinical presentation, and predictors of clinical restenosis in coronary bioresorbable scaffolds. JACC Cardiovasc Interv 2017;10(18):1819–27.

62. Anadol R, Lorenz L, Weissner M, et al. Characteristics and outcome of patients with complex coronary lesions treated with bioresorbable scaffolds: three-year follow-up in a cohort of consecutive patients. EuroIntervention 2018;14(9):e1011–9.

63. Anadol R, Dimitriadis Z, Polimeni A, et al. Bioresorbable everolimus-eluting vascular scaffold for patients presenting with non STelevation-acute coronary syndrome: a three-years follow-up1. Clin Hemorheol Microcirc 2018;69(1–2):3–8.

64. Anadol R, Schnitzler K, Lorenz L, et al. Three-years outcomes of diabetic patients treated with coronary bioresorbable scaffolds. BMC Cardiovasc Disord 2018;18(1):92.

65. Polimeni A, Anadol R, Munzel T, et al. Predictors of bioresorbable scaffold failure in STEMI patients at 3years follow-up. Int J Cardiol 2018;268:68–74.

66. Sorrentino S, De Rosa S, Ambrosio G, et al. The duration of balloon inflation affects the luminal diameter of coronary segments after bioresorbable vascular scaffolds deployment. BMC Cardiovasc Disord 2015;15:169.

67. Dimitriadis Z, Polimeni A, Anadol R, et al. Procedural predictors for bioresorbable vascular scaffold thrombosis: analysis of the individual components of the "PSP" technique. J Clin Med 2019;8(1):93.

68. Gori T, Weissner M, Gonner S, et al. Characteristics, predictors, and mechanisms of thrombosis in coronary bioresorbable scaffolds: differences between early and late events. JACC Cardiovasc Interv 2017;10(23):2363–71.

69. Polimeni A, Gori T. Bioresorbable vascular scaffold: a step back thinking of the future. Postepy Kardiol Interwencyjnej 2018;14(2):117–9.

70. Gori T, Polimeni A, Indolfi C, et al. Predictors of stent thrombosis and their implications for clinical practice. Nat Rev Cardiol 2019;16(4):243–56.

71. Kozuma K, Tanabe K, Hamazaki Y, et al. Long-term outcomes of absorb bioresorbable vascular scaffold vs. everolimus-eluting metallic stent- a randomized

comparison through 5 years in Japan. Circ J 2020; 84(5):733–41.

72. Stone GW, Kimura T, Gao R, et al. Time-varying outcomes with the absorb bioresorbable vascular scaffold during 5-year follow-up: a systematic meta-analysis and individual patient data pooled study. JAMA Cardiol 2019;4(12):1261–9.

73. Haude M, Ince H, Abizaid A, et al. Sustained safety and performance of the second-generation drug-eluting absorbable metal scaffold in patients with de novo coronary lesions: 12-month clinical results and angiographic findings of the BIOSOLVE-II first-in-man trial. Eur Heart J 2016; 37(35):2701–9.

UNITED STATES POSTAL SERVICE®
Statement of Ownership, Management, and Circulation
(All Periodicals Publications Except Requester Publications)

1. Publication Title	2. Publication Number	3. Filing Date
CARDIOLOGY CLINICS	000 – 701	9/18/2020

4. Issue Frequency	5. Number of Issues Published Annually	6. Annual Subscription Price
FEB, MAY, AUG, NOV	4	$352.00

7. Complete Mailing Address of Known Office of Publication (Not printer) (Street, city, county, state, and ZIP+4®)

ELSEVIER INC.
230 Park Avenue, Suite 800
New York, NY 10169

Contact Person
Malathi Samayan
Telephone (Include area code)
91-44-4299-4507

8. Complete Mailing Address of Headquarters or General Business Office of Publisher (Not printer)

ELSEVIER INC.
230 Park Avenue, Suite 800
New York, NY 10169

9. Full Names and Complete Mailing Addresses of Publisher, Editor, and Managing Editor (Do not leave blank)

Publisher (Name and complete mailing address)

DOLORES MELONI, ELSEVIER INC.
1600 JOHN F KENNEDY BLVD. SUITE 1800
PHILADELPHIA, PA 19103-2899

Editor (Name and complete mailing address)

JOANNA COLLETT, ELSEVIER INC.
1600 JOHN F KENNEDY BLVD. SUITE 1800
PHILADELPHIA, PA 19103-2899

Managing Editor (Name and complete mailing address)

PATRICK MANLEY, ELSEVIER INC.
1600 JOHN F KENNEDY BLVD. SUITE 1800
PHILADELPHIA, PA 19103-2899

10. Owner (Do not leave blank. If the publication is owned by a corporation, give the name and address of the corporation immediately followed by the names and addresses of all stockholders owning or holding 1 percent or more of the total amount of stock. If not owned by a corporation, give the names and addresses of the individual owners. If owned by a partnership or other unincorporated firm, give its name and address as well as those of each individual owner. If the publication is published by a nonprofit organization, give its name and address.)

Full Name	Complete Mailing Address
WHOLLY OWNED SUBSIDIARY OF REED/ELSEVIER, US HOLDINGS	1600 JOHN F KENNEDY BLVD. SUITE 1800 PHILADELPHIA, PA 19103-2899

11. Known Bondholders, Mortgagees, and Other Security Holders Owning or Holding 1 Percent or More of Total Amount of Bonds, Mortgages, or Other Securities. If none, check box ▶ ☐ None

Full Name	Complete Mailing Address
N/A	

12. Tax Status (For completion by nonprofit organizations authorized to mail at nonprofit rates) (Check one)
The purpose, function, and nonprofit status of this organization and the exempt status for federal income tax purposes:
☒ Has Not Changed During Preceding 12 Months
☐ Has Changed During Preceding 12 Months (Publisher must submit explanation of change with this statement)

PS Form **3526**, July 2014 [Page 1 of 4 (see instructions page 4)] PSN: 7530-01-000-9931   PRIVACY NOTICE: See our privacy policy on www.usps.com.

---

13. Publication Title	14. Issue Date for Circulation Data Below
CARDIOLOGY CLINICS	MAY 2020

15. Extent and Nature of Circulation			Average No. Copies Each Issue During Preceding 12 Months	No. Copies of Single Issue Published Nearest to Filing Date
a. Total Number of Copies (Net press run)			174	156
b. Paid Circulation (By Mail and Outside the Mail)	(1)	Mailed Outside-County Paid Subscriptions Stated on PS Form 3541 (include paid distribution above nominal rate, advertiser's proof copies, and exchange copies)	85	79
	(2)	Mailed In-County Paid Subscriptions Stated on PS Form 3541 (include paid distribution above nominal rate, advertiser's proof copies, and exchange copies)	0	0
	(3)	Paid Distribution Outside the Mails Including Sales Through Dealers and Carriers, Street Vendors, Counter Sales, and Other Paid Distribution Outside USPS®	52	43
	(4)	Paid Distribution by Other Classes of Mail Through the USPS (e.g., First-Class Mail®)	0	0
c. Total Paid Distribution [Sum of 15b (1), (2), (3), and (4)]		▶	137	122
d. Free or Nominal Rate Distribution (By Mail and Outside the Mail)	(1)	Free or Nominal Rate Outside-County Copies included on PS Form 3541	21	17
	(2)	Free or Nominal Rate In-County Copies included on PS Form 3541	0	0
	(3)	Free or Nominal Rate Copies Mailed at Other Classes Through the USPS (e.g., First-Class Mail)	0	0
	(4)	Free or Nominal Rate Distribution Outside the Mail (Carriers or other means)	0	0
e. Total Free or Nominal Rate Distribution (Sum of 15d (1), (2), (3) and (4))		▶	21	17
f. Total Distribution (Sum of 15c and 15e)		▶	158	139
g. Copies not Distributed (See Instructions to Publishers #4 (page #3))			16	17
h. Total (Sum of 15f and g)		▶	174	156
i. Percent Paid (15c divided by 15f times 100)			86.7%	87.86%

* If you are claiming electronic copies, go to line 16 on page 3. If you are not claiming electronic copies, skip to line 17 on page 3.

16. Electronic Copy Circulation	Average No. Copies Each Issue During Preceding 12 Months	No. Copies of Single Issue Published Nearest to Filing Date
a. Paid Electronic Copies ▶		
b. Total Paid Print Copies (Line 15c) + Paid Electronic Copies (Line 16a) ▶		
c. Total Print Distribution (Line 15f) + Paid Electronic Copies (Line 16a) ▶		
d. Percent Paid (Both Print & Electronic Copies) (16b divided by 16c × 100) ▶		

☒ I certify that 50% of all my distributed copies (electronic and print) are paid above a nominal price.

17. Publication of Statement of Ownership
☒ If the publication is a general publication, publication of this statement is required. Will be printed in the NOVEMBER 2020 issue of this publication. ☐ Publication not required.

18. Signature and Title of Editor, Publisher, Business Manager, or Owner

Malathi Samayan   Date 9/18/2020

Malathi Samayan - Distribution Controller

I certify that all information furnished on this form is true and complete. I understand that anyone who furnishes false or misleading information on this form or who omits material or information requested on the form may be subject to criminal sanctions (including fines and imprisonment) and/or civil sanctions (including civil penalties).

PS Form **3526**, July 2014 (Page 2 of 4)   PRIVACY NOTICE: See our privacy policy on www.usps.com